Recent Advances in Children's Motor Development: From Birth to Adolescence

Recent Advances in Children's Motor Development: From Birth to Adolescence

Guest Editors

Dario Colella
Domenico Monacis

MDPI Basel • Beijing • Wuhan • Barcelona • Belgrade • Novi Sad • Cluj • Manchester

Guest Editors

Dario Colella
DISTeBA, Department of
Biological and
Environmental Sciences
University of Salento
Lecce
Italy

Domenico Monacis
Department of Education and
Sports Sciences
Pegaso University
Napoli
Italy

Editorial Office
MDPI AG
Grosspeteranlage 5
4052 Basel, Switzerland

This is a reprint of the Special Issue, published open access by the journal *Children* (ISSN 2227-9067), freely accessible at: https://www.mdpi.com/journal/children/special_issues/U5169689BM.

For citation purposes, cite each article independently as indicated on the article page online and as indicated below:

Lastname, A.A.; Lastname, B.B. Article Title. *Journal Name* **Year**, *Volume Number*, Page Range.

ISBN 978-3-7258-7847-5 (Hbk)
ISBN 978-3-7258-7848-2 (PDF)
https://doi.org/10.3390/books978-3-7258-7848-2

Cover image courtesy of Domenico Monacis

Contents

About the Editors

Dario Colella

Dario Colella is a Full Professor of Methods and Didactics of Motor Activities at the Department of Biological and Environmental Sciences and Technologies, University of Salento in Lecce, Italy. Professor Colella is deeply engaged with the global academic community. He is an invited speaker at national and international congresses, a peer reviewer for numerous esteemed journals, and a member of several editorial boards. He has acted as a Guest Editor for prominent special issues, including "Physical Education, Exercise and Sport for a Sustainable Environment and Lifestyle", "Physical Education, Physical Activity and Health Promotion in Children and Adolescents" and "Recent Advances in Children's Motor Development: From Birth to Adolescence".

Domenico Monacis

Domenico Monacis is a Researcher in the Methods and Didactics of Motor Activities at the Department of Education and Sports Sciences, Pegaso Telematic University in Naples, Italy. He holds a degree in Motor and Sport Sciences and a Ph.D. in Culture, Education, and Communication. His research focuses on optimizing physical education through evidence-based didactics. Key areas of interest include teaching styles and motor learning, early childhood motor development, and the socio-cultural determinants of health promotion in adolescence. Furthermore, he investigates the effects of experimental methodological interventions on motor skill acquisition and explores the integration of modern technologies—such as Exergames and Active Videogames—into physical education curricula.

Preface

Motor development is a fundamental and multifaceted pillar of a child's developmental journey, serving as an essential foundation for optimizing physical, cognitive, emotional, and psychosocial well-being. However, driven by current complex socio-cultural transformations—primarily the pervasive integration of digital tools and devices in childhood—the ways in which children access knowledge and interact with their peers are changing rapidly.

This Reprint aims to address this topic in depth, exploring how motor experience supports children's growth in developmental age through recent scientific evidence and good practices. Within this work, a particular emphasis is placed on pedagogical and educational models related to lifespan motor development. In a historical moment of rapid transition, there is an urgent need to embrace models that reflect the complex, fluid, and context-dependent nature of developmental change.

The contributions included in this collection offer an innovative synthesis that emphasizes the deep interconnection between perception, action, cognition, and physical fitness, alongside factors related to the practice of physical activity. From novel advancements in motor development, this Reprint aims to tangibly showcase the links between scientific and methodological approaches applied in various contexts (i.e., sport, physical education, free time, and adapted physical activity). Ultimately, our hope is to provide scholars, teachers, and professionals with the tools to effectively translate theory into practice , fully enhancing the pervasive, foundational, and highly transformative nature that movement assumes at every stage of human growth.

Dario Colella and Domenico Monacis
Guest Editors

children

MDPI

Editorial

Tracking Current Evidence and Future Perspectives of Children's Motor Development

Domenico Monacis [1,*] and Dario Colella [2]

1 Department of Education and Sports Sciences, Pegaso University, 80143 Naples, Italy
2 Department of Biological and Environmental Sciences and Technologies, University of Salento, 73100 Lecce, Italy; dario.colella@unisalento.it
* Correspondence: domenico.monacis@unipegaso.it

Motor development is a fundamental and multifaceted pillar of a child's developmental journey, serving as a fundamental foundation for optimizing a child's physical, cognitive, emotional, and psychosocial well-being [1]. In today's social and healthcare landscape, characterized by a concerning prevalence of hypokinetic phenotypes and growing challenges related to the heterogeneous trajectories of neurodevelopment [2,3], the academic community is called upon to produce robust empirical evidence. This body of evidence is essential for guiding intervention strategies that promote Physical Literacy, active lifestyles, foster full inclusion, and maximize each individual's developmental potential, moving beyond purely compensatory or therapeutically approaches.

This Special Issue, titled *"Recent Advances in Children's Motor Development: From Birth to Adolescence,"* compiles nine high-profile scientific contributions, presenting a significant synergic and innovative epistemological framework. The primary added value of this Special Issue lies in the dense network of theoretical and methodological interconnections among the published studies, which, while investigating different populations and developmental stages, converge toward the overcoming of biomechanical reductionism in favor of a holistic, ecological, and embodied construct.

Within this context of epistemological renewal, physical experiences in the fields of physical education, extracurricular activities, and sports initiation are not merely an indispensable component of the educational curriculum, but a genuine ecosystem for interdisciplinary intervention [4]. However, driven by current socio-cultural transformations—primarily the pervasive integration of digital tools and devices in childhood—the ways in which children access knowledge and interact with their peers are changing rapidly. In this evolving landscape, the translation of developmental theory into educational practice often reveals methodological opacity, especially in managing the delicate transition from spontaneous movement to structured sports practice in the absence of solid pedagogical foundations [4]. Although the scientific literature of the past decade shows a growing focus on the prevention of hypokinesia, health promotion, and the optimization of motor learning processes, we are simultaneously witnessing a progressive fragmentation and decontextualization of best practices oriented toward motor development [5]. In a society that tends to compress, overstructure, or even suppress certain dimensions of motor development in favor of partial, formal, and adult-centered educational approaches, there is an urgent need to embrace pedagogical models that reflect the complex, fluid, and context-dependent nature of developmental change.

It is crucial to restore centrality to a motor experience that is intrinsically motivating, spontaneous, creative, and radically inclusive, specifically designed to enhance the deep interconnection between perception, action, cognition, and physical fitness [6]. Movement, in fact, represents a pervasive, foundational, and highly transformative phenomenon in a child's ontogenesis. It acts as an irreplaceable medium for navigating different contexts (e.g., school, sports, and leisure time) and for translating theory into practice, long before motor actions take on the conventional, strictly utilitarian, and rational connotations typical of adulthood [4,5].

In perfect alignment with the aims of this Special Issue, it is crucial to reaffirm the educational value of movement-based experiences, with a particular emphasis on pedagogical and health-related models to lifespan motor development, catalyzing and nurturing those cognitive–motor, affective, and relational interconnections that constitute the very essence of harmonious and holistic development [7,8].

Below, we offer a critical and cross-cutting examination of the contributions, highlighting their innovative contribution to the advancement of research on motor development.

1. *The Developmental Ecosystem: Early Determinants and School Dynamics*

A central pillar of this Special Issue is the adoption of an ecological paradigm, which posits that the acquisition of motor skills is inextricably linked to environmental variables. The study by An and Libertus provides the foundation for this perspective, demonstrating, through an Integrated Ecological Model, how parental constructs (beliefs, attitudes, and expectations) significantly modulate the very earliest neuromotor trajectories of the newborn.

This fundamental focus on the developmental ecosystem finds its natural extension in the context of formal education through the study by Luptáková et al., which analyzes the effectiveness of co-teaching models (Team Teaching) in primary physical education classes. Both studies suggest significant pedagogical implications for driving educational interventions: the optimization of children's motor development cannot be separated from the structuring of qualified learning environments and the training of caregivers (parents and teachers). To evaluate the effectiveness of such settings, an ecologically valid psychometric assessment tool was needed. In this regard, Iannaccone et al. provide the cross-cultural validation of the CAPL-2 questionnaire for the Italian children, allowing for the assessment of Physical Literacy by integrating the performance of motor tasks with affective–cognitive dimensions, such as motivation and perceived competence.

2. *Neurocognitive Synergies: Epistemological Continuity Between Developmental Disorders and High Performance*

The most innovative heuristic approach in this Special Issue emerges from a joint examination of Han et al.'s review on cluttering and Timea et al.'s controlled trial on adolescent athletes. Although situated at opposite ends of the spectrum of functional abilities, these studies share a primary neurophysiological focus: the intrinsic interdependence between executive functions and motor control.

Han and colleagues reconceptualize alterations in verbal fluency not as a mere mechanical deficit, but rather as a specific vulnerability in motor–cognitive integration that manifests under conditions of high executive load. Similarly, Timea et al. address the same cognitive–motor interface in the context of elite athletic performance: the implementation of the SmartACT hybrid protocol (integrating mindfulness, cognitive flexibility, and visual–motor reaction technologies) demonstrates that training in executive functions and the mitigation of psychological stress are direct predictors of optimized agility and reaction times. A significant paradigm shift emerges from these findings: the cognitive–motor interface constitutes the primary target for intervention, whether aimed at supporting neurotypical development, managing atypical conditions, or enhancing performance.

 https://doi.org/10.3390/children13040492

3. *Movement as an Immersive Medium for Inclusion and Systemic Adaptation*

A third thematic strand reinforces the view of movement as a vehicle for global adaptation, focusing on the quality of the motor experience rather than its mere quantification. The contributions by Lev-Ari et al. and by Lotan and Weiss, centered on individuals with Autism Spectrum Disorder (ASD), deconstruct isolated approaches in favor of immersive ecosystems. The practice of Capoeira (Lev-Ari et al.) and hydrotherapy protocols (Lotan and Weiss) emerge as complex socio-sensory environments capable of best promoting postural regulation, balance, and socio-communicative engagement, acting as powerful inclusive catalysts.

This conceptualization of movement as a promoter of systemic health finds full analytical support in the study by Monacis et al. Developing both mediation and moderation models in secondary schoolchildren (aged 11–14 years old), the authors corroborate the hypothesis that Physical Activity Levels (PALs) act as essential mediators between Body Mass Index (BMI) and physical fitness development. The key finding is that structured and consistent physical engagement has the capacity to mitigate the potential functional limitations associated with excess weight. Underlying these optimization processes is the need for proper stratification of neuromotor risk: in this regard, the contribution by Podstawski et al. on the use of the Vojta method reaffirms the importance of early identification of central coordination disorders, an indispensable prerequisite for the timely initiation of harmonious motor development pathways.

4. *Concluding Reflections and Future Research Perspectives*

The nine studies presented here confirm that the motor development process must be investigated as a complex dynamic system, resulting from the continuous interaction between the organism's neurobiological constraints, the affordances of the physical and relational environment, and the task constraints of specific human activities.

In order to improve our understanding of recent advancements in motor development, future research should focus on the following strategic areas:

1. Longitudinal and multicenter designs: Tracking motor development trajectories over the long term and investigating how early determinants and parenting styles predict adherence to physical activity and motor competence in adulthood;
2. Technology assessment tools: advances in wearable technologies and artificial intelligence must be leveraged to collect kinematic and behavioral data in real-world settings, overcoming the inherent limitations of laboratory evaluations and self-report measures;
3. Transdisciplinary synergy: promoting a research framework that structurally integrates cognitive neuroscience, movement sciences, and educational disciplines, in order to validate multi-component interventions that support the well-documented link between motor skills, executive functions, and emotional domains;
4. Translation into health policy and education paradigms: the robust evidence emerging from this Special Issue must be translated into stringent policy guidelines, incentivizing structural presence of movement specialists starting in elementary school and promoting the integration of inclusive motor experiences (such as adapted martial arts or aquatic activities) into the Essential Levels of Care (LEAs) and public health promotion programs.

In closing, as Guest Editors, we want to thank the authors for sharing their research.

We also want to thank the peer reviewers for checking this research; their feedback was very helpful. We also thank the Editorial Board of *Children* for always helping us. We think this collection of research will be very useful for scholars, teachers and the international academic community.

https://doi.org/10.3390/children13040492

Conflicts of Interest: The authors declare no conflicts of interest.

List of Contributions:

1. An, R.; Libertus, K. Parental Perspectives and Infant Motor Development: An Integrated Ecological Model. *Children* **2025**, *12*, 724. https://doi.org/10.3390/children12060724.
2. Han, W.; Zhou, L.; Lu, J.; Pill, S. Cluttering in Children and Adolescents: Speech Motor Development, Neurocognitive Mechanisms, and Allied Health Implications. *Children* **2026**, *13*, 97. https://doi.org/10.3390/children13010097.
3. Iannaccone, A.; Cudicio, A.; Falese, L.; Federico, B.; Crotti, M.; Lovecchio, N.; Digennaro, S.; Agosti, V. Validation of the Italian Translation and Cultural Adaptation of the Canadian Assessment of Physical Literacy-2 (CAPL-2) Questionnaire for Children. *Children* **2025**, *12*, 1290. https://doi.org/10.3390/children12101290.
4. Lev-Ari, R.; Lotan, M.; Korn, L. The Role of Capoeira in Improving Motor and Social Skills in Children with Autism. *Children* **2025**, *12*, 1305. https://doi.org/10.3390/children12101305.
5. Lotan, M.; Weiss, M. Balance and Coordination Improvements in Children and Adolescents with Autism Spectrum Disorder (ASD), Resulting from a Hydrotherapy Intervention. *Children* **2026**, *13*, 94. https://doi.org/10.3390/children13010094.
6. Luptáková, G.; Argajová, J.; Balga, T.; Augustovičová, D.; Sobotová, P.; Balint, G.; Antala, B. Team Teaching Models in Primary Physical Education: Effects on Basic Motor Competencies and Self-Reported Physical Literacy. *Children* **2025**, *12*, 1595. https://doi.org/10.3390/children12121595.
7. Monacis, D.; Sannicandro, I.; Colella, D. Exploring Self-Reported Physical Activity Levels and Physical Fitness in Italian Children: A Mediation and Moderation Analysis. *Children* **2025**, *12*, 204. https://doi.org/10.3390/children12020204.
8. Podstawski, R.; Balewska-Juras, K.; Borysławski, K.; Szabo, A.; Snarska, J. An Assessment of Motor Skills in Infants at Risk of Atypical Psychomotor Development Using the Vojta Method. *Children* **2025**, *12*, 976. https://doi.org/10.3390/children12080976.
9. Timea, B.M.; Carmen, C.-B.; Nicolae, O.M.; Nicola, M.; Teodor, G.V.; Maria, S.A.; Cornelia, P.; Hervás-Gómez, C.; Florina, G.E.; Dan, M. Effects of the SmartACT Intervention on Motor and Psychological Variables in Adolescent Athletes: A Controlled Trial Using BlazePod and Microgate. *Children* **2025**, *12*, 1338. https://doi.org/10.3390/children12101338.

References

1. Adolph, K.E.; Hoch, J.E. Motor Development: Embodied, Embedded, Enculturated, and Enabling. *Annu. Rev. Psychol.* **2019**, *70*, 141–164. [CrossRef] [PubMed]
2. Green, D.; Lingam, R.; Mattocks, C.; Riddoch, C.; Ness, A.; Emond, A. The Risk of Reduced Physical Activity in Children with Probable Developmental Coordination Disorder: A Prospective Longitudinal Study. *Res. Dev. Disabil.* **2011**, *32*, 1332–1342. [CrossRef] [PubMed]
3. Dapp, L.C.; Gashaj, V.; Roebers, C.M. Physical Activity and Motor Skills in Children: A Differentiated Approach. *Psychol. Sport Exerc.* **2021**, *54*, 101916. [CrossRef]
4. Getchell, N.; Schott, N.; Brian, A. Motor Development Research: Designs, Analyses, and Future Directions. *J. Mot. Learn. Dev.* **2020**, *8*, 410–437. [CrossRef]
5. Hulteen, R.M.; Morgan, P.J.; Barnett, L.M.; Stodden, D.F.; Lubans, D.R. Development of Foundational Movement Skills: A Conceptual Model for Physical Activity Across the Lifespan. *Sports Med.* **2018**, *48*, 1533–1540. [CrossRef] [PubMed]
6. Salvatierra-Calderón, V.; Romero-Pérez, E.M.; Lemes, V.; Sadarangani, K.P.; Reyes-Molina, D.; Delgado-Floody, P.; Soto-Sánchez, J.; Ferrari, G.; Brand, C.; Cristi-Montero, C. The Multiple Mediation Impact of Adolescents' Physical Fitness and Cognitive Perceptions on Their Objective Measures—The Cogni-Action Project. *Psychol. Sport Exerc.* **2024**, *75*, 102721. [CrossRef] [PubMed]
7. Martins, C.; Valentini, N.C.; Sääkslahti, A.; Africa, E.K.; Webster, E.K.; Nobre, G.; Robinson, L.E.; Duncan, M.; Tortella, P.; Bandeira, P.F.; et al. Motor Competence as Key to Support Healthy Development of 3-to 5-Year-Old Children: An Expert Statement on Behalf of the International Motor Development Research Consortium. *J. Mot. Learn. Dev.* **2024**, *12*, 437–454. [CrossRef]
8. Wang, X.; Zhou, B. Motor Development-Focused Exercise Training Enhances Gross Motor Skills More Effectively than Ordinary Physical Activity in Healthy Preschool Children: An Updated Meta-Analysis. *Front. Public Health* **2024**, *12*, 1414152. [CrossRef] [PubMed]

https://doi.org/10.3390/children13040492

children

MDPI

Review

Parental Perspectives and Infant Motor Development: An Integrated Ecological Model

Ran An * and Klaus Libertus

Department of Psychology, University of Pittsburgh, Pittsburgh, PA 15260, USA; klaus.libertus@pitt.edu
* Correspondence: raa122@pitt.edu

Abstract: Infant motor development has traditionally been studied through child-centered frameworks that often overlook the vital role parents play in shaping early outcomes. This paper provides a renewed ecological approach, foregrounding parental perspectives—knowledge, beliefs, attitudes, theories, and expectations—and examining how they directly and indirectly guide infants' motor trajectories. Drawing on cross-cultural evidence, we illustrate how differences in parental priorities and caregiving behaviors can either accelerate or delay the emergence of crucial motor skills. We also highlight the reciprocal relationship between parent and child: while parental views shape caregiving practices, children's developing abilities and behaviors can, in turn, alter their parents' perspectives. Building on existing theories, including Bronfenbrenner's ecological systems theory and dynamic systems theory, our integrated model situates the parent–child dyad within broader socioeconomic, cultural, and environmental contexts. This model shows the dynamic, ever-evolving interplay between parents and children and demonstrates the importance of aligning parental cognition with targeted interventions to optimize motor development. By examining how cultural norms, individual experiences, and contextual factors converge, this paper offers both a theoretical framework and practical implications for supporting infants' growth. This paper will inform future research by encouraging parent-focused developmental studies and guiding practitioners to design culturally informed interventions in the field of motor development.

Keywords: motor development; infant development; parental influence; parental beliefs; parental cognitions; ecological systems theory

1. Introduction

Child development is a multifaceted process that involves a dynamic interplay between children and their environment. Among the many factors influencing this process, parents play a particularly profound role in shaping early learning [1]. Researchers have long emphasized the importance of maternal care during infancy, as the quality of this care can either facilitate or hinder a child's development [2]. When infants enter the world, they are entirely dependent on their caregivers, in many cases, their parents. As a child grows, parents play multiple roles, including feeding, protecting, educating, disciplining, and bonding with their children [3]. Through daily interactions, parents shape their children's development both directly and indirectly. At the same time, parents also develop a sense of efficacy in their caregiving roles and establish expectations for their children [4]. Therefore, a deeper examination of parents' roles during infancy is crucial for understanding the complexities of early childhood development.

One significant and often overlooked component of parental influence is the role of parental perspectives. In this paper, we use the term parental perspectives as a comprehensive concept that integrates a range of cognitive and affective constructs—including knowledge, beliefs, attitudes, theories, and expectations. While each of these components has been explored in past literature, there is no single term that adequately captures their combined influence on parenting behavior, especially within dynamic and culturally diverse contexts. We intentionally chose perspectives to reflect the holistic nature of how parents view development, themselves, and their children. This broader term allows us to account for both the explicitly held beliefs and tacit assumptions, which collectively shape caregiving behaviors. These perspectives act as guiding principles, determining which activities are introduced, how feedback is given, and how much effort is invested in caregiving [5]. These beliefs are active and evolving, in response to a parent's own experiences, cultural background, and direct interactions with their child. Ultimately, parental perspectives create a framework that guides behavior and helps shape a child's developmental journey across multiple domains, including motor skills.

The objectives of this paper are to (1) review the theoretical and empirical literature on the role of parental perspectives in motor development, (2) identify gaps in the existing frameworks, and (3) propose a novel integrated ecological model that positions parents as dynamic agents within child development. We begin by examining the foundational and contemporary theories that address motor development and the role of parents. Drawing from this theoretical foundation, we then review the empirical studies on how parental perspectives, caregiving behaviors, and environmental contexts shape motor trajectories. Based on the insights and gaps identified in these areas, we introduce a new ecological model that places the parent–child dyad at the center of the model. Finally, we reflect on the implications of this model for future research and intervention efforts, emphasizing the need to recognize parents as active, contextually embedded agents in shaping early motor outcomes.

1.1. Parental Perspectives in Academic Domains

Research has shown that parental perspectives significantly influence children's developmental trajectories. This phenomenon has been primarily studied in the context of academic achievement. For example, children whose parents value math tend to perform better in that subject [6,7]. The mechanisms through which parental beliefs shape children's math skills are important to understand. One proposed mechanism is that parents' beliefs about the importance of math influence the types of activities they engage in with their children. Studies suggest that parents who place a high value on math are more likely to engage in math-related activities, such as counting and sorting, with their preschool and school-age children, thereby promoting their children's math development [8–12]. Conversely, parental anxiety about their own math abilities is negatively associated with their children's math performance [13].

Similar patterns emerge in literacy development. Parents who hold strong beliefs about the importance of literacy are more likely to provide early literacy experiences [14] and engage in positive interactions during joint book reading activities [15]. Through these home literacy practices, parents can foster both reading skills and motivation to read in their children [16]. Children whose parents believe reading is a source of entertainment show more interest in reading [17]. More generally, parents' academic expectations and school readiness-related beliefs contribute to the quantity and quality of parenting practices and, in turn, influence children's school readiness [18]. Interestingly, even non-academic beliefs can influence early learning. For example, parents who emphasize the importance of play are more likely to support activities that foster creativity, problem-solving, and social–

emotional skills [19,20]. Additionally, maternal self-efficacy beliefs have been associated with toddlers' cognitive outcomes and affection towards their mothers [21].

Collectively, these studies show that parental perspectives, whether specific to academic subjects or more generally, can shape children's development by influencing the behaviors and environments that support learning. While much of this research has focused on cognitive skills like math and reading, other domains of development—particularly motor development—have received far less attention.

1.2. Importance of Motor Development

Motor development is critical for children's overall growth and lays the foundation for other domains, such as language, social, and cognitive development [22,23]. Children are intrinsically drawn to move their bodies and discover new motor possibilities. These skills open new opportunities for children to explore their surroundings and engage in more social interactions, which in turn influences their further development [24–27].

For instance, the development of reaching skills in early infancy allows children to grasp and manipulate objects, facilitating object exploration and problem-solving skills [28]. Later, the emergence of locomotion skills, such as walking, enables infants to travel greater distances, experience new visual perspectives, interact with objects in various ways, and communicate more with caregivers [29]. This interconnection among motor skills, environment, and other domains of development is often explained through the concept of 'developmental cascades', where advancements in one area can elicit positive responses from the environment that promote further development [30,31]. For example, as a child learns to crawl, their parents may praise and encourage them, which gradually facilitates language learning and helps them make meaningful connections with their surroundings. This, in turn, promotes overall development. Therefore, understanding motor development is essential, as it acts as the building blocks for infant development.

While all infants achieve motor milestones as they grow, caregivers' support is essential in this process. They contribute by providing physical space, engaging in play, and creating safe yet challenging environments for their children [3]. Understanding how parental perspectives influence motor development can reveal insights into these dynamics. Unlike cognitive domains, motor development research has historically received less attention regarding parental perspectives, though it is equally vital [23]. To contextualize motor development within a broader developmental framework, it is necessary to review the theoretical perspectives that have guided the research in this area. The following section will evaluate these theories to highlight their contributions and gaps, ultimately building the foundation for a renewed model. While this model emphasizes the relational and environmental influences on motor development, we acknowledge that child development arises from a complex interplay between innate biological factors and contextual experiences. Genetic predispositions and neuromotor readiness also play a vital role in shaping early motor skills.

2. Review of Theoretical Models

The theories on motor development provide frameworks for understanding how infants acquire motor skills and interact with their environments. Four prominent theories provide insights into motor development: the maturational theory, Bronfenbrenner's ecological systems theory, Vygotsky's sociocultural theory, and dynamic systems theory. Each of these frameworks offers a unique lens.

2.1. Maturational Theory

Traditionally, motor development has been studied through a biological lens, as exemplified by the maturational perspectives put forward by Arnold Gesell and others in the early 1900s [32–35]. Maturational views have remained popular and found widespread adoption in therapeutic settings. A key principle of the maturational theories of motor development is that motor development follows a biologically predetermined sequence of maturation, and environmental factors are considered to play only a minor role. Accordingly, infants are expected to follow a strict developmental sequence based primarily on internal readiness, regardless of external stimuli [36]. While this theory provides a foundational understanding of the biological underpinnings of motor development, its biologically determined view overlooks the significant role of experiences guided by parental engagement [37]. For example, maturational theories fail to explain cross-cultural differences in infant motor skill attainment [38].

2.2. Dynamic Systems Theory

A second theory that has found widespread adoption in the motor development literature is the dynamic systems theory. Dynamic systems views address the shortcomings of maturational perspectives by shifting the focus from fixed developmental sequences to the complex interplay of biological, environmental, and task-related factors that shape motor development [39–41]. According to this theory, children's behaviors are organized into dynamic patterns that exhibit both stability and flexibility. By emphasizing self-organization and the adaptive nature of motor skill acquisition, this theory provides a valuable point of view regarding the complexity of developmental changes. However, dynamic systems theory has been criticized for its vague conceptualization of systems and its lack of specificity in identifying the causes of developmental change. This broad focus can make it difficult to predict or identify specific causal mechanisms [42]. In this theory, systems are rather abstract entities that exert some influence on a child (also known as the developing system). However, little attention is paid to these systems themselves. Specifically, while dynamic systems views acknowledge that parents dynamically and reciprocally influence their child, the theory does not address the parent's own behavior, goals, or beliefs–the dynamic systems theory does not try to explain why the systems act the way they do.

2.3. Sociocultural Theory

Although not exclusively focused on motor development, other broader theories, such as sociocultural theory and ecological systems theory, are also relevant. Lev Vygotsky's sociocultural theory offers profound insights into how social interactions and cultural norms shape individual development [43]. A central concept of Vygotsky's theory is the Zone of Proximal Development (ZPD), which highlights the difference between what a child can achieve independently and what he/she can achieve under the guidance of a more knowledgeable other, such as a caregiver, peer, or teacher. This process of scaffolding allows children to integrate new knowledge into their existing mental structures. Vygotsky's framework emphasizes the importance of social and cultural contexts in learning. However, the theory may not be universally applicable, as different social groups may employ diverse learning methods, and each individual's social experience is unique [44].

2.4. Ecological Systems Theory

While Vygotsky's theory underlines social interactions and cultural contexts, Urie Bronfenbrenner's ecological systems theory provides a more comprehensive view of the bidirectional influences of the environment on child development. The ecological systems theory [45–47] complements other theories by situating the child within a complex system of relationships across multiple environmental levels. These interconnected systems range from the immediate family and close friends (microsystem) to broader cultural and societal influences (macrosystem). The exosystem, mesosystem, and chronosystem provide additional layers that contribute to a child's upbringing. Despite its wide application, ecological systems theory has faced some criticism. For instance, some scholars have argued that culture is deeply integrated into daily activities and should not be placed in a separate, distal system [48].

Despite the theoretical advancements, gaps remain in understanding the role of parental perspectives in infant motor skill development. The ecological systems theory and sociocultural theory may not fully apply to all social groups, as caregiving practices and interactions between parents and children can vary widely across cultures and communities. Therefore, the dynamics between parents and children can differ significantly, limiting the universality of these theories. Moreover, while these theories provide valuable insights, they are not specifically tailored to motor development during infancy. Factors, such as school and peers, may not be applicable.

In terms of the theories that do focus on motor development, the maturational theory neglects the influence of environmental factors, suggesting that development is driven primarily by internal biological processes. On the other hand, the dynamic systems theory acknowledges the role of environmental variables, but its vague conceptualization of systems and subsystems makes it difficult to apply to specific contexts. Most importantly, all of the previous theories position the child at the center of the developmental model. While this perspective is critical, it has failed to look into the essential role that parents play, especially during infancy.

2.5. Other Theories

Although our model is grounded in behavioral and ecological perspectives, we acknowledge that theories, such as Neuronal Group Selection Theory (NGST), offer a complementary neurobiological perspective. NGST proposes that motor development involves the selection of efficient neural networks through a process of variation and experience-driven adaptation [49,50]. Although NGST is more focused on internal neurodevelopmental processes, its emphasis on variability and experience aligns broadly with our model's attention to contextual influences. While NGST offers an important framework for understanding motor variability at the neural systems level, it is beyond the scope of this paper.

Similarly, the Developmental Niche framework [51,52] has informed the structure of our ecological layer. This model highlights how a child's development is shaped by three interrelated systems: the physical and social settings of the child, the culturally structured caregiving practices, and the caretaker's psychology. While this framework offers a culturally grounded lens and emphasis on the child's developmental context, including their parents, it does not focus specifically on observable child behaviors as developmental outcomes. Our model builds upon this framework by integrating its cultural and relational components into a system that centers the parent–child dyad and explicitly links parental perspectives, behaviors, and child motor development within an ecological structure.

3. Review of Empirical Studies

The empirical research provides valuable insights into the mechanisms through which parental perspectives and behaviors influence infant motor development. Prior research examining whether and how parental perspectives may influence child development can be categorized into explicit parental perspectives, implicit caregiving behaviors, and intervention-driven changes. Together, these studies illuminate the pathways by which parental perspectives shape behaviors, how these behaviors directly impact motor outcomes, and how contextual factors influence both perspectives and practices.

3.1. Explicit Assessments of Parental Perspectives on Motor Development

The research on explicit parental perspectives provides a window into how parents conceptualize motor development and the ways these conceptualizations shape their caregiving behaviors. Parental perspectives are influenced by cultural norms, socioeconomic conditions, and personal experiences, creating significant variability in the practices that ultimately affect infant motor outcomes. However, research that focuses on parental perspectives in the motor development domain remains scarce. The few studies that have focused on the role of parental perspectives have been completed mainly outside of the United States.

In Brazil, the research has shown that parental attitudes toward motor development can shape parenting practices and infant outcomes. For example, Gomes et al. [53] asked parents about their beliefs and practices. It was observed that parents exhibited different approaches based on their beliefs. Parents who valued motor stimulation were more likely to actively encourage motor stimulation, offering toys and spending time on the floor with their children to practice sitting and walking. Additionally, a more recent study by Graciosa et al. [54] demonstrated that parents who viewed motor development as a natural process tended to have children with later-emerging independent walking skills. Together, these two studies show that parental beliefs or practices may accelerate or slow down motor skill development.

In England, a series of studies by Hopkins & Westra [55,56] compared Jamaican mothers living in England with their English counterparts. The results of these studies revealed surprising contrasting patterns. The Jamaican mothers expected their children to achieve sitting and walking earlier than the English mothers. These expectations were quite accurate, as the Jamaican infants did reach these milestones earlier. Interestingly, 3 English infants progressed from sitting to walking without having crawled, while 12 Jamaican infants achieved walking alone without crawling. These observations may be related to differences in beliefs. The Jamaican mothers viewed sitting and walking as significant steps toward independence and success, whereas crawling was seen as primitive and hazardous. These views were not held by the British mothers, resulting in different motor development trajectories across the two groups.

In Isreal, infants have been observed to reach certain motor milestones earlier than their American peers, while Dutch infants tend to reach them later [57,58]. These developmental differences correspond with the distinct parental beliefs and caregiving strategies in each culture. Israeli parents tend to place significant importance on motor development and often engage in stimulating practices, such as prone positioning and floor play. In contrast, Dutch parents generally emphasize rest, regularity, and allowing development to unfold at a child's own pace. These patterns have been confirmed by recent cross-cultural research, which identified two contrasting cultural models of parenting beliefs: one emphasizing active facilitation as a parent in Israel, and the other prioritizing autonomy and supportive caregiving in the Netherlands [59,60]. Together, these findings highlight how observed developmental outcomes are shaped by underlying parental belief systems and broader cultural values.

The research on several African communities provides additional context. In these communities, infants often achieve motor milestones significantly earlier than their American and European counterparts [61]. This advancement is often attributed to broader societal factors. In these communities, motor skills are often encouraged from an early age, with parents employing hands-on methods to promote skills like sitting and standing [62]. For example, Yoruba mothers have reported that the age at which babies attain motor milestones depends on how they are reared. Some mothers have even suggested that children will not achieve these milestones without active teaching. These beliefs are coupled with cultural traditions. Yoruba caregivers often prop infants into sitting positions and place them in cardboard boxes or basins, believing these practices help foster independent sitting [63].

The reviewed studies highlight the significant variability in parental beliefs and behaviors, not only across cultures but also within them, revealing the complexity of the relationship between caregiving practices and motor development. In Brazil, the research demonstrates that even within the same cultural context, parental attitudes toward motor development can vary widely. Some parents actively promote motor stimulation, engaging in practices, such as floor play and the use of toys, to encourage sitting and walking [53]. In contrast, others adopt a more hands-off approach, viewing motor development as a natural process that unfolds without the need for direct intervention [54]. These differing perspectives align with distinct caregiving strategies and are potentially associated with variations in the timing of motor milestones, such as the emergence of independent walking. Cultural contrasts across countries further emphasize the influence of parental values on caregiving practices. Jamaican mothers prioritize sitting and walking, connecting these milestones with independence and maturity, while Israeli parents emphasize prone positioning to encourage the development of early physical skills [55–57]. In contrast, Dutch parents adopt a self-paced developmental philosophy, linked with a slower attainment of motor milestones [58]. These studies collectively reveal the nuanced relationships among parental perspectives, caregiving behaviors, and motor outcomes, demonstrating variability both within and across cultural contexts. They raise important questions about the factors that influence these relationships and challenge assumptions of uniformity in caregiving practices and beliefs, even within a shared cultural framework.

3.2. *Implicit Assessments of Parental Perspectives on Motor Development*

While explicit assessments provide insights into the indirect influences of parental perspectives, implicit assessments reveal the direct connections between caregiving practices and motor development. These studies often examine how parenting behaviors, shaped by cultural values and societal norms, impact infants' motor trajectories. Although these practices may not always reflect consciously articulated beliefs, they provide critical information about the parent–child dyad.

Research conducted in Kokwet highlighted how societal norms shape proactive caregiving. Super [64] observed that over 80% of mothers reported actively teaching their children skills, such as sitting and standing, demonstrating a deeply embedded cultural emphasis on fostering motor development. Similarly, in Zambia, parents engage in culturally specific techniques to encourage motor skills, such as tossing infants to increase their arousal and muscle tone or placing them in slings to promote postural stability [65,66]. These practices are associated with advanced skills, such as sitting and standing, but with delayed crawling compared to Euro-American infants, reflecting differing cultural values about which motor milestones are prioritized. In contrast, Euro-American parents view crawling as an essential milestone, linking it to early locomotor ability, autonomy, and environmental mastery [67]. To promote these abilities, they encourage independent locomotor efforts and reinforce quadrupedal movements [38].

The delayed development of certain skills due to caregiving practices is another theme in implicit assessments. For instance, in rural Chinese communities, parents often do not emphasize motor milestones and engage minimally in interactive play with their infants.

Wang et al. [68] observed that this lack of emphasis is associated with delayed motor skills and other developmental domains, suggesting that parental behaviors significantly influence developmental outcomes. A more striking example comes from Tajikistan, where the use of the "gahvora"—a traditional cradle that binds infants for prolonged periods—limits movement and leads to delayed milestones, such as crawling and walking [69,70]. In a recent comparative study, Wang et al. [71] extended these findings by examining motor restriction and infant locomotion in three culturally distinct societies: Tajikistan, Aka, and Tanna. They found that infants in Tajikistan experienced the longest durations of physical restriction due to cradle use, while Aka and Tanna infants were given far more opportunities to move around their neighborhoods and explore. Altogether, these findings illustrate how implicit caregiving practices, informed by cultural traditions, can both nurture and constrain opportunities for movement.

Within-cultural variations in parenting behaviors provide additional insights. In the United States, the "Back to Sleep" campaign, which promoted supine sleeping to reduce sudden infant death syndrome (SIDS), led many parents to restrict the use of prone sleeping positions [72]. Davis et al. [73] found that this shift was associated with delayed motor milestones, such as rolling and crawling. However, infants who regularly participated in tummy time or were placed in prone positions during waking hours demonstrated significantly higher locomotion scores [74]. These findings suggest that while parental practices may not always explicitly prioritize certain motor activities, these implicit decisions have measurable effects on infants' motor development.

Cultural priorities regarding motor milestones also highlight the variability in implicit caregiving practices. For example, in Euro-American families, where crawling is viewed as a critical developmental step, parents may unconsciously encourage behaviors that facilitate independent mobility. Conversely, in communities where early sitting or standing is emphasized, practices like tossing or propping infants reflect an implicit belief in the importance of fostering postural control and balance.

Altogether, these examples demonstrate that caregiving practices are shaped by cultural values, societal norms, and individual parenting strategies. They show how parental behaviors influence motor trajectories by creating opportunities or imposing limitations. While these behaviors may not directly reflect parents' conscious perspectives, they provide a valuable lens for understanding how implicit priorities and beliefs drive caregiving decisions and, consequently, infant development.

3.3. Research on Intervention Programs for Parents Points to Changes in Parental Behaviors

Intervention programs provide critical insights into how parental perspectives and behaviors can be influenced to support infant motor development. These programs target either the explicit and implicit aspects of parenting by addressing parental beliefs, modifying caregiving practices through structured activities, or fostering new skills. By engaging parents as active participants, interventions highlight the mechanisms through which parent-focused approaches can foster both immediate and long-term developmental outcomes.

Programs designed to explicitly modify parental perspectives demonstrate how changes in beliefs can influence caregiving behaviors and child outcomes. The Newborn Individualized Developmental Care and Assessment Program (NIDCAP) exemplifies this approach. By educating parents about infant behavioral cues and caregiving techniques, the NIDCAP aims to reduce parental stress and enhance parent–infant interactions. Participants have reported improved confidence in interpreting their infant's needs and greater adaptability in caregiving strategies, leading to better motor outcomes for their children [75]. Another program by Moxley-Haegert and Serbin [76] supports this notion. In this study, a home treatment program was implemented to help developmentally delayed children. The caregivers who received parent education were more knowledgeable and had a better understanding of their children's development than the no-education control group. Their children also had better motor outcomes as well. Moreover, at the follow-up visit a year later, the caregivers who received education participated more in treatment programs and were more motivated than those in the control group. Their children also showed continued advancement in their motor skills. These changes seemed to be long-lasting, demonstrating the benefit of support and education for parents.

The implicit influences on parental perspectives that indirectly shape behaviors have been observed in both clinical and non-clinical settings. Clinical programs targeting infants at risk of developmental delays have demonstrated the importance of parental involvement for achieving positive outcomes. For instance, interventions emphasizing motor-enhancing exercises rely heavily on parents' active participation, and studies have shown that greater parental involvement correlates with improved motor milestones [77,78]. These findings suggest that interventions not only improve infant outcomes but also enhance parents' understanding of their role as facilitators of development. Importantly, parents involved in such programs have often reported lasting changes in their caregiving behaviors, even after the intervention concluded [79].

Non-clinical interventions illustrate the transformative potential of parent-led practices integrated into daily routines. For example, Lobo and Galloway [80] demonstrated that parents trained in enhanced handling and positioning techniques for three weeks observed significant improvements in their infants' gross and fine motor skills. Similarly, "sticky mittens" interventions, where parents guide infants in enriched reaching sessions, resulted in increased manual exploration, better coordination, and stronger parent–infant engagement [81,82]. These interventions influence parental behaviors by embedding motor skill practices into naturalistic interactions, ensuring that the changes are practical and sustainable.

The mechanisms driving changes in parental perspectives and behaviors are multifaceted. Education programs directly influence explicit beliefs by equipping parents with knowledge about developmental processes and caregiving techniques. For instance, by learning the importance of tummy time or handling exercises, parents may adopt more structured motor-stimulating behaviors. Behavior-focused interventions rely on experiential learning, where parents see tangible improvements in their child's development, reinforcing the value of their caregiving practices. These experiences create positive feedback loops, where successful engagement strengthens parental confidence and commitment to motor-focused caregiving.

Whether these changes last depend on several factors, including the intensity and frequency of the intervention, the support available to parents post-intervention, and how well the practices align with parents' cultural and ecological contexts. Studies like those by Lobo and Galloway [80] have demonstrated that when interventions are integrated into daily routines and supported by follow-up resources, parents are more likely to sustain the changes over time.

Collectively, these examples illustrate that interventions targeting both parental perspectives and behaviors can influence caregiving practices and create lasting impacts on infant motor development. By providing parents with practical skills, reinforcing positive outcomes, and addressing cultural and contextual factors, these programs equip families with the tools necessary to sustain nurturing caregiving environments.

4. New Integrated Model

While the existing theories and empirical studies offer valuable insights into motor development, significant gaps remain in understanding how parental perspectives dynamically influence caregiving behaviors and motor outcomes within diverse ecological contexts. The existing theoretical models, such as Bronfenbrenner's ecological systems theory and dynamic systems theory, recognize the importance of environmental and interactive factors, but they often overlook the active role of parents, particularly how their beliefs and behaviors dynamically influence motor outcomes. These frameworks lack an integration of parental perspectives as the central agents of developmental change, especially during infancy.

To address the existing gaps, we propose a new integrated model that situates the parent–child dyad within an ecological framework, emphasizing the dynamic interplay among parental perspectives, parental behaviors, and infant motor development (see Figure 1). By consolidating the existing theories, the model is structured around three core components: parental perspectives, parental behaviors, and children's behaviors. These interactions are embedded within an ecological layer that represents the unique contexts of both parents and children. This structure is conceptually informed by the Developmental Niche framework [51,52], which identifies the physical and social settings of the child, culturally regulated caregiving, and caregiver psychology as the key organizing systems in development. Our model draws on these subsystems but departs from the Developmental Niche framework by placing a stronger emphasis on parental perspectives as active drivers, and by focusing explicitly on motor behavior as a developmental outcome.

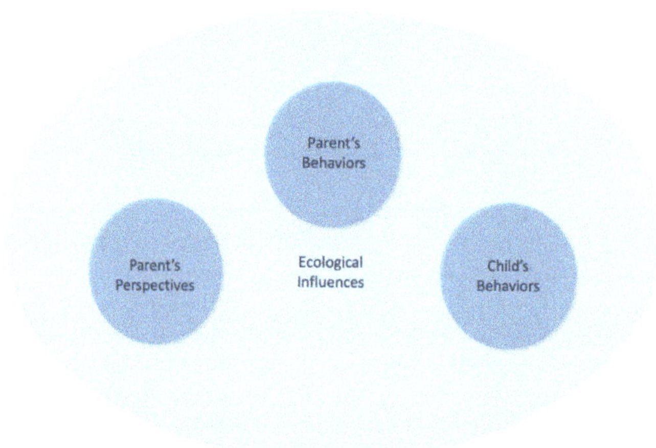

Figure 1. Integrated model of parent–child dyad in motor development. *Note*: This figure illustrates the new integrated model that places the parent–child dyad within an ecological framework, emphasizing the dynamic interplay among parental perspectives, parental behaviors, and children's behaviors. It highlights the evolving nature of these interactions and demonstrates the importance of environmental contexts in shaping motor outcomes.

The model recognizes that parental perspectives and behaviors evolve through interactions with their children and their broader environment. It also draws attention to the importance of cultural and socioeconomic contexts in shaping these perspectives and practices, providing a comprehensive understanding of how parents influence their children's development. By focusing on the reciprocal nature of the parent–child dyad and the contextual factors that shape these interactions, this model offers new insights into the mechanisms through which parental perspectives affect motor outcomes.

Model Components

At the heart of this model are parental perspectives—a wide range of cognitive constructs that parents hold regarding their children, themselves, the course of development, and child-rearing practices. These perspectives encompass knowledge, beliefs, attitudes, theories, and expectations. The existing research has explored aspects of parental perspectives under the term "parental cognitions", which refers to parenting knowledge, beliefs, expectations, perceptions, and satisfaction [5,83]. Parents acquire information about child development through their daily experiences, such as babysitting siblings; through communicating with others, such as friends and family; and through education, such as parenting classes. For example, when a father sees his daughter turning her head side-to-side, he may know that she is hungry because he learned this from a parenting book. Additionally, parents form beliefs, theories, and ethnotheories [84] based on their own experiences, cultural backgrounds, and interactions with their children. For instance, a parent who experienced physical play during childhood may believe that physical play is essential for child development. Parents also develop expectations regarding their children's developmental milestones. For example, a mother may expect her daughter to start walking around 12 months based on observations of other children. These perspectives guide parental behaviors, which, in turn, influence children's behaviors (see Figures 2a and 3a). Our model builds on the previous literature by unifying these constructs under the umbrella of parental perspectives to better capture their interaction with infant development and environmental contexts.

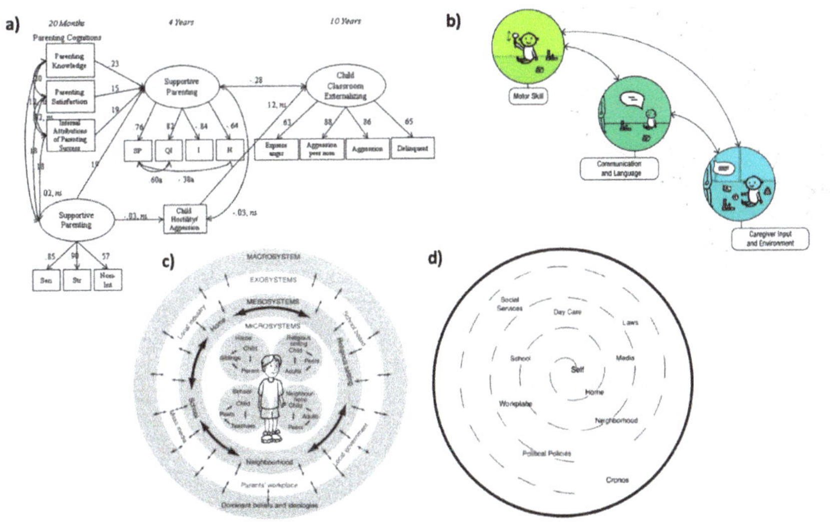

Figure 2. Illustrations informing the integrated framework. *Note*: This figure presents four illustrations that inspired the development of the proposed integrated framework. (**a**) is taken from Bornstein and colleagues [5], and demonstrates how parental cognition shapes parenting practices, which in turn influence child outcomes. (**b**) is taken from Iverson [30], and illustrates the developmental cascade model, where a child's motor development influences their surroundings, including parental behaviors. (**c**) is taken from Bronfenbrenner's ecological systems theory [45], and situates a child within a series of systems, from immediate family to broader societal norms, all of which impact the child's development bidirectionally. Finally, (**d**) is taken from Vélez-Agosto and colleagues [48], and includes the revised ecological model, which moves cultural factors into the microsystem. These models together serve as the theoretical foundation for the proposed model.

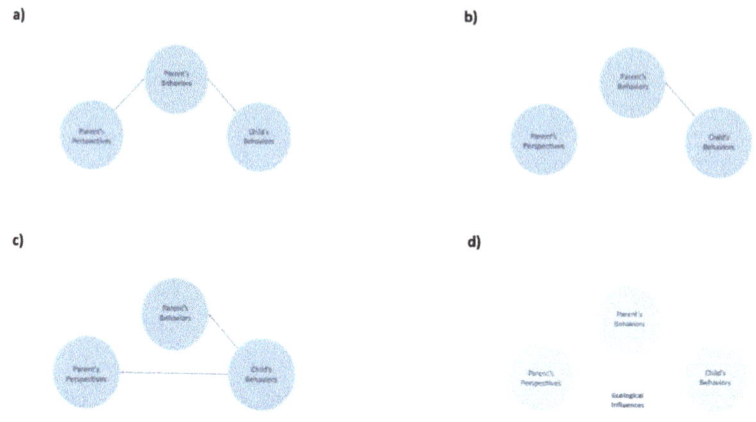

Figure 3. Components of the integrated model and ecological influences. *Note*: This figure series builds cumulatively to depict the integrated model. Each subfigure (**a**–**d**) introduces a distinct element, clarifying how parental perspectives, behaviors, child behaviors, and ecological context interact progressively. (**a**) shows how parental perspectives shape parental behaviors and indirectly influence children's behaviors. (**b**) reveals the direct impact of parental behaviors on children's motor development not directed by their perspectives. (**c**) focuses on children's behaviors, emphasizing the reciprocal nature of the parent–child relationship, where children's actions can influence parental behaviors and perspectives. (**d**) introduces the ecological layer, which is unique to each parent–child dyad, illustrating how these broader environmental contexts affect them.

Parental behaviors refer to the actions, responses, and methods parents use in child-rearing. These behaviors are shaped by parents' knowledge, theories, attitudes, and beliefs [85]. For example, when a father sees his hungry daughter turning her head, he draws from his knowledge and responds by feeding her. A mother who believes motor stimulation is beneficial might reinforce tummy time with her son. Parents' expectations also influence how they interact with their children. For example, a mother who expects her child to walk early may provide more opportunities to practice walking. It is also important to note that parental perspectives do not always align with actual practices. A father may believe screen time is harmful for motor development while allowing his child to watch TV due to exhaustion. Nevertheless, parental behaviors play a crucial role in shaping children's motor development (see Figure 3b).

Children's behaviors in this model refer to the observable motor actions that infants display through their interactions with caregivers and their environment. These behaviors include both immediate reactions to parental actions and the motor skills that develop over time. For instance, children whose parents encourage sitting may acquire sitting skills faster, and those whose parents restrict walking may develop walking skills slower. Due to the reciprocal nature of parent–child dynamics, children's behaviors can also influence their parents' behaviors and perspectives (see Figures 2b and 3c). While traditional models have viewed the child as a passive recipient of parental guidance, this model aligns with the concept of bidirectional influences between parents and children, as described by Relation Developmental Systems-Based models [86]. Our model also draws from Piaget's and Gibson's notion of children as active learners. Ref. [87] suggested that infants explore and experiment with motor actions to construct knowledge about their abilities and everything around them. Similarly, ref. [88]'s theory of perception emphasized that children are attuned to environmental cues, learning from the opportunities their surroundings provide. Together, these works indicate that children actively shape their own motor development through exploration, creating a feedback loop where their actions elicit meaningful responses from their caregivers. This bidirectional process also reflects the concept of developmental cascades, where a child's motor development sparks environmental responses, further shaping growth [30]. For example, if an infant does well during tummy time, the parent may continue the activity, which may alter the parent's perception of their child's abilities.

Parents and children alone do not fully encapsulate the complexity of child development. Integrating an ecological layer is crucial to account for the additional factors that affect this process. Drawing from Bronfenbrenner's ecological systems theory [45] and its revised version [48], we propose that parental perspectives, parental behaviors, and children's behaviors are embedded within an ecological layer (see Figures 2c,d and 3d). This layer includes, but is not limited to, factors such as neighborhoods, extended families, community networks, social trends, cultural contexts, public policies, socioeconomic status, and life events. More importantly, contemporary ecological factors, such as increased screen time, dual-working parents, shifting parenting norms, and access to developmental information through digital platforms, also shape parents, making them important contextual variables in modern motor development. These factors are incorporated into a flexible and inclusive ecological layer, acknowledging that not all families engage with every factor in the same way. These ecological factors influence parenting through a variety of mechanisms. For example, cultural norms shape what behaviors are encouraged or discouraged (e.g., prioritizing walking vs. crawling), while education systems and access to information affect parents' knowledge about developmental milestones. Social support networks—including extended family or community groups—can provide reinforcement or challenges to parents' child-rearing practices. Socioeconomic conditions may limit or expand the physical space, time, or safety available for motor play. Even national health policies or campaigns (such as supine sleep recommendations) can unintentionally alter daily caregiving routines. These contextual forces do not operate in isolation; they often interact with each other and with parents' own experiences to shape the perspectives they hold and the behaviors they enact. Thus, the ecological layer in our model functions not only as a backdrop, but as a dynamic set of influences that help explain the variability in parental decision-making across cultural and socioeconomic contexts.

The relationships among parental perspectives, parental behaviors, and children's motor development are conceptualized as correlational, dynamic, and bidirectional. Rather than assuming fixed causal pathways, our model highlights how these components mutually influence and reflect one another over time. These patterns unfold within broader ecological contexts, which shape and are shaped by the parent–child dyad. We do not claim that any of the model components directly determine motor outcomes. Instead, we propose that they are associated with and play an important part in infant motor development. This framework is testable using correlational and longitudinal designs, such as studies examining whether specific parental perspectives are associated with variations in motor milestones over time. While not prescriptive or predictive, the model offers a structure for generating empirically grounded questions about how parent and child factors interact within complex ecological systems. A comparative table of the proposed model and previous models can be found below (see Table 1).

Table 1. Comparison of our model with previous models.

Feature	Maturational Theory	Dynamic Systems Theory	Sociocultural Theory	Ecological Systems Theory	Proposed Integrated Model
Central Focus	Biological maturation of the child	Interplay of internal and external systems	Social interaction and guided learning	Multilayered environmental influences on the child	Parent-child dyad within ecological context
View of Parent	Peripheral, minor environmental influence	Implicit part of the system	"More knowledgeable other", but secondary to child	One of many microsystem agents	Active, reflective agent influencing development
Mechanism of Change	Genetically driven maturation	Self-organization and adaptation	Scaffolding within ZPD	Systemic and bidirectional influences	Reciprocal, evolving influence situated in the context
Parental Perspectives Addressed	No	No	Limited	Indirectly	Central and directly defined
Applicability to Motor Development	Yes, but limited to biological factors	Yes, but concept is too abstract	Not motor-specific	Not motor-specific	Specifically designed for infant motor development
Bidirectional Influence	No	Yes	Yes	Yes	Yes
Accounting for Variability in Developmental Context	Assumes universal biological sequence; minimal contextual sensitivity	Acknowledges context, but lacks specificity in application	Cultural learning varies, but often child-centered	Includes multiple systems, but model is generalized across groups	Context-sensitive and individualized; adapts to each family's unique ecological environment

Note: This table compares the key characteristics of the major developmental theories—maturational theory, dynamic systems theory, sociocultural theory, ecological systems theory—with the proposed model. It highlights the distinctive features of each framework across several dimensions, including their focus, treatment of parental roles, mechanisms of change, inclusion of parental perspectives, applicability to motor development, model direction, and considerations of varied developmental contexts.

5. Discussion

The proposed integrated model for understanding infant motor development provides a comprehensive framework that addresses parental perspectives, parental behaviors, and child behaviors within an ecological context. By emphasizing the evolving, reciprocal interactions among these components, this model offers a holistic perspective on the factors that influence motor development during infancy.

5.1. Summary of Proposed Model

Central to this model are parental perspectives, which play a key role in shaping how parents interact with their children and the behaviors they adopt. These perspectives also determine the opportunities and support children receive for motor development. Importantly, parental perspectives are not fixed; they change as parents gain new experiences, insights, and as they respond to their children's behaviors. These shifting perspectives, in turn, guide their actions and practices.

Equally important are children's behaviors, which encompass the observable motor actions and reactions that emerge as they engage with their environment and caregivers. These behaviors are influenced by parental perspectives and actions but also affect how parents respond. This aligns with developmental theories that have pointed out the active role children play in shaping their own development [87,88]. Rather than viewing parent–child interactions as a one-way process, this model highlights the cyclical nature of these exchanges, where children's actions continuously inform parental behaviors and beliefs [86].

The proposed model is also unique as it places parents in the inner circle, examining the factors influencing their perspectives and behaviors. Such an approach not only highlights the critical role parents play during infancy but also provides a deeper understanding of why parents engage in specific parenting behaviors. This understanding can inform targeted interventions, enabling us to better help parents so that they, in turn, can better support their children.

The ecological layer integrates various contextual factors into a flexible framework, recognizing that each family operates within a unique set of circumstances. As societal conditions evolve, so too do the environments that influence motor development. By incorporating elements of prior theories, this model underlines the changing nature of children's developmental contexts, while accounting for the distinct challenges and opportunities that families encounter [45,48]. Ultimately, the interactions among parents, children, and their surrounding environment jointly craft parenting practices and developmental outcomes.

5.2. Implications for Research and Practice

The integrated model has significant implications for both research and practice. Researchers can use this model to design studies that capture the complexity of environmental influences on motor development, employing methodologies that account for the interactions among different contextual factors. Observing and documenting changes in motor behaviors within various contexts will provide valuable insights into the developmental process and offer a clearer understanding of motor skill acquisition.

For practitioners, this model can guide the development of interventions that address multiple layers of influence, from direct parent–child interactions to broader community and societal supports. By focusing on enhancing parental perspectives and behaviors, interventions can create supportive environments that foster motor development. Understanding the unique circumstances of each family can also inform culturally sensitive and contextually relevant approaches.

5.3. Limitations and Future Directions

Despite its contributions, the model has a few limitations. It is based on correlational patterns and does not establish causal mechanisms. While this reflects the complexity of real-world development, it also limits its predictive precision. Additionally, the model does not explicitly account for factors, such as parental mental health, child temperament, and child genetic/innate processes, that may moderate or mediate parent–child dynamics and influence child motor outcomes. Its applicability to high-adversity contexts—such as children who are cared for by caregivers other than their parents—may be limited. Further, while it centers on parental perspectives and behaviors, it does not yet incorporate children's own beliefs, which may be relevant in older age groups and should be addressed.

The primary focus of the current review and proposed model is on motor development during infancy. However, the proposed model does not need to be limited to the motor domain. Examining the applicability of our proposed model to other developmental domains would be beneficial and should be entertained in future research. Further, longitudinal studies examining how parental perspectives evolve over time and how these changes correlate with children's motor trajectories would enhance our understanding of the reciprocal nature of child–parent interactions over time.

Finally, another important direction for future work involves understanding where parents' perspectives come from. One source is formal parenting education, which varies across countries and systems. A recent analysis by Lobo et al. [89] compared publicly available parent education materials and found that motor development was discussed quite often, yet the content varied by country. Future research should explore how their content and other parenting resources influence caregivers and, in turn, infants' motor behaviors.

6. Conclusions

Parental perspectives and behaviors shape and influence a child's development across domains. However, research on the impact of parental perspectives or behaviors on infant motor development remains rare. This may be due to the lack of a theoretical model that focuses on how parental perspectives and behaviors within a specific ecological context act to shape infant motor behaviors and development specifically. To address this gap, we propose a new holistic model centered on infants' observable motor behaviors and explicitly include parental perspectives and behaviors as factors shaping motor developmental outcomes. In contrast to prior models, the proposed model separates parental beliefs from their behaviors, situates parent–child interactions within a larger ecological context, and includes bidirectional relations between infant behavior and both parental beliefs and behaviors. We hope that the proposed model will be applied to prior research and will generate new hypotheses for future research on the complex factors shaping infant motor development.

Author Contributions: Conceptualization: R.A., Methodology: R.A., Resources: R.A. and K.L., Writing: R.A. and K.L. All authors have read and agreed to the published version of the manuscript.

Funding: This research has received no external funding.

Institutional Review Board Statement: Not applicable.

Informed Consent Statement: Not applicable.

Data Availability Statement: No new data were created or analyzed in this study.

Conflicts of Interest: The authors declare no conflict of interest.

References

1. Landry, S.H. The role of parents in early childhood learning. In *Encyclopedia on Early Childhood Development*; Centre of Excellence for Early Childhood Development: Montreal, QC, Canada, 2008.
2. Bornstein, M.H. Human Infancy . . . and the Rest of the Lifespan. *Annu. Rev. Psychol.* **2014**, *65*, 121–158. [CrossRef] [PubMed]
3. Mowder, B.A. Parent Development Theory: Understanding parents, parenting perceptions and parenting behaviors. *J. Early Child. Infant Psychol.* **2005**, *1*, 46–64.
4. Goldberg, S. Social Competence in Infancy: A Model of Parent-Infant Interaction. *Merrill Palmer Q. Behav. Dev.* **1977**, *23*, 163–177.
5. Bornstein, M.H.; Putnick, D.L.; Suwalsky, J.T.D. Parenting cognitions → parenting practices → child adjustment? The standard model. *Dev. Psychopathol.* **2018**, *30*, 399–416. [CrossRef]
6. Silver, A.M.; Elliott, L.; Libertus, M.E. When beliefs matter most: Examining children's math achievement in the context of parental math anxiety. *J. Exp. Child Psychol.* **2021**, *201*, 104992. [CrossRef]
7. Silver, A.M.; Chen, Y.; Smith, D.K.; Tamis-LeMonda, C.S.; Cabrera, N.; Libertus, M.E. Mothers' and fathers' engagement in math activities with their toddler sons and daughters: The moderating role of parental math beliefs. *Front Psychol.* **2023**, *14*, 1124056. [CrossRef]
8. Cannon, J.; Ginsburg, H.P. 'Doing the Math': Maternal Beliefs About Early Mathematics Versus Language Learning. *Early Educ. Dev.* **2008**, *19*, 238–260. [CrossRef]

9. LeFevre, J.-A.; Skwarchuk, S.-L.; Smith-Chant, B.L.; Fast, L.; Kamawar, D.; Bisanz, J. Home numeracy experiences and children's math performance in the early school years. *Can. J. Behav. Sci. Rev. Can. Des Sci. Comport.* **2009**, *41*, 55–66. [CrossRef]
10. Musun-Miller, L.; Blevins-Knabe, B. Adults' beliefs about children and mathematics: How important is it and how do children learn about it? *Early Dev. Parent.* **1998**, *7*, 191–202. [CrossRef]
11. Sonnenschein, S.; Galindo, C.; Metzger, S.R.; Thompson, J.A.; Huang, H.C.; Lewis, H. Parents' Beliefs about Children's Math Development and Children's Participation in Math Activities. *Child Dev. Res.* **2012**, *2012*, 1–13. [CrossRef]
12. Zippert, E.L.; Ramani, G.B. Parents' Estimations of Preschoolers' Number Skills Relate to at-Home Number-Related Activity Engagement: Parents' Estimates of Child's Number Skills. *Inf. Child. Dev.* **2017**, *26*, e1968. [CrossRef]
13. Maloney, E.A.; Ramirez, G.; Gunderson, E.A.; Levine, S.C.; Beilock, S.L. Intergenerational Effects of Parents' Math Anxiety on Children's Math Achievement and Anxiety. *Psychol. Sci.* **2015**, *26*, 1480–1488. [CrossRef]
14. Lynch, J.; Anderson, J.; Anderson, A.; Shapiro, J. Parents' Beliefs About Young Children's Literacy Development and Parents' Literacy Behaviors. *Read. Psychol.* **2006**, *27*, 1–20. [CrossRef]
15. Bingham, G.E. Maternal Literacy Beliefs and the Quality of Mother-Child Book-reading Interactions: Assoications with Children's Early Literacy Development. *Early Educ. Dev.* **2007**, *18*, 23–49. [CrossRef]
16. Baker, L.; Scher, D. Beginning Readers' Motivation for Reading in Relation to Parental beliefs and Home Reading Experiences. *Read. Psychol.* **2002**, *23*, 239–269. [CrossRef]
17. Baker, L.; Scher, D.; Mackler, K. Home and family influences on motivations for reading. *Educ. Psychol.* **1997**, *32*, 69–82. [CrossRef]
18. Puccioni, J. Parents' Conceptions of School Readiness, Transition Practices, and Children's Academic Achievement Trajectories. *J. Educ. Res.* **2015**, *108*, 130–147. [CrossRef]
19. Manz, P.H.; Bracaliello, C.B. Expanding home visiting outcomes: Collaborative measurement of parental play beliefs and examination of their association with parents' involvement in toddler's learning. *Early Child. Res. Q.* **2016**, *36*, 157–167. [CrossRef]
20. Rowe, M.L.; Casillas, A. Parental goals and talk with toddlers. *Infant Child Dev.* **2011**, *20*, 475–494. [CrossRef]
21. Coleman, P.K.; Karraker, K.H. Maternal self-efficacy beliefs, competence in parenting, and toddlers' behavior and developmental status. *Infant Ment. Health J.* **2003**, *24*, 126–148. [CrossRef]
22. Leonard, H.C.; Hill, E.L. Review: The impact of motor development on typical and atypical social cognition and language: A systematic review. *Child Adolesc. Ment. Health* **2014**, *19*, 163–170. [CrossRef] [PubMed]
23. Libertus, K.; Hauf, P. Editorial: Motor Skills and Their Foundational Role for Perceptual, Social, and Cognitive Development. *Front Psychol.* **2017**, *8*, 301. [CrossRef]
24. Franchak, J.M.; Kretch, K.S.; Adolph, K.E. See and be seen: Infant-caregiver social looking during locomotor free play. *Dev. Sci.* **2018**, *21*, e12626. [CrossRef]
25. Gibson, E.J.; Pick, A.D. *An Ecological Approach to Peptual Learning and Development*; Oxford University Press: Oxford, UK, 2000.
26. Marcinowski, E.C.; Tripathi, T.; Hsu, L.; McCoy, S.W.; Dusing, S.C. Sitting skill and the emergence of arms-free sitting affects the frequency of object looking and exploration. *Dev. Psychobiol.* **2019**, *61*, 1035–1047. [CrossRef] [PubMed]
27. Soska, K.C.; Adolph, K.E.; Johnson, S.P. Systems in development: Motor skill acquisition facilitates three-dimensional object completion. *Dev. Psychol.* **2010**, *46*, 129–138. [CrossRef]
28. Lobo, M.A.; Galloway, J.C. Postural and Object-Oriented Experiences Advance Early Reaching, Object Exploration, and Means-End Behavior. *Child Dev.* **2008**, *79*, 1869–1890. [CrossRef] [PubMed]
29. Adolph, K.E.; Tamis-LeMonda, C.S. The Costs and Benefits of Development: The Transition from Crawling to Walking. *Child Dev. Perspect.* **2014**, *8*, 6. [CrossRef]
30. Iverson, J.M. Developmental Variability and Developmental Cascades: Lessons from Motor and Language Development in Infancy. *Curr. Dir. Psychol. Sci.* **2021**, *30*, 228–235. [CrossRef]
31. Masten, A.S.; Cicchetti, D. Developmental cascades. *Dev. Psychopathol.* **2010**, *22*, 491–495. [CrossRef]
32. Gesell, A. *Infancy and Human Growth*; The Macmillan Company: New York, NY, USA, 1928.
33. Gesell, A. The Developmental Morphology of Infant Behavior Pattern. *Proc. Natl. Acad. Sci. USA* **1932**, *18*, 139–143. [CrossRef]
34. Gesell, A.; Amatruda, C. The Embryology of Behavior: The Beginnings of the Human Mind. In *Classics in Developmental Medicine*; MacKeith: London, UK, 1988.
35. McGraw, M.B. *The Neuromuscular Maturation of the Human Infant*; Columbia University Press: New York, NY, USA, 1943; p. 140.
36. Formiga, C.K.M.R.; Linhares, M.B.M. Motor Skills: Development in Infancy and Early Childhood. In *International Encyclopedia of the Social & Behavioral Sciences*; Elsevier: Amsterdam, The Netherlands, 2015; pp. 971–977. [CrossRef]
37. Sameroff, A. A Unified Theory of Development: A Dialectic Integration of Nature and Nurture. *Child Dev.* **2010**, *81*, 6–22. [CrossRef] [PubMed]
38. Cintas, H.L. Cross-Cultural Similarities and Differences in Development and the Impact of Parental Expectations on Motor Behavior.pdf. *Pediatr. Phys. Ther.* **1995**, *7*, 103–111. [CrossRef]
39. Smith, L.B.; Thelen, E. Development as a dynamic system. *Trends Cogn. Sci.* **2003**, *7*, 343–348. [CrossRef] [PubMed]
40. Thelen, E. Dynamic Systems Theory and the Complexity of Change. *Psychoanal. Dialogues* **2005**, *15*, 255–283. [CrossRef]

41. Thelen, E.; Smith, L.B. *A Dynamic Systems Approach to the Development of Cognition and Action*; The MIT Press: Cambridge, MA, USA, 1994. [CrossRef]
42. Spencer, J.P.; Perone, S.; Buss, A.T. Twenty Years and Going Strong: A Dynamic Systems Revolution in Motor and Cognitive Development: Dynamic Systems Revolution in Motor and Cognitive Development. *Child Dev. Perspect.* **2011**, *5*, 260–266. [CrossRef]
43. Vygotsky, L.S. *Mind in Society*; Harvard University Press: Cambridge, MA, USA, 1978. [CrossRef]
44. Liu, C.H.; Matthews, R. Vygotsky's philosophy: Constructivism and its criticisms examined. *Int. Educ. J.* **2005**, *6*, 386–399.
45. Bronfenbrenner, U. *The Ecology of Human Development: Experiments by Nature and Design*; Harvard University Press: Cambridge, MA, USA, 1979.
46. Bronfenbrenner, U.; Ceci, S.J. Nature-Nurture Reconceptualized in Developmental Perspective: A Bioecological Model. *Psychol. Rev.* **1994**, *101*, 568–586. [CrossRef]
47. Härkönen, U. *The Bronfenbrenner Ecological Systems Theory of Human Development*; Oxford University Press: Oxford, UK, 2007.
48. Vélez-Agosto, N.M.; Soto-Crespo, J.G.; Vizcarrondo-Oppenheimer, M.; Vega-Molina, S.; Coll, C.G. Bronfenbrenner's Bioecological Theory Revision: Moving Culture from the Macro into the Micro. *Perspect. Psychol. Sci.* **2017**, *12*, 900–910. [CrossRef]
49. Hadders-Algra, M. Early human motor development: From variation to the ability to vary and adapt. *Neurosci. Biobehav. Rev.* **2018**, *90*, 411–427. [CrossRef]
50. Hadders-Algra, M. The Neuronal Group Selection Theory: A framework to explain variation in normal motor development. *Develop. Med. Child. Neuro.* **2000**, *42*, 566–572. [CrossRef]
51. Harkness, S.; Super, C.M. Culture and human development: Where did it go? And where is it going? *New Dir. Child Adolesc. Dev.* **2020**, *2020*, 101–119. [CrossRef] [PubMed]
52. Harkness, S.; Super, C.M. The developmental niche: A theoretical framework for analyzing the household production of health. *Soc. Sci. Med.* **1994**, *38*, 217–226. [CrossRef] [PubMed]
53. Gomes, A.M.; Ribeiro, R.F.; Prat, B.V.; Magalhães, L.D.C.; Morais, R.L.D.S. Parental practices and beliefs on motor development in the first year of life. *Fisioter Mov.* **2017**, *30*, 769–779. [CrossRef]
54. Graciosa, M.D.; Ferronato, P.A.M.; Drezner, R.; De Jesus Manoel, E. Emergence of locomotor behaviors: Associations with infant characteristics, developmental status, parental beliefs, and practices in typically developing Brazilian infants aged 5 to 15 months. *Infant Behav. Dev.* **2024**, *76*, 101965. [CrossRef] [PubMed]
55. Hopkins, B.; Westra, T. Maternal Expectations of Their Infants' Development: Some Cultural Differences. *Develop. Med. Child. Neuro.* **1989**, *31*, 384–390. [CrossRef]
56. Hopkins, B.; Westra, T. Motor development, maternal expectations, and the role of handling. *Infant Behav. Dev.* **1990**, *13*, 117–122. [CrossRef]
57. Kohen-Raz, R. Mental and motor development of kibbutz, institutionalized, and home-reared infants in Israel. *Child Dev.* **1968**, *39*, 489–504. [CrossRef]
58. Steenis, L.J.P.; Verhoeven, M.; Hessen, D.J.; Van Baar, A.L. Performance of Dutch Children on the Bayley III: A Comparison Study of US and Dutch Norms. *PLoS ONE* **2015**, *10*, e0132871. [CrossRef]
59. Oudgenoeg-Paz, O.; Atun-Einy, O.; van Schaik, S.D.M. Two Cultural Models on Infant Motor Development: Middle Class Parents in Israel and the Netherlands. *Front. Psychol.* **2020**, *11*, 119. [CrossRef]
60. van Schaik, S.D.M.; Oudgenoeg-Paz, O.; Atun-Einy, O. Cross-cultural differences in parental beliefs about infant motor development: A quantitative and qualitative report of middle-class Israeli and Dutch parents. *Dev. Psychol.* **2018**, *54*, 999–1010. [CrossRef]
61. Geber, M.; Dean, R.F.A. The State of Development of Newborn African Children. *Lancet* **1957**, *269*, 1216–1219. [CrossRef] [PubMed]
62. Goodnow, J.J.; Collins, W.A. Development according to parents: The nature, sources, and consequences of parents' ideas. In *Essays in Developmental Psychology*; Lawrence Erlbaum Associates: Hove, UK, 1990.
63. Ejemen, O.P.; Bernard, O.E.; Oluwafemi, D.I. Socio-Cultural Context of Developmental Milestones in Infancy in South West Nigeria: A Qualitative Study. *Eur. Sci. J.* **2015**, *11*, 1–17.
64. Super, C.M. Environmental Effects on Motor Development: The Case of 'African Infant Precocity. *Dev. Med. Child Neurol.* **1976**, *18*, 561–567. [CrossRef]
65. Brazelton, T.B.; Koslowski, B.; Tronick, E. Neonatal Behavior among Urban Zambians and Americans. *J. Am. Acad. Child Psychiatry* **1976**, *15*, 97–107. [CrossRef]
66. Capute, A.J.; Shapiro, B.K.; Palmer, F.B.; Ross, A.; Wachtel, R.C. Normal Gross Motor Development: The Influences of Race, Sex And Socio-Economic Status. *Dev. Med. Child Neurol.* **2008**, *27*, 635–643. [CrossRef]
67. Lagerspetz, K.; Nygåkd, M.; Strandvik, C. The Effects of Training in Crawling on the Motor and Mental Development of Infants. *Scand. J. Psychol.* **1971**, *12*, 192–197. [CrossRef]

68. Wang, L.; Liang, W.; Zhang, S.; Jonsson, L.; Li, M.; Yu, C.; Sun, Y.; Ma, Q.; Bai, Y.; Abbey, C.; et al. Are infant/toddler developmental delays a problem across rural China? *J. Comp. Econ.* **2019**, *47*, 458–469. [CrossRef]
69. Karasik, L.B.; Tamis-LeMonda, C.S.; Ossmy, O.; Adolph, K.E. The ties that bind: Cradling in Tajikistan. *PLoS ONE* **2018**, *13*, e0204428. [CrossRef] [PubMed]
70. Karasik, L.B.; Adolph, K.E.; Fernandes, S.N.; Robinson, S.R.; Tamis-LeMonda, C.S. Gahvora cradling in Tajikistan: Cultural practices and associations with motor development. *Child Dev.* **2023**, *94*, 1049–1067. [CrossRef]
71. Wang, Y.; Karasik, L.; Hewlett, B.; MacGillivray, T. Cultural Diversity in Infant Motor Development: A Comparison of Early Locomotor Experience. *J. Cross-Cult. Psychol.* **2025**, 00220221251321089. [CrossRef]
72. AAP. Positioning and Sudden Infant Death Syndrome (SIDS): Update. *Pediatrics* **1996**, *98*, 1216–1218. [CrossRef]
73. Davis, B.E.; Moon, R.Y.; Sachs, H.C.; Ottolini, M.C. Effects of Sleep Position on Infant Motor Development. *Pediatrics* **1998**, *102*, 1135–1140. [CrossRef] [PubMed]
74. Hewitt, L.; Kerr, E.; Stanley, R.M.; Okely, A.D. Tummy Time and Infant Health Outcomes: A Systematic Review. *Pediatrics* **2020**, *145*, e20192168. [CrossRef]
75. Blauw-Hospers, C.H.; Hadders-Algra, M. A systematic review of the effects of early intervention on motor development. *Dev. Med. Child Neurol.* **2005**, *47*, 421–432. [CrossRef]
76. Moxley-Haegert, L.; Serbin, L.A. Developmental Education for Parents of Delayed Infants: Effects on Parental Motivation and Children's Development. *Child Dev.* **1983**, *54*, 1324–1331. [CrossRef] [PubMed]
77. Hughes, A.J.; Redsell, S.A.; Glazebrook, C. Motor Development Interventions for Preterm Infants: A Systematic Review and Meta-analysis. *Pediatrics* **2016**, *138*, e20160147. [CrossRef]
78. Riethmuller, A.M.; Jones, R.A.; Okely, A.D. Efficacy of Interventions to Improve Motor Development in Young Children: A Systematic Review. *Pediatrics* **2009**, *124*, e782–e792. [CrossRef]
79. Hamilton, M.; Goodway, J.; Haubenstricker, J. Parent-Assisted Instruction in a Motor Skill Program for At-Risk Preschool Children. *Adapt. Phys. Act. Q.* **1999**, *16*, 415–426. [CrossRef]
80. Lobo, M.A.; Galloway, J.C. Enhanced Handling and Positioning in Early Infancy Advances Development Throughout the First Year: Handling and Positioning Advance Development. *Child Dev.* **2012**, *83*, 1290–1302. [CrossRef]
81. Libertus, K.; Needham, A. Teach to reach: The effects of active vs. passive reaching experiences on action and perception. *Vis. Res.* **2010**, *50*, 2750–2757. [CrossRef]
82. Needham, A.; Barrett, T.; Peterman, K. A pick-me-up for infants' exploratory skills: Early simulated experiences reaching for objects using 'sticky mittens' enhances young infants' object exploration skills. *Infant Behav. Dev.* **2002**, *25*, 279–295. [CrossRef]
83. Cote, L.; Bornstein, M. Cultural and Parenting Cognitions in Acculturating Cultures. *J. Cross-Cult. Psychol.* **2003**, *34*, 323–349. [CrossRef]
84. Keller, H. Culture and Cognition: Developmental Perspectives. *J. Cogn. Educ. Psych.* **2011**, *10*, 3–8. [CrossRef]
85. Kochanska, G.; Kuczynski, L.; Radke-Yarrow, M. Correspondence between Mothers' Self-Reported and Observed Child-Rearing Practices. *Child Dev.* **1989**, *60*, 56–63. [CrossRef] [PubMed]
86. Lerner, R.M.; Johnson, S.K.; Buckingham, M.H. Relational Developmental Systems-Based Theories and the Study of Children and Families: Lerner and Spanier (1978) Revisited. *J. Fam. Theo. Revie.* **2015**, *7*, 83–104. [CrossRef]
87. Piaget, J. *The Origins of Intelligence in Children*; W W Norton & Co.: New York, NY, USA, 1952; p. 419. [CrossRef]
88. Gibson, E.J. Exploratory behavior in the development of perceiving, acting, and the acquiring of knowledge. *Annu. Rev. Psychol.* **1988**, *39*, 1–41. [CrossRef]
89. Lobo, M.A.; Orlando, J.M.; Cunha, A.B.; Atun-Einy, O.; Oudgenoeg-Paz, O.; de Toledo, A.M.; de Souza, R.M.; Alghamdi, Z.S.; Alhindi, E.; Klein, M. Analysis of Content About Infant Development from Formal Parent Education Sources in Different World Regions. *Dev. Psychobiol.* **2025**, *67*, e70021. [CrossRef]

children

MDPI

Article

Team Teaching Models in Primary Physical Education: Effects on Basic Motor Competencies and Self-Reported Physical Literacy

Gabriela Luptáková [1,*], Jaroslava Argajová [1], Tibor Balga [1], Dušana Augustovičová [1], Pavlína Sobotová [1], Gheorghe Balint [2] and Branislav Antala [1]

[1] Faculty of Physical Education and Sport, Comenius University in Bratislava, Nábr. arm. gen. L. Svobodu 9, 81469 Bratislava, Slovakia; jaroslava.argajova@uniba.sk (J.A.); tibor.balga@uniba.sk (T.B.); dusana.augustovicova@uniba.sk (D.A.); sobotova30@uniba.sk (P.S.); branislav.antala@uniba.sk (B.A.)

[2] Faculty of Movement, Sports and Health Sciences, "Vasile Alecsandri" University of Bacău, Calea Marasesti, no. 157, 600115 Bacău, Romania; gbalint@ub.ro

* Correspondence: gabriela.luptakova@uniba.sk

Highlights:

What are the main findings?

- No single configuration proved statistically superior across all groups; however, models including a PE specialist achieved the strongest within-group gains in both motor competence and self-perceived physical literacy.
- More frequent participation in organized out-of-school physical activity was significantly associated with higher basic motor competence.

What are the implications of the main findings?

- The Generalist Teacher + Coach model presents a paradox (improved motor skills but negatively impacted self-perceived physical literacy); therefore, PET-involved team teaching is recommended at the primary level for reliable gains in both objective motor skills and physical literacy self-perceptions.
- Objective motor competence and self-perceptions are positively correlated but capture distinct dimensions; effective physical literacy policy requires measuring both the objective skill and the affective domain.

Abstract: Background/Objectives: To address the inconsistent provision of specialist physical education (PE) in primary schools, this study investigated the comparative efficacy of distinct team teaching configurations. The objective was to compare these instructional models' impact on students' basic motor competencies (MC) and self-reported physical literacy (PL). **Methods:** This cluster-randomized trial involved $N = 266$ students (grades 1–4) in Slovakia, assigned to one of five instructional models (PE teacher; GT+PET; PET+AT; GT+C; and GT+AT). The five-month intervention included two 45 min PE lessons weekly. Given the cluster design and non-normal data, the Wilcoxon singed-rank test and Kruskal–Wallis H-test were applied to assess the differences, and Cohen's r was applied to determine effect size. **Results:** Comparative analysis showed no significant differences across teaching models for Self-Movement ($p = 0.544$), Object-Movement ($p = 0.138$), or PL ($p = 0.219$). Significant within-group MC gains were found in 4 teaching models, yet the practical effect size was generally weak to moderate (r ranging from 0.21 to 0.69). The strongest practical improvement was observed in the AT+PET Self-Movement group (r = 0.69). In contrast, the GT+PET configuration achieved no significant MC gain. For PL, only the AT+PET and GT+PET models showed significantly positive but moderate changes (r = 0.32 and 0.37). Conversely, the GT+C model resulted in a moderately significant decline in PL ($\Delta = -9.16$,

https://doi.org/10.3390/children12121595

r = 0.43). A positive but practically weak correlation emerged between the MC subscales and PL (ρ ranging from 0.135 to 0.238, $p < 0.05$), with the highest limited association for Catching (ρ = 0.377, $p < 0.01$). The frequency of organized out-of-school physical activity was positively correlated with MC subscales (ρ = 0.195–0.282, $p < 0.01$) but not significantly correlated with PL. **Conclusions:** No single teaching model proved superior for improving overall motor competence or self-perceived physical literacy. While most effective configurations yielded moderate practical gains, the GT+C model presents a key paradox: while effective for objective skills, it proved detrimental to self-perceived physical literacy. These findings lead to explicit policy and implementation recommendations focused on strengthening collaborative instruction. Policymakers should consider strategies to support the integration of specialist PE teachers (PETs), such as establishing co-teaching as a recommended practice and allocating dedicated resources for funding and collaborative planning time to leverage the specialized knowledge they bring. Furthermore, schools are encouraged to focus on the effective implementation of PET-involved team teaching approaches (e.g., AT+PET and GT+PET). These models are not only effective but also support the co-professionalization of the generalist teacher, which is essential for ensuring that high-quality, evidence-based PE practices are consistently embedded.

Keywords: physical education; team teaching; motor competence; physical literacy; primary school

1. Introduction

The concept of team teaching (also known as co-teaching or tandem teaching) is a collaborative instructional model in which two professionals instruct students in a single setting, based on mutual goals and shared responsibility [1–3]. Recognized as a component of educator professionalism, this partnership enhances instructional choices and promotes "activating learning" [4–6], offering richer learning experiences, increased curriculum access, and more personalized attention, fostering an inclusive culture [7–12]. The approach has gained significant traction in primary Physical Education (PE) internationally [13–18]. This shift is fueled by widespread concern that generalist teachers (GTs) are often inadequately equipped to deliver high-quality PE, citing insufficient knowledge of basic motor skills and inadequate training for progressive motor development [14,19–24]. This deficit is critical, as teacher competence is the strongest predictor of PE lesson quality and student outcomes [25,26]. Consequently, policymakers are increasingly turning to team teaching arrangements involving trained PE specialists (PETs) to ensure evidence-based pedagogical approaches [17,18,27–29], which in primary PE often takes the form of a "generalist plus one" [13,30].

Crucially, however, there is a methodological issue regarding the frequent conflation of "coach" and "specialist", underscoring a vital distinction in expertise that affects instructional outcomes [31,32]. While perceptual evidence supports the value of specialist-involved team teaching, citing increased physical activity and student motivation [16,33,34], the overall effectiveness of various configurations remains inconclusive due to a persistent "empirical information deficit" [35,36]. Therefore, rigorous experimental designs are required to compare the impact of different expert-driven models on student development [37]. To fully address this gap, it is vital to establish the key outcome variables for student development. The first variable, basic motor competencies (MC), also known as Actual Motor Competence, refers to the ability to skillfully perform physical skills and movement patterns [38]. MC is critical, as low motor skill competence may make a child less inclined to participate in physical activities. However, MC alone is insufficient to describe lifelong engagement with physical activity, leading this study to also assess Physical Literacy (PL), which is a broader construct encompassing motivation, confidence, physical competence (MC), knowledge, and understanding to value and take responsibility for engagement in physical activities for life [38].

The self-reported PL measure is used to capture the subjective dimension of physical literacy, which includes Perceived Motor Competence alongside affective and cognitive domains. This relationship is complex and often weak, particularly at a young age, as the ability to accurately perceive motor competence increases with grade [38]. The low to moderate agreement between objective and perceived competence [39] highlights the necessity of measuring both domains. Specifically, we focused on the self-reported domains of PL because these dimensions—such as motivation and confidence—are hypothesized to be strongly and directly influenced by the instructional behavior and feedback provided within diverse team teaching configurations. It is acknowledged, however, that self-report measures are inherently limited by potential social desirability bias and subjective interpretation, necessitating their use as a complement to, rather than a replacement for, objective assessment.

The current study addresses the critical gap by employing a comprehensive quasi-experimental design to compare a broader range of instructional models, including those with varying levels of specialization and co-teacher roles, against a single PE teacher control group. Teaching configurations are visualized in Figure 1.

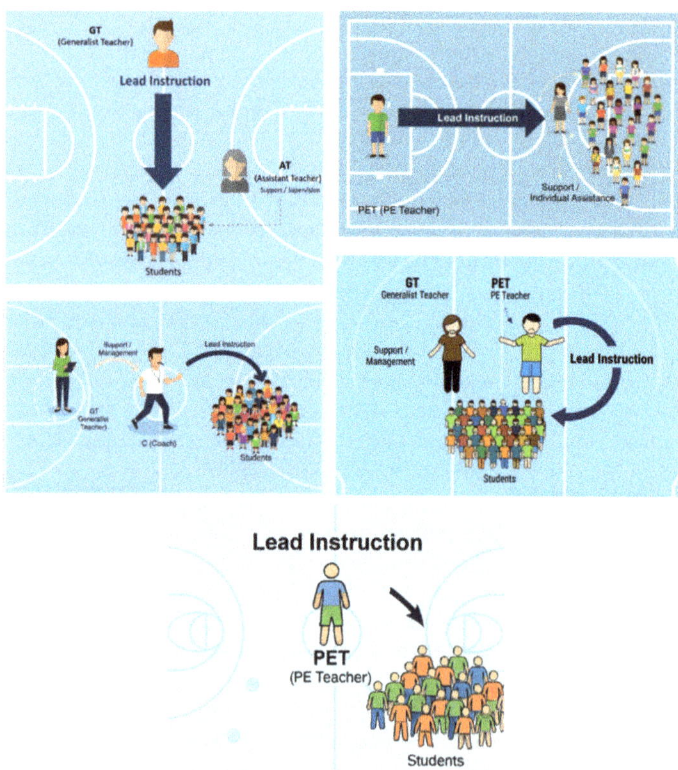

Figure 1. Schematic Representation of the Five Instructional Models Investigated in Primary Physical Education.

The primary aim of this study was to investigate the comparative efficacy of distinct team teaching configurations and single PE teacher instruction on primary school students' basic motor competencies (MC) and self-perceived physical literacy (PL). Furthermore, the study aimed to analyze the interrelationship between these two key outcome variables and investigate the associations between organized out-of-school physical activity and both MC and PL outcomes.

Research Hypotheses

H1 (Comparative Efficacy): *Team teaching configurations involving a PE specialist will result in significantly greater gains in basic motor competencies and self-perceived physical literacy compared to the single PE teacher model and non-specialist models.*

H2 (Variable Correlation): *A significant positive correlation will exist between students' objectively measured motor competencies and their self-perceived physical literacy following the intervention.*

H3 (Covariate Association): *Higher frequency and competitive involvement in out-of-school organized physical activity will be positively associated with higher scores in both motor competencies and self-perceived physical literacy.*

2. Materials and Methods

2.1. Study Design and Participants

This study utilized a quasi-experimental design where pre-existing classes were the unit of analysis, often referred to as a cluster-based approach. Pre-existing classes at three primary schools in the Bratislava region were selected based on availability and willingness to participate in the five-month PE intervention. Assignment to one of the five teaching configurations was performed at the class level to maintain the integrity of the instructional environment. The assignment of classes to one of the five configurations was conducted using simple random assignment. Class clusters were assigned without stratification. We confirm that no balancing (e.g., matching groups based on pre-test results, socio-economic status, or gender ratios) or explicit stratification was applied. This approach was selected to maintain the highest possible objectivity in the randomization process and avoid introducing researcher selection bias, which is a standard procedure for cluster-randomized trials where the intervention is delivered at the school level. Classes were pre-existing organizational units, and entire classes—not individual pupils—were allocated to instructional configurations to preserve ecological validity. This naturalistic cluster allocation avoided contamination between groups but inevitably introduced minor baseline heterogeneity.

Before commencement, written informed consent was obtained from the parents or legal guardians of all participating students (minors). The study was conducted in accordance with the Declaration of Helsinki and received ethical approval from the Ethics Committee of the Faculty of Physical Education and Sports, Comenius University in Bratislava, Slovakia (Approval no. 10/2024, dated 21 June 2024).

To investigate how instructional structure influences physical literacy and motor development, pre-existing classes were assigned to one of four distinct team teaching models or single PE teacher instruction. The five instructional configurations were structurally based on a Complementary Co-Teaching Model, where the expertise of each partner was intended to be leveraged to enhance instruction. The participant demographics for each configuration are detailed in Table 1, and the composition, qualifications, and intended roles are presented in Table 2.

Table 1. Participant Demographics by Instructional Configuration.

Configuration Name	*n* (Students)	Mean Age (Years)	SD
Physical Education (PE) teacher	48	7.44	1.27
Generalist teacher + Coach	48	6.58	0.54
Generalist teacher + PE teacher	44	7.66	1.54
PE teacher + Assistant teacher	82	7.70	1.21
Generalist teacher + Assistant teacher	44	7.68	0.64

Table 2. Operational Definitions of Instructional Configurations.

Configuration Name	Teacher Composition	Key Teacher Qualifications	Intended Roles
PET	Single Certified PE Teacher	Master's in PE; single-teacher control group.	PET (All instructional roles)
GT+C	Generalist Teacher (GT) + Sports Coach (C)	GT (Primary Ed Master's); Coach (Sport Science/License; national program).	Lead: Coach (skill execution). Support: GT (classroom management/pedagogy).
GT+PET	Generalist Teacher (GT) + PE Teacher (PET)	GT (Primary Ed Master's); PET (PE Master's).	Lead: PET (motor skill development). Support: GT (pedagogy/class management).
AT+PET	Assistant Teacher (AT) + PE Teacher (PET)	AT (Pedagogical Sciences; after-school); PET (PE Master's).	Lead: PET (motor skill development). Support: AT (management/tindividual assistance).
GT+AT	Generalist Teacher (GT) + Assistant Teacher (AT)	GT (Primary Ed Master's); AT (Pedagogical Sciences; after-school).	Lead: GT (lesson delivery). Support: AT (supervision/behavior management).

The intervention utilized the standard state-mandated PE curriculum for the primary level in Slovakia. Crucially, the specific lesson content and pedagogical choices were not standardized, mandated, or monitored by the research team across the five instructional groups. The study aimed to investigate the efficacy of the different teacher configurations operating in their typical, naturalistic environment. This decision reflects a commitment to ecological validity, but it must be acknowledged that lesson content variability represents an uncontrolled confounding factor in the interpretation of the subsequent results.

Prior to the intervention, all participating teachers (PETs, GTs, Coaches, and ATs) were individually or collectively briefed by the research team regarding the study's requirements. This communication focused on the research rationale, the importance of adhering to the intervention timeline, and general guidance on leveraging specialized expertise consistent with the intended roles in Table 2. This informal briefing served to orient teachers to the study's parameters, but it did not constitute a formalized training session and did not include standardized role-playing or team-building exercises. Consequently, specific co-teaching roles were neither formally prescribed nor monitored, meaning that the instructional fidelity of the co-teaching process remains an unmeasured variable in this study.

2.2. Data Collection

Data collection occurred at baseline (T1) in October 2024, preceding the intervention, and post-intervention (T2) in April 2025, following the five-month experimental period.

Basic motor competencies were assessed at T1 and T2 using the Motor Competence Assessment (MOBAK) test instrument, which is designed to evaluate fundamental motor competencies and uses age-appropriate versions: MOBAK 1–2 (Grades 1–2) [40] and MOBAK 3–4 (Grades 3–4) [41]. The test measures two main categories: Self-movement (balancing, jumping, sidestepping/running, rolling) and Object movement (throwing, catching, dribbling, bouncing). All tests were administered by trained research assistants to ensure consistency. Scores for each competence area (Self-movement and Object movement) were initially recorded as raw sum scores (0–8 points) according to the MOBAK scoring protocol.

Self-reported physical literacy was assessed at T1 and T2 using the Physical Literacy Assessment for Youth-Self (PLAYself) questionnaire [42]. The PLAYself questionnaire was specifically chosen as a complementary measure to the objective MOBAK assessment. While MOBAK addresses the need for objective motor skill assessment (functionally equivalent to the physical competence dimension, such as PLAYfun), the PLAYself measure is essential for capturing the affective and psychological components of physical literacy (e.g., self-efficacy, motivation, and confidence). This dual-assessment strategy allows us to rigorously investigate the interplay between skill development and self-perception, which is one of the key aims of the study and central to determining the holistic efficacy of the different instructional models. The Physical Literacy Self-Description subscale, which measures a child's self-efficacy related to physical activity participation, was used for analysis. The questionnaire was translated into Slovak using a rigorous forward–backward translation method to ensure conceptual equivalence. This process followed the established protocol by Chráska [43], involving (1) a forward translation into Slovak by two independent translators, (2) reconciliation into a unified version, (3) a blinded backward translation back into English, and (4) a final expert review to resolve any discrepancies. In line with standard psychometric principles for scale development, where $\alpha \geq 0.70$ is the accepted threshold for acceptable internal consistency in research settings, an internal consistency of α 0.70 was considered acceptable [43]. The internal consistency for the scale was $\alpha = 0.72$. The questionnaire was teacher-administered for students in Grades 1 and 2, and self-administered for students in Grades 3 and 4.

To complement the results obtained in the school setting, Out-of-School Physical Activity (OOSPA) was assessed post-intervention (T2) using a context-specific questionnaire administered by teachers. This instrument was systematically derived from established regional and international physical activity recall protocols and tailored to the cultural and curricular context of Slovak primary education, thereby exhibiting strong ecological validity for this specific population. Questions focused on: (1) Frequency of Organized Physical Activity; (2) Competitive Involvement; and (3) Sport Type (individual or collective sports). These OOSPA data serve as a critical covariate in the statistical analysis, directly addressing our Hypothesis H3, and are essential for controlling the influence of external physical activity on both MC and PL outcomes to ensure the internal validity of our comparison between the teaching models.

2.3. Data Analysis

Data analysis was performed using IBM SPSS Statistics 21 for Windows. Given the fixed sample size ($N = 266$), post hoc sensitivity analysis using G*Power indicated 80% power ($\alpha = 0.05$, two-tailed) to detect at least medium effects ($r \approx 0.30/\eta^2 \approx 0.06$). Smaller effects may have remained undetected. All data distributions were tested for normality using the Shapiro–Wilk test. Since a lack of normality was observed in the change scores and the study used a quasi-experimental, cluster-randomized design, non-parametric tests and appropriate contextual reporting were employed. The statistical significance threshold was set at $\alpha = 0.05$ (two-tailed). To control the family-wise error rate, p-values from pairwise post hoc tests were adjusted using the Holm–Bonferroni procedure. Missing data were <5% for all variables and handled by listwise deletion. Sensitivity checks with multiple imputation ($m = 20$) yielded comparable results.

The main objective of comparing the efficacy of the five instructional groups was addressed in two steps:

- Within-Group Change: To assess development within each configuration, the non-parametric Wilcoxon Signed-Rank Test was used to compare T1 and T2 scores for MOBAK Self-Movement, MOBAK Object-Movement, and Perceived Physical Literacy. The mean difference (Δ) and the 95% Confidence Interval (CI) for each difference were reported. Statistical significance for within-group change was determined if the 95% CI did not include zero and/or the Wilcoxon test yielded a $p < 0.05$.
- Between-Group Comparison: To statistically assess whether overall group differences in the T1 to T2 change scores were significant, a non-parametric Kruskal–Wallis H-test was conducted across the five instructional groups for each outcome measure. The Kruskal–Wallis test was chosen due to the lack of normality and the ordinal nature of the dependent variables.

To explore the relationship between the measured constructs and provide essential contextual data, Spearman's rank-order correlations (ρ) were calculated:

- Correlations were calculated between children's self-reported physical literacy and their objectively assessed motor competence (MOBAK subscale scores) at both initial (T1) and final (T2) testing to examine changes in self-awareness.
- Correlations were calculated between Out-of-School Physical Activity (OOSPA) variables (frequency, competitive involvement, and sport type) and the primary outcome measures (MOBAK subscales and self-reported physical literacy). This was carried out to quantify the potential influence of external activity on the study outcomes.

Effect sizes were reported for all inferential tests: for within-group changes, $r = Z/\sqrt{N}$; for Kruskal–Wallis tests, ε^2 was computed. Effect sizes and Spearman correlation coefficients were interpreted using conventional cut-offs (0.10 = weak, 0.30 = moderate, 0.50 = strong), following Cohen's guidelines [44].

3. Results

3.1. Changes in Basic Motor Competences by Instructional Group

Most importantly, the results indicated no statistically significant differences across teaching groups for Self-Movement ($H(4) = 3.09$, $p = 0.544$) or Object-Movement ($H(4) = 6.96$, $p = 0.138$). Although the Object-Movement test approached significance, these findings suggest that while within-group improvements occurred across several configurations, the comparative efficacy across the five groups was not statistically distinct.

To assess the students' development in basic motor competencies, changes in the MOBAK Self-Movement and Object-Movement scores across different instructional groups were analyzed, as seen in Table 3. To visually depict distributional change, compact boxplots of pre- and post-scores for each instructional model were added (Figures 2 and 3). In addition, Δ-change barplots illustrate the mean gain (T2-T1) for each outcome measure (MOBAK subscales) across the five instructional configurations (Figures 4 and 5). Table 4 presents the *p*-values and effect sizes of within-group changes between T1 and T2.

In the Self-Movement subscale, the AT+PET group showed moderate improvement (Δ = +0.79, 95% CI = [0.45, 1.13]), which indicates a moderate effect (r = 0.32), closely followed by the GT+C group (Δ = +0.65, 95% CI = [0.18, 1.12]), also indicating a moderate effect (r = 0.30). Similarly, the PET-only (Δ = +0.40, $p < 0.05$, r = 0.38) and GT+AT (Δ = +0.30, $p < 0.05$, r = 0.43) groups showed statistically significant improvements with moderate effects, while the GT+PET group's change (Δ = +0.19, CI crossing zero) was not statistically significant (r = 0.14), indicating a weak effect.

Table 3. Changes in Basic Motor Competences by Instructional Group.

	Teaching Model	Median	Mean	95% Confidence Interval for Mean		Std. Deviation	Min	Max	IQR
				Lower Bound	Upper Bound				
Self-movement [score]	Physical Education Teacher	0	0.4	−0.15	0.95	0.99	−1	2	1
	Generalist Teacher & Coach	1	0.65	0.18	1.12	1.16	−1	3	2
	Generalist Teacher & Physical Education Teacher	0	0.19	−0.26	0.63	1.23	−2	4	1.75
	Assistant Teacher & Physical Education Teacher	0.5	0.79	0.45	1.13	1.04	−1	3	2
	Generalist Teacher & Assistant Teacher	0	0.30	0.00	0.61	0.70	−1	1	1
Object movement [score]	Physical Education Teacher	1	1.07	0.19	1.94	1.58	−3	4	1
	Generalist Teacher & Coach	1	0.92	0.31	1.54	1.52	−2	4	2
	Generalist Teacher & Physical Education Teacher	0	0.22	−0.34	0.77	1.54	−2	5	2
	Assistant Teacher & Physical Education Teacher	0.5	0.53	0.04	1.01	1.47	−2	4	3
	Generalist Teacher & Assistant Teacher	1	0.43	−0.07	0.94	1.16	−2	3	1

Note. IQR = Interquartile Range.

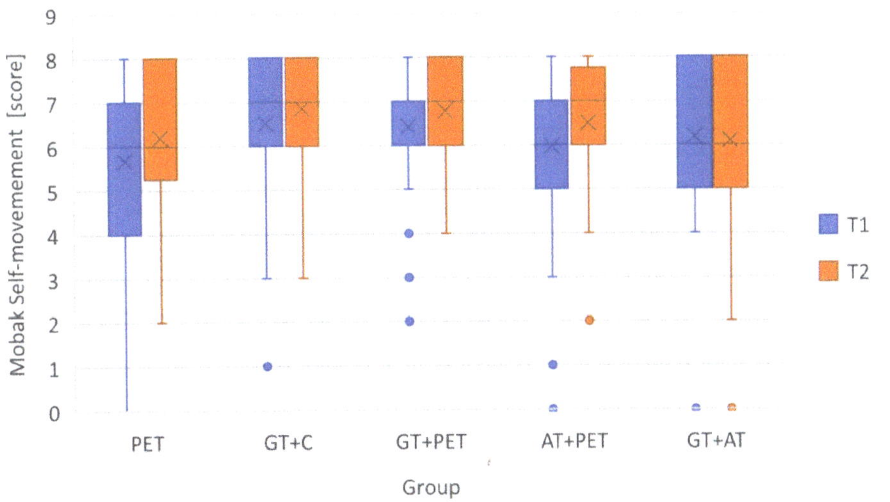

Figure 2. Within-group Changes in MOBAK Self-movement score between T1 and T2.

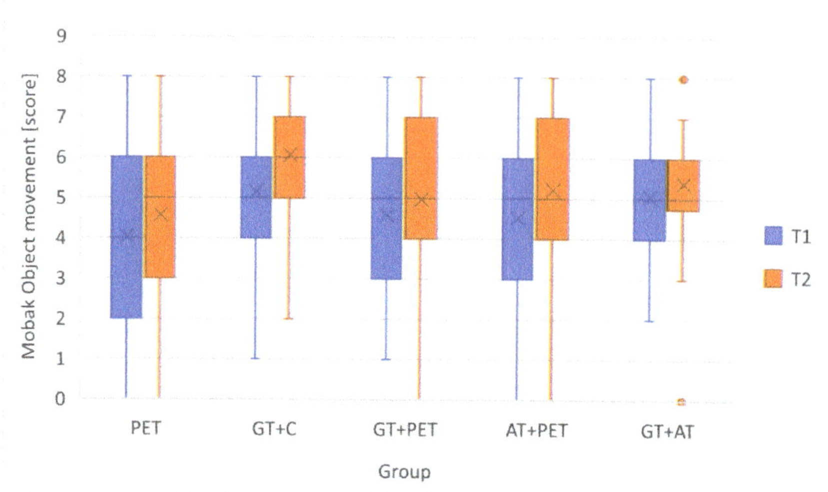

Figure 3. Within-group Changes in MOBAK Object-movement score between T1 and T2.

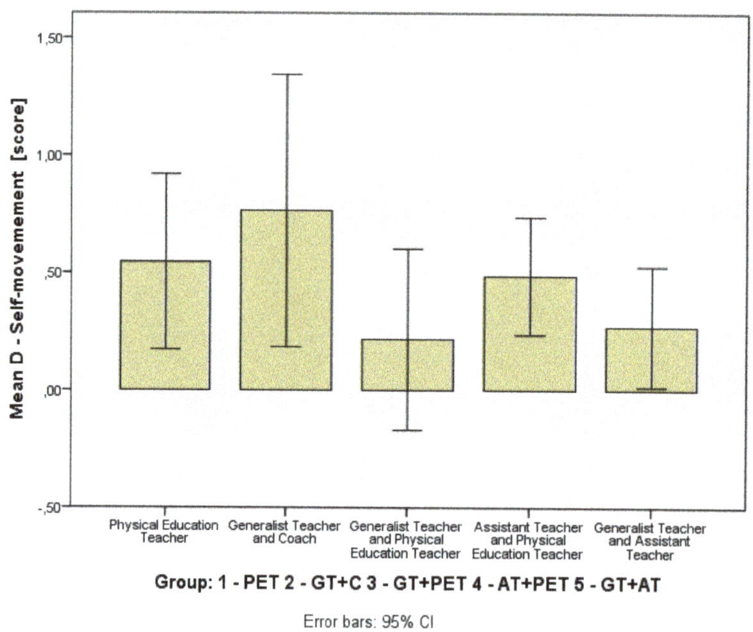

Figure 4. Mean Gain (T2–T1) in Basic Motor Competences: MOBAK Self-Movement Scores by Instructional Group.

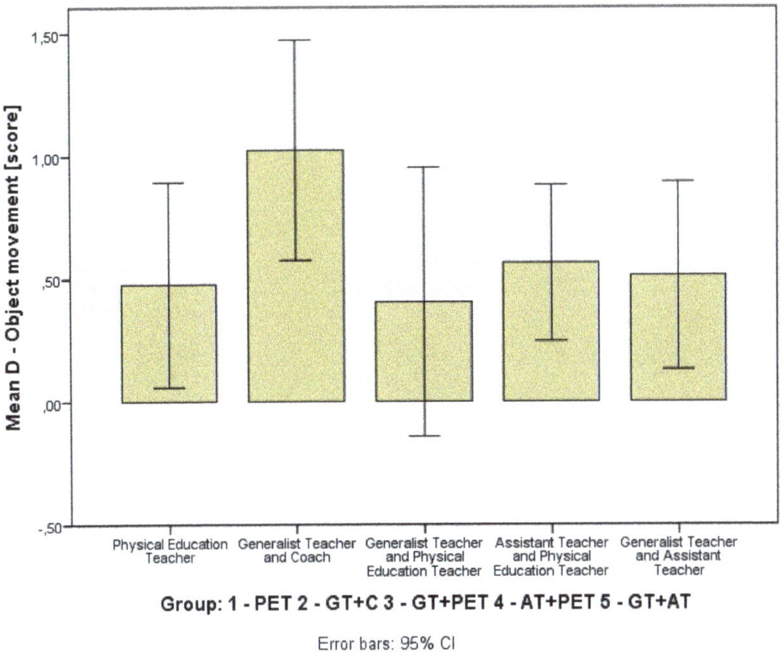

Figure 5. Mean Gain (T2–T1) in Basic Motor Competences: MOBAK Object-Movement Scores by Instructional Group.

Table 4. Within-group Statistical and Practical Significance in Motor Competence and Self-reported Physical Literacy.

	PET			GT+C			GT+PET			PET+AT			GT+AT		
	OM	SM	PS	OM	SM	PS	OM	SM	PS	OM	SM	PS	OM	SM	PS
Z	−2.293	−2.784	−0.578	−3.593	−2.241	−3.609	−1.217	−1.013	−3.252	−3.235	−3.508	−3.026	−2.441	−2.27	−0.487
p	0.022	0.005	0.563	0.000	0.025	0.000	0.224	0.311	0.001	0.001	0.000	0.002	0.015	0.023	0.626
r	0.28	0.38	0.07	0.44	0.30	0.43	0.14	0.14	0.37	0.30	0.69	0.32	0.40	0.43	0.05

Note. PET = Physical Education teacher, GT+C = Generalist teacher + Coach, GT+PET = Generalist teacher + Physical Education teacher, PET+AT = Physical Education teacher + Assistant teacher, GT+AT = Generalist teacher + Assistant teacher, OM = Object-movement, SM = Self-movement, PS = Self-reported physical literacy, Z = Wilcoxon Signed-Rank Test Z-score, p = statistical significance, r = Cohens r (effect size).

In the Object-Movement subscale, the PET-only group exhibited the largest increase (Δ = +1.07, CI = [0.19, 1.94]), a statistically significant improvement but with a weak effect (r = 0.28). The GT+C (Δ = +0.92, CI = [0.31, 1.54], r = 0.44), AT+PET (Δ = +0.53, CI = [0.04, 1.01], r = 0.30) and GT+AT (Δ = +0.43, p = 0.015, r = 0.40) groups showed statistically significant progress with moderate effects. In contrast, the GT+PET (Δ = +0.22, p = 0.224, r = 0.14), indicating a weak effect, had non-significant gains with confidence intervals that included zero.

Furthermore, Figure 6 suggests that the students' ability to perform object-movement skills was only moderately or weakly correlated with their ability to perform self-movement skills within this specific sample, indicating that these subskills may be relatively independent or measured distinctly.

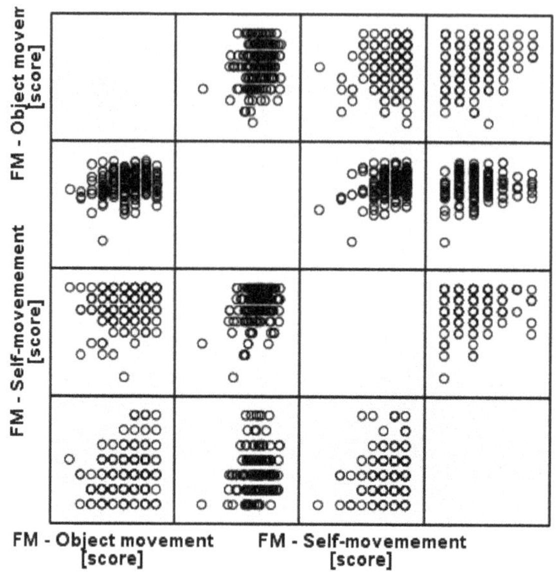

Figure 6. Correlation Matrix of Fundamental Movement (FM) Subscales: Object Movement vs. Self-Movement Scores.

3.2. Changes in Self-Perceived Physical Literacy by Instructional Group

To evaluate the effect of different instructional teams on the students' self-perceived physical literacy, changes in PLAYself total scores were analyzed across five teaching configurations (Table 5). To visually depict distributional change, a compact boxplot of pre- and post-scores for each instructional model was added (Figure 7). The Δ-change barplot illustrates the mean gain (T2-T1) for PL across the five instructional configurations (Figure 8). Table 4 presents the *p*-values and effect sizes of within-group changes between T1 and T2 (see Section 3.1).

Table 5. Changes in Self-perceived Physical Literacy by Instructional Group.

Teaching Model		Mean	Median	95% Confidence Interval for Mean		Std. Deviation	Min	Max	IQR
				Lower Bound	Upper Bound				
PlaySelf [score]	Physical Education Teacher	−3.42	4.37	−18.14	11.29	26.58	−79.67	26.89	30.16
	Generalist Teacher & Coach	−9.16	−12.04	−13.50	−4.81	10.76	−28.41	17.26	12.77
	Generalist Teacher & Physical Education Teacher	5.65	3.83	1.88	9.43	10.47	−16.81	25.33	16.51
	Assistant Teacher & Physical Education Teacher	5.82	5.69	2.47	9.16	10.17	−15.11	36.70	13.68
	Generalist Teacher & Assistant Teacher	2.72	−1.56	−5.54	10.99	19.12	−22.26	68.93	21.48

Note. IQR = Interquartile Range.

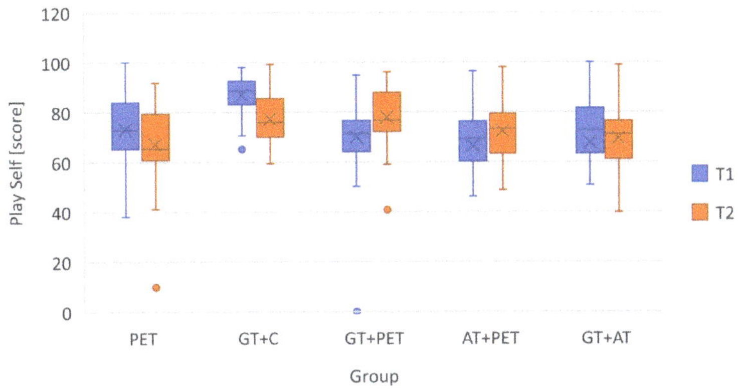

Figure 7. Within-group Changes in PLAYSelf score between T1 and T2.

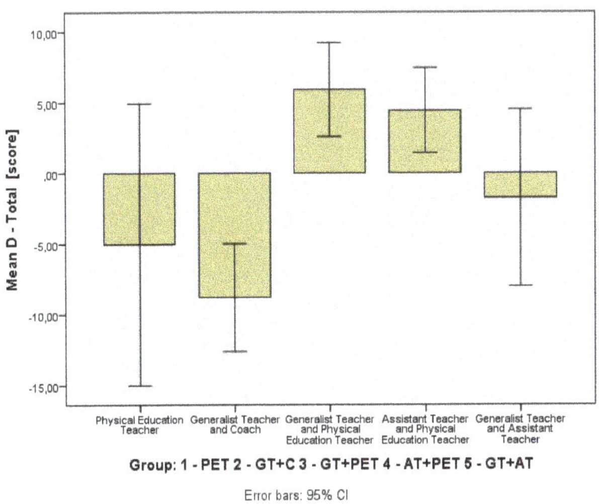

Figure 8. Mean Gain (T2–T1) in self-reported physical literacy: PLAYSelf Total Scores by Instructional Group.

The GT+PET ($\Delta = +5.65$, r = 0.37, $p = 0.001$) showed statistically significant gains with a moderate effect. The AT+PET ($\Delta = +5.82$, r = 0.69, $p = 0.002$) groups showed positive gains in self-perceived physical literacy. This change was statistically significant and reflected a strong effect size, suggesting a strongly significant improvement in self-perceptions.

In contrast, the GT+C ($\Delta = -9.16$, r = 0.43, $p = 0.000$) exhibited a statistically significant decline with a moderate negative effect size. The GT+AT group showed a non-significant increase of +2.72 (r = 0.05, $p = 0.626$), indicating a very weak effect, and PET-only non-significant decrease in PL ($\Delta = -3.42$, r = 0.07, $p = 0.563$), also indicating a very weak effect.

Despite observable trends, a Kruskal–Wallis test comparing all five groups indicated that the differences were not statistically significant overall, $H(4) = 5.75$, $p = 0.219$. This suggests that while the use of specific instructional models (GT+PET and AT+PET) resulted in significant within-group gains in perceived physical literacy, there was no statistically significant difference in the magnitude of change when comparing the five models.

3.3. Associations Between Self-Perceived Physical Literacy and Motor Competence

To investigate the alignment between students' subjective and objective competencies, Spearman's rank-order correlations (ρ) were calculated between the PLAYself Total Score and the MOBAK subscales pre- and post-intervention (Tables 6 and 7). A scatterplot illustrates the correlation between all relevant variables (MOBAK vs. PLAYSelf at T1 and T2) to visually support the findings of Hypothesis H2 (Figure 9).

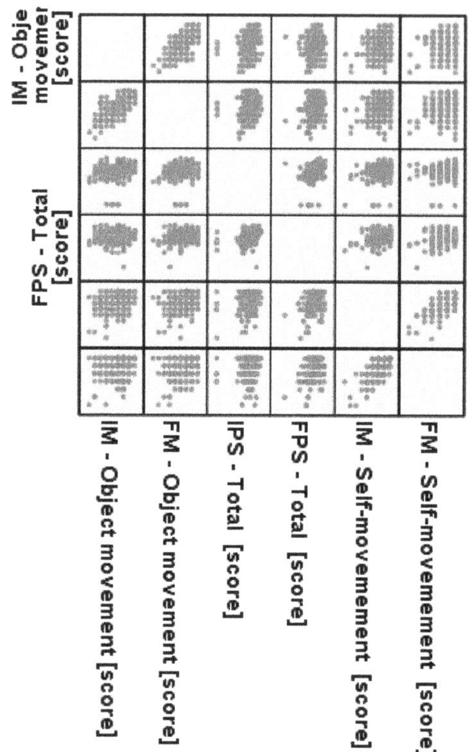

Figure 9. Correlation Between Objective Motor Competence (MOBAK) and Self-Reported Physical Literacy (PLAYSELF) at Pre- (T1) and Post-Intervention (T2).

Table 6. Associations Between Self-Perceived Physical Literacy and Motor Competence—Initial performance (T1).

Correlation Coefficient	Balancing [Score]	Rolling [Score]	Jumping [Score]	Running [Score]	Self-Movement [Score]	Throwing [Score]	Catching [Score]	Dribbling [Score]	Bouncing [Score]	Object Movement [Score]	PlaySelf—Total [Score]
Balancing [score]	1	0.099	0.159 *	0.171 **	0.450 **	0.105	0.165 *	0.11	−0.04	0.11	0.066
Rolling [score]	0.099	1	0.217 **	0.197 **	0.558 **	−0.001	0.108	0.111	0.083	0.099	−0.039
Jumping [score]	0.159 *	0.217 **	1	0.1	0.734 **	0.202 **	0.317 **	0.026	0.106	0.222 **	0.12
Running [score]	0.171 **	0.197 **	0.1	1	0.533 **	0.046	0.181 **	0.226 **	0.163 *	0.234 **	0.147 *
Self-movement [score]	0.450 **	0.558 **	0.734 **	0.533 **	1	0.172 **	0.307 **	0.166 *	0.11	0.265 **	0.135 *
Throwing [score]	0.105	−0.001	0.202 **	0.046	0.172 **	1	0.312 **	0.161 *	0.158 *	0.590 **	0.098
Catching [score]	0.165 *	0.108	0.317 **	0.181 **	0.307 **	0.312 **	1	0.169 **	0.251 **	0.630 **	0.223 **
Dribbling [score]	0.11	0.111	0.026	0.226 **	0.166 *	0.161 *	0.169 **	1	0.303 **	0.655 **	0.03
Bouncing [score]	−0.04	0.083	0.106	0.163 *	0.11	0.158 *	0.251 **	0.303 **	1	0.672 **	0.088
Object movement [score]	0.11	0.099	0.222 **	0.234 **	0.265 **	0.590 **	0.630 **	0.655 **	0.672 **	1	0.183 **
PlaySelf—Total [score]	0.066	−0.039	0.12	0.147 *	0.135 *	0.098	0.223 **	0.03	0.088	0.183 **	1

Note. * Correlation is significant at the 0.05 level (2-tailed). ** Correlation is significant at the 0.01 level (2-tailed).

Table 7. Associations Between Self-Perceived Physical Literacy and Motor Competence—Final performance (T2).

Correlation Coefficient	Balancing [Score]	Rolling [Score]	Jumping [Score]	Running [Score]	Self-Movement [Score]	Throwing [Score]	Catching [Score]	Dribbling [Score]	Bouncing [Score]	Object Movement [Score]	PlaySelf—Total [Score]
Balancing [score]	1	0.162 *	0.124	0.295 **	0.456 **	0.087	0.003	0.02	0.106	0.076	0.145 *
Rolling [score]	0.162 *	1	0.155 *	0.267 **	0.556 **	0.013	0.097	0.09	0.201 **	0.149 *	0.062
Jumping [score]	0.124	0.155 *	1	0.109	0.766 **	0.189 **	0.272 **	0.138 *	0.036	0.234 **	0.214 **
Running [score]	0.295 **	0.267 **	0.109	1	0.521 **	0.04	0.271 **	0.117	0.210 **	0.217 **	0.193 **
Self-movement [score]	0.456 **	0.556 **	0.766 **	0.521 **	1	0.146 *	0.261 **	0.157 *	0.134 *	0.256 **	0.238 **
Throwing [score]	0.087	0.013	0.189 **	0.04	0.146 *	1	0.262 **	0.155 *	0.202 **	0.644 **	0.038
Catching [score]	0.003	0.097	0.272 **	0.271 **	0.261 **	0.262 **	1	0.194 **	0.236 **	0.613 **	0.377 **
Dribbling [score]	0.02	0.09	0.138 *	0.117	0.157 *	0.155 *	0.194 **	1	0.263 **	0.596 **	0.018
Bouncing [score]	0.106	0.201 **	0.036	0.210 **	0.134 *	0.202 **	0.236 **	0.263 **	1	0.663 **	0.111
Object movement [score]	0.076	0.149 *	0.234 **	0.217 **	0.256 **	0.644 **	0.613 **	0.596 **	0.663 **	1	0.182 *
PlaySelf—Total [score]	0.145 *	0.062	0.214 **	0.193 **	0.238 **	0.038	0.377 **	0.018	0.111	0.182 *	1

Note. * Correlation is significant at the 0.05 level (2-tailed). ** Correlation is significant at the 0.01 level (2-tailed).

At initial testing (T1), self-perceived physical literacy demonstrated weak but statistically significant positive correlations with objectively measured motor competence. As shown in Table 6, self-reported literacy was significantly associated with MOBAK Object-Movement (ρ = 0.183, $p < 0.01$) and MOBAK Self-Movement (ρ = 0.135, $p < 0.05$). At the individual skill level, the strongest, but still weak, association was observed between self-perception and catching (ρ = 0.223, $p < 0.01$), followed by running (ρ = 0.147, $p < 0.05$) (a weak correlation).

At final testing (T2), these relationships persisted, and in the case of self-movement, strengthened (see Table 7). The self-reported physical literacy maintained a weak, but significant positive correlation with MOBAK Object-Movement (ρ = 0.182, $p < 0.05$). Notably, the relationship with MOBAK Self-Movement became stronger and more significant (ρ = 0.238, $p < 0.01$) compared to the baseline, however, was still weak. Among individual skills, catching remained the strongest correlate (ρ = 0.377, $p < 0.01$) with a moderate level of correlation, suggesting that the children's self-perception of literacy in this sample was most closely aligned with their proficiency in manipulative skills.

3.4. Associations Between Organized Out-of-School Physical Activity Participation and Basic Motor Competencies

Associations between organized out-of-school physical activity (OOSPA) and basic motor competencies are presented in Table 8. The analysis used bivariate correlations to provide contextual information regarding the students' external physical activity levels. As part of the background assessment, children reported the type of organized sport they engaged in outside school. Overall, 43.0% participated in collective sports, 39.5% in individual sports, 1.2% in both, and 16.3% reported no participation. Frequency of participation in organized sport (OOSPA-Frequency) showed significant but weak positive correlations with both subscales of basic motor competence:

Table 8. Associations Between Organized Out-of-School Physical Activity Participation and Basic Motor Competencies.

Correlation Coefficient	Frequency of Organized Physical Activity [Scale 1–6]	Competitive Involvement: 1—Regularly, 2—Sometimes, 3—Never	Sport Type: 0—None, 1—Collective, 2—Individual, 3—Both	Self-Movement [Score]	Object Movement [Score]
Frequency of Organized Physical Activity [scale 1–6]	1	−0.539 **	0.394 **	0.195 **	0.282 **
Competitive Involvement: 1—Regularly, 2—Sometimes, 3—Never	−0.539 **	1	−0.277 **	−0.061	−0.145 *
Sport Type: 0—None, 1—Collective, 2—Individual, 3—Both	0.394 **	−0.277 **	1	0.095	0.001
Self-movement [score]	0.195 **	0.061	0.095	1	0.256 **
Object movement [score]	0.282 **	−0.145 *	0.001	0.256 **	1

Note. * Correlation is significant at the 0.05 level (2-tailed). ** Correlation is significant at the 0.01 level (2-tailed).

Object Movement (ρ = 0.282, $p < 0.01$), suggesting that students who engage more frequently in organized activity outside of school tend to display greater proficiency in skills like throwing, catching, dribbling, and bouncing.

Self-Movement (ρ = 0.195, $p < 0.01$), indicating a positive link between participation frequency and fundamental motor skills such as running, jumping, balancing, and rolling.

The variable Competitive Involvement was coded so that higher values (1 to 3) reflect less frequent participation in competitive settings (1 = Regularly; 3 = Never). Therefore, the negative correlation observed indicates that more frequent competitive involvement is positively associated with better outcomes. Specifically, higher competitive involvement (lower numerical code) was significantly, albeit weakly, linked to Object Movement ($\rho = -0.145$, $p < 0.05$). No significant association was found between competitive involvement and Self-Movement skills ($\rho = -0.061$).

The variable Sport Type (Collective, Individual, Both, or None) showed no statistically significant correlation with either the Self-Movement ($\rho = 0.095$) or Object Movement ($\rho = 0.001$) competencies.

3.5. *Associations Between Organized Out-of-School Physical Activity Participation and Self-Reported Physical Literacy*

Associations between the three dimensions of OOSPA and self-reported physical literacy are presented in Table 9. The results indicate that the relationship between organized sport participation and self-perception of physical literacy was weak, non-significant, and primarily driven by the frequency of participation.

Table 9. Associations Between Organized Out-of-School Physical Activity Participation and Self-Perceived Physical Literacy.

Correlation Coefficient	Frequency of Organized Physical Activity [Scale 1–6]	Competitive Involvement: 1—Regularly, 2—Sometimes, 3—Never	Sport Type: 0—None, 1—Collective, 2—Individual, 3—Both	PlaySelf [Score]
Frequency of Organized Physical Activity [scale 1–6]	1	−0.539 **	0.394 **	0.133
Competitive Involvement: 1—Regularly, 2—Sometimes, 3—Never	−0.539 **	1	−0.277 **	−0.061
Sport Type: 0—None, 1—Collective, 2—Individual, 3—Both	0.394 **	−0.277 **	1	0.111
PlaySelf [score]	0.133	−0.061	0.111	1

** Correlation is significant at the 0.01 level (2-tailed).

Frequency of organized physical activity showed a weak positive association with self-perceived physical literacy ($\rho = 0.133$), which approached, but did not reach, statistical significance. This weak correlation suggests a marginal trend where students who participate more often in organized sports tend to report slightly higher self-efficacy related to physical activity.

There was no statistically significant association between competitive involvement and self-perceived physical literacy ($\rho = -0.061$), indicating a negligible association. Similarly, sport type (collective/individual) showed no statistically significant association with perceived physical literacy ($\rho = 0.111$), indicating a weak association.

In summary, none of the dimensions of OOSPA demonstrated a statistically significant correlation with self-reported physical literacy at the $\alpha < 0.05$ level, suggesting that a child's external involvement in organized sports was not strongly predictive of their self-reported physical literacy in this sample.

4. Discussion

4.1. Comparative Instructional Efficacy

The primary aim of this study was to assess the comparative efficacy of various team teaching configurations against single-teacher instruction on the development of basic motor competencies (MC) and self-reported physical literacy (PL). Contrary to our hypotheses that a specific co-teaching model would prove statistically superior, the main finding indicated no statistically significant difference in the magnitude of change among the five instructional configurations for either MC or PL. This null comparative finding suggests that over a standard five-month curriculum, the mere presence of an additional teacher or specialist, irrespective of their defined role, was not a sufficient condition to create a statistically distinct comparative advantage between the groups. This result aligns with the "empirical information deficit" highlighted in previous quantitative research [35,45], as a significant body of evaluative studies has similarly failed to establish a clear, statistically superior co-teaching model, particularly when assessing academic outcomes [37].

This outcome must be interpreted in light of the methodological challenges inherent to quasi-experimental designs in educational settings. As Veteska et al. [6] argue, the true impact of team teaching is determined primarily by how it is put into practice, rather than the theoretical configuration itself. Differences in teacher collaboration quality, fidelity of planning, and lesson-to-lesson instructional choices—all factors that differed across the five unique configurations—likely served as confounding variables. This underlying complexity made it difficult to detect a specific superior configuration, ultimately leading to the observed null comparative finding.

4.2. The Crucial Role of Specialist Expertise

While the analysis did not yield statistically significant differences between the five instructional configurations, the detailed descriptive data revealed a critical pattern: the largest and most consistent significant gains in basic motor competencies were confined to the configurations that included a certified PE teacher. Specifically, the PET-only group achieved the largest gains in Object-Movement, and the AT+PET configuration showed the largest team-based improvement in Self-Movement. The finding that PET involvement was the major driving factor behind students achieving statistically significant individual development directly supports the established literature that identifies perceived teacher competence as the strongest predictor of PE lesson quality [26]. The PET's specialized training, which emphasizes correct performance and skill application [46], likely enabled them to provide the precise, evidence-based pedagogical approach necessary to move students beyond simple participation toward genuine motor skill mastery [28]. The ability of the single-teacher PET and the PET in the AT+PET model to generate superior within-group gains in MOBAK directly reinforces previous experimental findings where groups taught by specialized kinesiologists statistically outperformed control groups taught by generalist teachers [29].

In our study, the absence of statistically significant differences across groups for both subscales is a key finding. It suggests that the instructional structure (i.e., whether a Generalist Teacher, Assistant Teacher, or Coach was present) was secondary to the presence of quality pedagogical expertise. The certified PE teacher, regardless of their co-teaching partner, was consistently associated with the largest within-group improvements, reinforcing the notion that the quality and expertise of the instructor is the primary driver of motor competence development, rather than the mere organizational structure of the teaching configuration.

Therefore, despite the absence of a statistically superior model across all outcome measures, the data consistently indicate that specialist PE teacher expertise is the essential ingredient for generating statistically meaningful motor skill development. These results strongly endorse the current policy trends in various international contexts that mandate the inclusion of certified professionals in primary PE.

4.3. Differential Impact on Self-Perception

The results for self-perceived physical literacy (PL) demonstrated a complex differential impact. The configurations leveraging certified PE teachers—specifically AT+PET and GT+PET—both achieved significant positive gains in student self-efficacy. This success suggests that the blending of pedagogical and specialized PE expertise may effectively foster a competence-supportive environment, a key factor within Self-Determination Theory. Indeed, the adoption of motivational teaching behaviors is recognized as a critical determinant of students' quality of experience in PE [47], and these PET-inclusive groups appeared successful in cultivating such a climate.

Conversely, the most complex finding was the GT+C paradox: this group achieved moderate objective gains in Object-Movement skills but experienced a significant decline in perceived physical literacy. This striking inverse relationship is likely attributed to the instructional style employed by the specialist coach, which typically prioritizes direct, technical correction and performance standards. Given the GT+C cohort's young age (M = 6.58), this type of feedback likely accelerated the developmental shift toward a more realistic, performance-contingent assessment of their abilities, moving away from the inflated, non-contingent self-perceptions common in early primary grades [48]. While this process resulted in improved objective motor skills, the observed psychological deflation poses a risk, as high perceived motor competence is a potent, independent predictor of engagement in physical activity [39]. This underscores that simply increasing the expertise in the room is insufficient; the pedagogical approach must actively foster psychological needs through mastery-oriented feedback, reinforcing that instructional style, rather than just structure, has a crucial bearing on student motivation and self-perception [34,49].

4.4. Interpretation of the Association Between Self-Perceived Physical Literacy and Motor Competence

Another key finding was the weak correlation between students' objectively measured motor competence (MOBAK) and their self-perceived physical literacy (PLAYself). Although the observed correlation was statistically significant at initial testing (T1), this weak alignment highlights the inherent challenges associated with measuring an abstract construct like physical literacy using self-report instruments in young populations.

The limited correspondence is typical in this age group and reflects both developmental and methodological limitations. Children in early primary grades often struggle to accurately interpret and report on abstract constructs like overall physical literacy, which is further complicated by the risk of social desirability bias where participants tend to over-report positive traits [48]. Furthermore, self-report measures like PLAYself, while crucial for capturing the affective dimension of physical literacy, inherently capture perceived competence rather than objectively demonstrated ability, leading to known issues with validity and reliability when compared to performance-based measures [38,39].

This weak initial alignment contrasts with studies suggesting a complete mismatch in young children [38,39]. Crucially, the relationship persisted, and in the case of Self-Movement, strengthened over the five-month intervention. This emergence of stronger alignment suggests that prolonged, structured physical education—regardless of the specific instructional model—began to facilitate a more accurate internalized self-assessment. Washburn and Kolen [38] support this interpretation, noting that children's ability to accurately perceive their motor competence tends to improve with age and consistent exposure. The strengthening relationship reinforces that fostering accurate self-perception is a developmental process actively supported in educational settings [50].

The fact that the strongest moderate correlation at final testing was observed for catching suggests that Object-Movement skills lend themselves more readily to external, measurable feedback, helping students to gauge their performance relative to peers, a process vital for developing accurate self-perception [38]. Ultimately, our results contribute to the evidence base confirming that promoting both competence and accurate self-perception is essential for encouraging active lifestyles [39], while simultaneously underscoring the necessity for future research to address the methodological disconnect between objective performance and subjective self-report in young children.

4.5. Associations Between Organized Out-of-School Physical Activity and Motor Competence

The analysis of Organized Out-of-School Physical Activity (OOSPA) participation provided crucial contextual information regarding the external factors influencing motor development in this sample. This study highlights the fact that the higher the participation in organized sports outside of school, the better the overall basic motor competence. Furthermore, the outcomes indicate that more frequent competitive involvement is positively associated with better Object-Movement outcomes.

To synthesize the findings, a critical pattern emerged when comparing the effects of internal (school-based) versus external (OOSPA) factors. The primary finding—that there were no statistically significant differences in motor competence gains between the five instructional configurations—suggests a limit to the influence of the school-based instructional model alone. This is particularly relevant given that school physical education typically comprises only 2 × 45 min per week, a limited time window in which to drive profound, comparative changes in complex motor skills.

When this limited instructional time is juxtaposed with the finding that OOSPA frequency showed a significant positive correlation with both Object-Movement ($\rho = 0.282$, $p < 0.01$) and Self-Movement ($\rho = 0.195$, $p < 0.01$) skills, the data highlight the potentially greater role of external variables.

Therefore, the study implies that the sheer volume and consistency of practice derived from organized out-of-school physical activity might be a more potent, or at least an equally important, driver for developing basic motor competence than the specific school-based instructional configuration or type of teacher. While the quality of instruction (as seen in the PET-led descriptive gains) is vital, the limited time dedicated to PE in the curriculum means that the overall volume of practice outside of school may exert the dominant influence on skill acquisition for children in this age group.

4.6. Limitations and Future Directions

The interpretation of the current study's findings, particularly the non-significant comparative effects, must be framed by several methodological limitations inherent to the quasi-experimental design and the ecological setting.

Firstly, the study employed a quasi-experimental, cluster-randomized design, meaning that students were not individually randomized but were nested within pre-existing classes, which served as the unit of intervention assignment. This non-independence of observations violates a key assumption of certain inferential statistics (such as the non-parametric Kruskal–Wallis test used for group comparisons) and may lead to an underestimation of standard errors and inflated Type I error rates. Consequently, our findings were interpreted conservatively. Future research should apply multi-level modeling to properly account for nested data (students within classes) and estimate random effects attributable to cluster variability.

Secondly, a critical limitation is the non-randomized nature of the cluster assignment, which resulted in groups that were not fully equivalent at the baseline, specifically concerning sample size and age. The instructional configurations varied substantially in group size, reducing statistical power for detecting effects in smaller cohorts. More importantly, the GT+C configuration was associated with students who were significantly younger (Mean Age: M = 6.58) compared to the remaining groups (M $\approx$ 7.7). This chronological age disparity introduced a developmental confound, particularly for the PL measure.

Thirdly, the lack of gender-specific analysis represents a limitation, as potential differential instructional impacts on boys' versus girls' outcomes may have been obscured by the pooled data. For instance, previous research suggests that gender may moderate the effect of instructional style on self-perception, with girls often being more sensitive to the type and quality of instructor feedback. Future studies should prioritize stratifying the analysis by gender to determine whether certain co-teaching configurations yield distinct outcomes for different sexes.

Fourthly, regarding assessment fidelity, all MOBAK assessments were conducted by a single, highly trained researcher to eliminate inter-rater variability. However, the lack of a formalized inter-rater reliability (IRR) check—such as parallel scoring by a second expert or video-based scoring—is a limitation. While this design choice ensured consistency (intra-rater reliability), it prevented external verification of the scoring fidelity and any potential drift in the researcher's application of the rubric over the assessment period.

Fifthly, the assessment of self-perceived physical literacy relied on the self-report questionnaire. This tool is susceptible to social desirability bias and halo effects, where children may potentially over-report their confidence. This limitation is exacerbated by the age disparity in the GT+C group; their younger age corresponds to a developmental stage of potentially inflated self-assessments, which is a crucial explanatory factor for the inverse relationship observed in perceived physical literacy.

Sixthly, in the pursuit of ecological validity, the study deliberately opted not to standardize or monitor specific lesson content, pedagogical choices, or the fidelity of the co-teaching implementation. Consequently, the observed outcomes reflect the combined effect of the intended structural configuration and the uncontrolled contextual variability arising from the teachers' planning quality, communication, and real-time execution of their defined roles. This lack of fidelity monitoring is a significant limitation and prevents a definitive isolation of the structural model's direct impact. Compounding this issue, the voluntary nature of the teachers' participation introduces a potential self-selection bias, where only highly motivated teachers—or those in schools already prioritizing PE—may have opted to participate. This restricts the generalizability of the findings to less motivated school environments. Future studies should incorporate direct behavioral observation to quantify the teaching style and quality of feedback provided within each configuration.

Additionally, the five-month (two 45 min lessons per week) intervention period may represent an insufficient time dose to elicit statistically significant comparative changes between the different instructional groups. This is especially relevant given the baseline variability and the complexity of developing both objective motor competence and PL simultaneously. A longer intervention duration or having more PE lessons per week is necessary to adequately assess the long-term, structural efficacy of these co-teaching models.

Finally, the assessment of Out-of-School Physical Activity (OOSPA) relied on a non-validated, context-specific questionnaire administered only at the post-intervention (T2) time point. While a validated tool would have been ideal, this specific questionnaire was retained in the main methodology because it captured ecologically relevant participation data essential to understanding the local contextual factors influencing skill development in this particular sample. However, the lack of prior psychometric validation (reliability and validity) is a clear limitation, and the OOSPA data should thus be interpreted conservatively. Furthermore, the single time-point assessment prevented its use as a true baseline covariate to statistically control for prior physical activity habits, which were shown to correlate significantly with motor competencies in the results.

5. Conclusions

This five-month intervention, comparing five distinct team teaching configurations, revealed no statistically significant differences in overall student development for either basic motor competence (MC) or self-perceived physical literacy (PL) across the instructional groups. This null comparative finding suggests that instructional structure alone may not yield a statistical advantage. However, analysis of within-group change scores indicated that configurations utilizing certified PE teacher expertise were the most successful in generating reliable gains in MC. The data further showed differential effects based on team composition, notably the significant decline in self-perceived PL observed solely within the Generalist Teacher + Coach configuration. Collectively, these findings suggest that the quality and expertise of the instructor remain the primary factor for meaningful motor skill development and positive self-perception. These results support the continued importance of involving certified specialist PE teachers in primary physical education instruction and underscore the value of ensuring that teacher training places sufficient focus on pedagogical approaches, such as competence-supportive strategies, to ensure that instruction promotes psychological well-being alongside technical skill acquisition.

Author Contributions: Conceptualization, G.L. and B.A.; methodology, G.L.; validation, J.A., D.A. and G.L.; formal analysis, D.A. and G.B.; investigation, G.L., J.A., P.S., B.A. and T.B.; data curation, J.A. and P.S.; writing—original draft preparation, G.L. and J.A.; writing—review and editing, G.L. and T.B.; visualization, G.L.; supervision, G.L.; project administration, B.A.; funding acquisition, B.A. and G.B. All authors have read and agreed to the published version of the manuscript.

Funding: This research and its associated article processing charges (APC) were funded by the VEGA grant, No. 1/0127/23, titled "Tandem teaching of physical and sports education at the primary school level and its impact on students' motor, cognitive, and affective development". The study sponsors had no role in the design and conduct of the study, the analysis and interpretation of data, or in the preparation, review, or approval of the manuscript.

Institutional Review Board Statement: The study was conducted in accordance with the Declaration of Helsinki and approved by the Ethics Committee of the Faculty of Physical Education and Sport, Comenius University in Bratislava, Slovakia (protocol code 10/2024, 21 June 2024).

Informed Consent Statement: Informed consent was obtained from all of the subjects' guardians involved in the study.

Data Availability Statement: The original data presented in the study are openly available in Zenodo at DOI: 10.5281/zenodo.17474303.

Conflicts of Interest: The authors declare no conflicts of interest. The funders had no role in the design of the study; in the collection, analyses, or interpretation of data; in the writing of the manuscript; or in the decision to publish the results.

Abbreviations

The following abbreviations are used in this manuscript:

PE	Physical Education
PL	Self-reported Physical Literacy
MC	Basic Motor Competencies
PET	Physical Education teacher

AT	Assistant teacher
GT	Generalist teacher
C	Sports Coach
OOSPA	Organized out-of-school physical activity
MOBAK	Test battery of basic motor competencies
T1	Initial Testing (Time Point 1/Pre-intervention)
T2	Final Testing (Time Point 2/Post-intervention)

References

1. Cook, L.; Friend, M. Co-teaching: Guidelines for creating effective practices. *Focus Except. Child.* **1995**, *28*, 1–16.
2. Cook, L.; Friend, M. *Co-Teaching: Principles, Practices, and Pragmatics*; New Mexico Public Education Department Quarterly Special Education Meeting; New Mexico Public Education Department: Santa Fe, NM, USA, 2004.
3. Hargreaves, A.; O'Connor, M.T. Solidarity with solidity: The case for collaborative professionalism. *Phi Delta Kappan* **2018**, *100*, 20–24. [CrossRef]
4. Strogilos, V.; King-Sears, M.E.; Tragoulia, E.; Voulagka, A.; Stefanidis, A. A meta-synthesis of co-teaching students with and without disabilities. *Educ. Res. Rev.* **2023**, *38*, 100504. [CrossRef]
5. Abrami, P.C.; Bernard, R.M.; Borokhovski, E.; Waddington, D.I.; Wade, C.A.; Persson, T. Strategies for teaching students to think critically: A meta-analysis. *Rev. Educ. Res.* **2015**, *85*, 275–314. [CrossRef]
6. Veteska, J.; Kursch, M.; Svobodova, Z.; Tureckiova, M.; Paulovcakova, L. Longitudinal Co-teaching Projects: Scoping Review. In *Orchestration of Learning Environments in the Digital World*; Ifenthaler, D., Isaías, P., Sampson, D.G., Eds.; Springer: Cham, Switzerland, 2022; pp. 37–51. [CrossRef]
7. Friend, M.; Cook, L.; Hurley-Chamberlain, D.; Shamberger, C. Co-Teaching: An illustration of the complexity of collaboration in special education. *J. Educ. Psychol. Consult.* **2010**, *20*, 9–27. [CrossRef]
8. Baeten, M.; Simons, M. Student teachers' team teaching: Models, effects, and conditions for implementation. *Teach. Teach. Educ.* **2014**, *41*, 92–110. [CrossRef]
9. Cook, S.C.; McDuffie-Landrum, K. Integrating effective practices into co-teaching: Increasing outcomes for students with disabilities. *Interv. Sch. Clin.* **2019**, *55*, 221–229. [CrossRef]
10. Gardiner, W. Mentoring two student teachers: Mentors' perceptions of peer placements. *Teach. Teach. Educ.* **2010**, *21*, 233–246. [CrossRef]
11. Simons, M.; Coetzee, S.; Baeten, M.; Vlerick, P. Measuring learners' perceptions of a team-taught learning environment: Development and validation of the Learners' Team Teaching Perceptions Questionnaire (LTTPQ). *Learn. Environ. Res.* **2020**, *23*, 45–58. [CrossRef]
12. Strogilos, V.; King-Sears, M.E. Co-teaching is extra help and fun: Perspectives on co-teaching from middle school students and co-teachers. *J. Res. Spec. Educ. Needs* **2019**, *19*, 92–102. [CrossRef]
13. Jones, L.; Green, K. Who teaches primary PE? Change and transformation through the eyes of subject leaders. *Sport Educ. Soc.* **2015**, *22*, 759–771. [CrossRef]
14. Dockerty, F.; Pritchard, R. Reconsidering models-based practice in primary physical education. *Education 3-13* **2023**, *53*, 1273–1284. [CrossRef]
15. Ní Chróinín, D.; O'Brien, N. Primary school teachers' experiences of external providers in Ireland: Learning lessons from physical education. *Ir. Educ. Stud.* **2019**, *38*, 327–341. [CrossRef]
16. Luptáková, G.; Balga, T.; Antala, B.; Cihová, I.; Argajová, J.; Dovičák, M.; Složik, M.; Gurský, T.; Macháček, J. Collaborative instruction with external providers in primary physical education: A three-year comparative analysis of generalist teacher perspective. *Kinesiol. Slov.* **2025**, *31*, 21–34. [CrossRef]
17. Luptáková, G.; Popeska, B.; Ristevska, H.; Balga, T.; Klincarov, I.; Antala, B. Tandem teaching for quality physical education: Primary teachers' preparedness and professional growth in Slovakia and North Macedonia. *Educ. Sci.* **2025**, *15*, 1397. [CrossRef]
18. Klincarov, I.; Popeska, B.; Mitevski, O.; Nikovski, G.; Mitevska-Petrusheva, K.; Majeric, M. Tandem teaching in physical and health education classes from teacher's perspective. In Proceedings of the 3rd International Scientific Conference Research in Physical Education, Sport, and Health, Skopje, North Macedonia, 31 May–2 June 2018; Velickovska, L.A., Ed.; Ss. Cyril and Methodius University in Skopje, Faculty of Physical Education, Sport, and Health: Skopje, North Macedonia, 2018; pp. 255–262.
19. Duncombe, R.; Cale, L.; Harris, J. Strengthening 'the foundations' of the primary school curriculum. *Educ. 3-13 Int. J. Prim. Elem. Early Years Educ.* **2018**, *46*, 76–88. [CrossRef]
20. Spittle, S.; Spittle, M.; Encel, K.; Itoh, S. Confidence and motivation to teach primary physical education: A survey of specialist primary physical education pre-service teachers in Australia. *Front. Educ.* **2022**, *7*, 1061099. [CrossRef]

21. D'Isanto, T.; D'Elia, F. Body, movement, and outdoor education in pre-school during the COVID-19 pandemic: Perceptions of teachers. *J. Phys. Educ. Sport* **2021**, *21*, 709–713. [CrossRef]
22. D'Isanto, T.; D'Elia, F. Primary school physical education outdoors during the COVID-19 pandemic: The perceptions of teachers. *J. Hum. Sport Exerc.* **2021**, *16*, S1521–S1535. [CrossRef]
23. Milić, M.; Radić Hozo, E.; Maulini, C.; De Giorgio, A.; Kuvačić, G. What is the place of physical education among the teaching priorities of primary school teachers? An empirical study on importance, qualification and perceived teachers' competence. *Educ. Sci.* **2022**, *12*, 613. [CrossRef]
24. Miholić, S. Kinesiological Competences of Primary Education Teachers in the Republic of Croatia. Ph.D. Dissertation, University of Zagreb, Faculty of Kinesiology, Zagreb, Croatia, 2017.
25. Francesco, C.; Coco, D.; Frattini, G.; Vago, P.; Andrea, C. Effective teaching competences in physical education. *J. Phys. Educ. Sport* **2019**, *19*, 1806–1813. [CrossRef]
26. Petračić, T. The Relationship Between Factors and the Quality of Physical Education Teaching in Primary School. Ph.D. Dissertation, University of Zagreb, Faculty of Kinesiology, Zagreb, Croatia, 2023.
27. Popeska, B. *Tandem Teaching in Physical Education: Current Experiences and Possibilities for Improvement*; Goce Delcev University: Stip, North Macedonia, 2022. Available online: https://eprints.ugd.edu.mk/31137/ (accessed on 8 September 2025).
28. Aliberti, S.; Kaçurri, A.; Kasa, A.; Giardullo, G. Stakeholders' opinions on teaching movement education in primary schools: A cross-sectional study. *J. Phys. Educ. Sport* **2025**, *25*, 423–431. [CrossRef]
29. Gerovac, A.; Emeljanovas, A.; Petrusic, T.; Novak, D. Generalist vs physical education specialist elementary school teacher: Do teacher characteristics matter? *Kinesiol. Slov. Sci. J. Sport* **2025**, *31*, 84–99. [CrossRef]
30. Antala, B. *Didaktika Telesnej a Športovej Výchovy pre Základné a Stredné Školy: Vybrané Kapitoly (Didactics of Physical and Sports Education for Primary and Secondary Schools: Selected Chapters)*; Slovenská Vedecká Spoločnosť pre Telesnú Výchovu a Šport: Bratislava, Slovakia, 2024.
31. Randall, V. 'We want to, but we can't': Pre-service teachers' experiences of learning to teach primary physical education. *Oxf. Rev. Educ.* **2023**, *49*, 209–228. [CrossRef]
32. McEvilly, N. What is PE and who should teach it? Undergraduate PE students' views and experiences of the outsourcing of PE in the UK. *Sport Educ. Soc.* **2022**, *27*, 662–675. [CrossRef]
33. Balga, T.; Luptáková, G.; Cihová, I.; Dovičák, M. Evaluating the impact of tandem teaching with coaches and generalist teachers on primary school students' perceptions in physical education. *Coll. Antropol.* **2024**, *48*, 161–166. [CrossRef]
34. Domville, M.; Watson, P.; Richardson, D.; Graves, L. Children's perceptions of factors that influence PE enjoyment: A qualitative investigation. *Phys. Educ. Sport Pedagog.* **2019**, *24*, 577–590. [CrossRef]
35. Gökbulut, Ö.D.; Akçamete, G.; Güneyli, A.; Toper, Ö. Impact of co-teaching approach in inclusive education settings on the development of reading skills. *Int. J. Whole Sch.* **2020**, *16*, 26–42. [CrossRef]
36. Qualls, L.W.; Arastoopour Irgens, G.; Hirsch, S.E. Co-Teaching as a dynamic system to support students with disabilities: A case study. *Educ. Sci.* **2025**, *15*, 733. [CrossRef]
37. Luptáková, G.; Antala, B.; Seman, F.; Popluhárová, M. Effects of teacher specialization on physical fitness and motor skills in tandem-taught physical education in elementary school. In *Zbornik Radova/Proceedings*; Croatian Kinesiology Association: Zagreb, Croatia, 2025; pp. 426–431.
38. Washburn, R.; Kolen, A. Children's self-perceived and actual motor competence in relation to their peers. *Children* **2018**, *5*, 72. [CrossRef] [PubMed]
39. Chai, H.; Xue, R.; Yao, L.; Miao, M.; Han, B. Configurations of actual and perceived motor competence among elementary school children in China: Differences in physical activity. *Front. Public Health* **2023**, *11*, 1280643. [CrossRef]
40. Herrmann, C.; Seelig, H. *MOBAK–1: Motorische Basiskompetenzen in der 1. Klasse: Testmanual (MOBAK-1: Basic Motor Competencies in First Grade: Testmanual)*; Departement für Sport, Bewegung und Gesundheit (DSBG), Universität Basel: Basel, Switzerland, 2014. Available online: https://kanton.baselland.ch/bildungs-kultur-und-sportdirektion/bildung-handbuch/unterricht/lehrplan-volksschule-bl/dokumente-lehrplan-volksschule-1/mobak_1_testmanual_august-2014.pdf (accessed on 8 September 2025).
41. Herrmann, C.; Seelig, H. *MOBAK–3: Basic Motor Competencies in Third Grade: Testmanual*; Department of Sport, Exercise and Health (DSBG), University of Basel: Basel, Switzerland, 2015; Available online: https://is.muni.cz/th/iu7x5/Anglicka_verze_prirucky_MOBAK_3.pdf (accessed on 8 September 2025).
42. Physical Literacy Canada. PLAYself Workbook. 2023. Available online: https://physicalliteracy.ca/wp-content/uploads/2023/09/PLAYself_workbook_2023_EN_WEB.pdf (accessed on 25 August 2025).
43. Chráska, M. *Metódy Pedagogického Výskumu—Základy Kvantitatívneho Výskumu (Research Methods in Pedagogy—Basics of Quantitative Research)*; Grada: Bratislava, Slovakia, 2007.
44. Cohen, J. *Statistical Power Analysis for the Behavioral Sciences*, 2nd ed.; Lawrence Erlbaum Associates: Mahwah, NJ, USA, 1988.
45. King-Sears, M.E.; Jenkins, M.C.; Brawand, A. Co-teaching perspectives from middle school algebra co-teachers and their students with and without disabilities. *Int. J. Incl. Educ.* **2020**, *24*, 427–442. [CrossRef]

46. Tsangaridou, N.; Charalambous, C.Y.; Kyriakides, E. Preservice classroom teachers' views and experiences of teaching physical education: Does taking a physical education specialization matter? *Eur. Phys. Educ. Rev.* **2024**, *30*, 265–282. [CrossRef]
47. Franco, E.; Coterón, J.; Spray, C. Antecedents of teachers' motivational behaviours in physical education: A scoping review utilising achievement goal and self-determination theory perspectives. *Int. Rev. Sport Exerc. Psychol.* **2025**, *18*, 1123–1162. [CrossRef]
48. Harter, S. *The Construction of the Self: A Developmental Perspective*; The Guilford Press: New York, NY, USA, 1999.
49. Monacis, D.; Annoscia, S.; Limone, P.; Colella, D. Examining the effects of reproductive and productive teaching styles interventions on primary schoolchildren: What implications for physical education teachers? *Phys. Educ. Theory Methodol.* **2023**, *23*, 839–849. [CrossRef]
50. Costa, R.Z.F.; Marques, I.; de Santo, D.L.; Medina-Papst, J. Relationship between children's competence self-perception, academic performance and motor performance. *J. Phys. Educ.* **2019**, *30*, 3034. [CrossRef]

children

Article

Validation of the Italian Translation and Cultural Adaptation of the Canadian Assessment of Physical Literacy-2 (CAPL-2) Questionnaire for Children

Alice Iannaccone [1,2,*,†], Alessandro Cudicio [3,†], Lavinia Falese [1,2], Bruno Federico [1,2], Matteo Crotti [3], Nicola Lovecchio [3], Simone Digennaro [1,2] and Valeria Agosti [4]

1 Department of Human Sciences, Society and Health, University of Cassino and Southern Lazio, Via Sant'Angelo, Loc. Folcara, 03043 Cassino, Italy; l.falese@unicas.it (L.F.); b.federico@unicas.it (B.F.); s.digennaro@unicas.it (S.D.)
2 European University of Technology EUt+, European Union
3 Department of Human and Social Sciences, University of Bergamo, 24129 Bergamo, Italy; alessandro.cudicio@unibg.it (A.C.); matteo.crotti@unibg.it (M.C.); nicola.lovecchio@unibg.it (N.L.)
4 Department of Humanities, Philosophy and Education, University of Salerno, 84084 Fisciano, Italy; vaagosti@unisa.it
* Correspondence: alice.iannaccone@unicas.it
† These authors equally contributed to this work.

Highlights:

What are the main findings?

- The Italian version of the CAPL-2 questionnaire demonstrated excellent internal consistency in the Motivation and Confidence domain (Cronbach's α: 0.88–0.97), aligning with international validation studies.
- The questionnaire showed high predictive validity for identifying children who meet WHO recommendations for physical activity, with AUC values of 0.95 (5 days) and 0.89 (6 days).

What is the implication of the main finding?

- The validated CAPL-2 offers Italian educators and researchers a culturally adapted, reliable tool to assess children's physical literacy in school and sport contexts.
- This tool can support early interventions promoting physical activity and lifelong health, in line with Italy's recent educational reforms and international public health goals.

Abstract: Background/Objectives: Physical literacy is a holistic concept promoting lifelong health by considering an individual's lived experience within their cultural context. This necessitates context-specific conceptualizations and pedagogies, highlighting the need for valid assessment tools for physical and sport educators. The Canadian Assessment of Physical Literacy (CAPL-2) is a well-known validated tool. This study aimed to validate the Italian translation and cultural adaptation of the CAPL-2 questionnaire for children aged 8–12. Methods: The CAPL-2 questionnaire was translated using a forward–backward procedure by bilingual experts. Subsequently, 111 Italian children (57 females, mean BMI 17.9 kg/m^2) completed the adapted CAPL-2 questionnaire twice over 10 days under supervision. The internal consistency of CAPL-2 was assessed with Cronbach's alpha. ROC curve analysis and AUC evaluated the CAPL-2's ability to predict adherence to WHO physical activity guidelines based on self-reported activity. Results: Results showed high internal consistency for the motivation and confidence domain (Cronbach's α: 0.88–0.97) but lower consistency for the knowledge and understanding domain (Cronbach's α: 0.20–0.34). Despite this, the CAPL-2 questionnaire demonstrated high predictive performance in identifying children active for at least 5 days (AUC: 0.95) or 6 days (AUC: 0.89). Conclusions:

The Italian version of CAPL-2 is a reliable tool for assessing physical literacy in Italian children aged 8 to 12, addressing key aspects such as motivation, confidence, physical skills, understanding of physical activity, and daily habits. It offers a valuable and culturally adapted instrument for trainers, teachers and educators in physical activity and sport contexts.

Keywords: assessment; cross-cultural adaptation; children; physical literacy; physical education; physical activity; sport; active lifestyle; lifelong; health

1. Introduction

The youngest generations are increasingly dedicating their time to sedentary activities, such as browsing social media, which has negative consequences for their overall well-being [1–3]. This is particularly troubling in relation to their development of identity, body image, and emotional intelligence. The rise in sedentary behaviour results in lower levels of physical activity, potentially worsening the adverse effects of unhealthy lifestyles [4–6]. Conversely, regular physical activity (PA) is associated with substantial physical and mental health benefits [7–9]. Among children and adolescents, physical activity (PA) supports healthy musculoskeletal development, particularly bone health, motor skill acquisition, and cognitive development. Despite these benefits, physical inactivity remains a global epidemic: 81% of boys and girls aged 11–17 years spend less than one hour a day performing moderate-to vigorous-intensity physical activity (MVPA) [7,9]. To address this public health challenge, global targets set by the WHO aim to reduce physical inactivity by 10% in 2025 and 15% in 2030 compared to 2010 levels, highlighting the urgency for multisectoral strategies due to projected healthcare costs potentially reaching USD 27 billion annually [10,11]. The findings from the recent national Health Behaviour in School-Aged Children (HBSC) survey in Italy reveal critical insights into the physical activity levels of adolescents. Specifically, the survey indicates that a mere 10.8% of male adolescents and 5.4% of female adolescents are meeting the recommended guidelines for MVPA [2].

In the context of promoting physical activity and addressing high rates of physical inactivity, the concept of physical literacy (PL) is globally emerging as a valuable theoretical construct around which to structure effective interventions [10,11]. There is increasing evidence that holistic approaches, such as multicomponent interventions targeting different factors (motivation, knowledge, competence, and self-perception), lead to greater improvements in physical activity than single-factor interventions [12,13].

For instance, Farias et al. [14] conducted a retrospective analysis to investigate the enduring impacts of a Sport Education curriculum on students' physical literacy (PL) reporting notable changes in students' motivation, perspectives, and behaviours concerning physical education (PE) and sports. The results revealed that students cultivated empathetic attitudes, developed resilience against discriminatory behaviour, and demonstrated a commitment to fair participation. These skills transcended the school setting, fostering the development of lifelong PL.

PL was described as an inclusive and holistic concept, conceived from its inception to promote lifelong health and well-being by centering on the person-in-the-world and their lived experience within their cultural context [15,16]. More recently, PL was emphasized as a lifelong journey characterized by evolving interactions between motivation, competence, knowledge, and the social and cultural context, highlighting the necessity of culturally appropriate assessment tools to foster physical activity effectively throughout life [15,16].

This concept is now increasingly recognized as a multidimensional construct, encompassing four domains: physical competence, motivation, confidence, knowledge, and behaviors necessary for lifelong engagement in physical activity [17,18], enabling people to participate meaningfully in physical and sport activities across their lifespan, thus aligning with strategies to combat sedentary lifestyles and foster lifelong health [19,20]. By fostering PL from an early age, individuals can develop a foundation that supports sustained physical and sport activity and well-being in adulthood and older age [21]. From these perspectives, PL is not confined to childhood but evolves continuously, adapting to the changing abilities and contexts throughout life [22,23]. Developing robust PL skills early in life helps individuals establish personal strategies to sustain active lifestyles throughout their lifespan [24].

Recognizing that diverse cultures, governance structures, geographical locations, and physical environments necessitate tailored conceptualizations and pedagogies to effectively foster PL [25,26], a recent Global Physical Literacy (GloPL) Action Framework [27] was established to unify this complex dimension in objectives and principles, as well as to delineate effective strategies for advancing PL on a global scale [28].

Standardized assessments of PL that take into account its complex dimensions are crucial to evaluate PL levels in the population and to support PL development [22,24]. The Canadian Assessment of Physical Literacy—Second Edition (CAPL-2) [29] has emerged as a comprehensive tool effective in evaluating multiple aspects of PL and a key instrument for understanding how PL develops and evolves across childhood [22,29,30] within different international contexts [31]. The CAPL-2 assessment comprises three Physical Competence protocols, two Daily Behavior protocols, and a 22-item questionnaire assessing the domains of Motivation and Confidence, and Knowledge and Understanding. Regarding the 22-item questionnaire, crucial for evaluating the cognitive and affective aspects of PL, extensive research has highlighted the necessity of tailoring the CAPL-2 questionnaire to reflect the linguistic nuances and cultural contexts of target populations, ensuring the assessment's validity and reliability into various languages and contexts [17,20,30,32–35].

Recognizing the unique cultural and educational characteristics of Italy, where recent investments have been made to enhance primary school physical education by introducing specialized physical education teachers in grades four and five (Legge 234/2021) [36], reflecting increased awareness of the inactivity pandemic [33], this study aims to validate and culturally adapt the CAPL-2 for Italian children, ensuring the instrument's appropriateness and reliability within the Italian context.

2. Materials and Methods

2.1. Sample and Procedures

A total of 111 children (54 males; 57 females) aged 8 to 12 years participating in a national summer camp in Italy were recruited (Table 1).

Table 1. Sample size and demographic characteristics.

Variable	Mean	Standard Deviation	Min	Max
Weight (kg)	34.64	9.38	19.9	64.4
Height (cm)	137.86	10.27	119.4	159.2
BMI (kg/cm^2)	17.93	3.08	13.21	26.98
Active days (days/week)	5.69	1.36	1	7

The convenience sample was recruited during a national summer camp attended by children from multiple Italian regions (including Northern, Central, Southern areas, and an island), ensuring heterogeneity in socio-cultural and socio-economic backgrounds and thus providing a broad representation of the national territory. The summer camp context was intentionally chosen because it allowed for continuous attendance of participants, close supervision by trained research assistants, and standardized administration procedures. In addition, this setting provided the optimal opportunity to administer the questionnaire twice within the required 10-day interval for the test-retest reliability assessment, under consistent and controlled conditions.

Eligibility criteria were the ability to speak Italian and an age between 8 and 12 years, consistent with the target population of the CAPL-2 and with previous validation studies of physical literacy questionnaires [29,37]. Importantly, children were not selected on the basis of competitive sport participation or prior knowledge/skills, making the sample representative of the general population of Italian children within this age range.

All research assistants underwent standardized training sessions before data collection, ensuring consistency in questionnaire administration, data collection procedures, and interaction with children. This study was conducted in accordance with the Declaration of Helsinki and approved by the Ethics Committee of the University of Cassino and Southern Lazio—IRB Department of Human Sciences, Society and Health (Approval number: 4R; Approval date: 11 September 2024).

To assess the internal consistency and reliability of the Italian version, the questionnaire was administered to the same group of children on two separate occasions, with a ten-day interval between the first and second administrations. To enhance the confidentiality of assessment results and to ensure the integrity of the test–retest process, each child was assigned a unique identification number, which was used to accurately record the scores obtained. Participants completed the questionnaire under the supervision of trained research assistants, who provided detailed instructions and responded to any inquiries that arose during the process. In accordance with the CAPL-2 guidelines, responses were collected anonymously on paper and subsequently entered into a secure database for analysis by a designated researcher.

2.2. CAPL-2 Measures

The current questionnaire is part of the comprehensive protocol developed by the Canadian Assessment of Physical Literacy-2 (CAPL-2) [29,37], designed to accurately and reliably assess a wide array of skills and abilities that define a child's level of physical literacy.

Specifically, the CAPL-2 questionnaires consist of two key domains of PL (i.e., motivation and confidence; knowledge and understanding domain) and four subscales.

Importantly, according to the CAPL-2 manual, self-reported MVPA is not a separate domain but is included within the broader daily behaviour domain of the CAPL-2 protocol, which encompasses both objective (e.g., pedometer-based) and subjective (self-report) indicators of physical activity.

The first domain, motivation and confidence, assesses children's confidence in their ability to be physically active and their motivation to participate in physical activity. The total score for this domain is derived from four subscales: Predilection and Adequacy items ("What's most like me?"), Intrinsic Motivation ("Why are you active?"), and Physical Activity Competence ("How do you feel about being active?"), each consisting of three items. According to the manual, the subscale scores range from 1.5 (or 1.8) to 7.5, with the maximum possible score for the entire domain being 30 points.

The second domain, knowledge and understanding, assesses a child's knowledge of physical activity, skills and fitness. The assessment comprises four multiple-choice questions, each presenting one correct answer alongside three incorrect options. The second part features a gap-fill task that requires completion of sentences. Each correctly inserted word is worth one point, allowing for a maximum of six points in this section.

Overall, the total score for this assessment ranges from 0 to 10, with 10 representing the highest possible score.

In addition, the CAPL-2 questionnaire includes a self-report measure of children's engagement in at least 60 min of daily MVPA. This item prompts participants to indicate how often they usually achieve this daily activity target. While this self-reported measure represents only one component of the daily behaviour domain, its inclusion provides valuable complementary information and allows for the examination of associations between physical activity levels and other domains of physical literacy.

2.3. Translation and Cultural Adaptation

The translation of the CAPL-2 questionnaire into Italian was carried out in accordance with the methodology outlined by Walde & Vollm [38]. This approach ensures accuracy and consistency in the translation process, adhering to the highest standards of linguistic quality.

(1) Translation: The original document was translated into Italian by two researchers who are native speakers, each working independently to ensure accuracy and fidelity to the source material.
(2) Review: The two versions have been systematically compared and reviewed by a researcher with expertise in physical literacy.
(3) Adjudication: Following the feedback provided by the reviewer, a preliminary version of the Italian CAPL-2 questionnaire was finalized.
(4) Pretest: The pre-final version of the Italian questionnaire was administered to a sample of 10 participants to assess the clarity and comprehensibility of the questions. Participants were prompted to provide feedback regarding their understanding of the questionnaire items.
(5) Documentation: After carefully considering the feedback gathered during the pretest phase, the final version of the questionnaire has been officially approved.

A graphical representation of the translation and cultural adaptation process is shown in the Supplementary Material (Figure S1).

The final Italian version of the CAPL-2 questionnaire used for the research is attached as Supplementary Material S1.

2.4. Statistical Analysis

All collected data were systematically organized and stored into a database specifically developed for the purposes of this study. The threshold of $\alpha = 0.05$ was adopted as the level of statistical significance. All calculations were performed using STATA software (v 18, STATACorp, College Station, TX, USA).

The socio-demographic characteristics—such as age, sex, height, body weight, and body mass index (BMI)—and all variables utilized in the calculations were comprehensively detailed. The data were presented as means and standard deviations (SD) for both the test and retest. The normality of all examined variables was evaluated using the Kolmogorov-Smirnov test.

The internal consistency and reliability of the overall domain score, as well as the total scores for each subdomain and individual item outcomes, were assessed using Cronbach's alpha [39,40]. Furthermore, Spearman's correlation was employed to examine the relationship between each item and the overall scores for every domain and subdomain.

The assessment of test–retest reliability, or reproducibility, was conducted by calculating the intraclass correlation coefficient (ICC) along with a 95% confidence interval (95% CI). A two-way random effects model was utilized to analyze single measures and absolute agreement, demonstrating the concordance between the initial test and the retest. The interpretation of ICC values adhered to the benchmarks set forth by Landis and Koch [41]: <0.20, slight agreement; 0.21 to 0.40, fair; 0.41 to 0.60, moderate; 0.61 to 0.80, substantial; and >0.80, almost perfect. Additionally, we computed the standard errors of measurement (SEM) and the minimum detectable change (MDC) to assess the error range for each item, subdomain, and domain. Moreover, to check the overall diagnostic performance of the Italian version of CAPL-2 Questionnaire we created a receiver operating characteristic (ROC) curve and evaluated the area under the curve (AUC).

In line with the statistical analysis procedures reported by Knisel et al. [33], two cut-points were selected within the CAPL-2 Questionnaire Manual (the ones that were closer to the World Health Organization PA recommendations for children [9]. The first cut-point concerned engaging in physical activity for at least 60 min for 5 days a week, while the second cut-point concerned engaging in physical activity for at least 60 min for 6 or 7 days a week. A ROC curve analysis was used to assess whether physical literacy scores are predictive of meeting the physical activity cut-points.

3. Results

Results showed good to excellent internal consistency for the motivation and confidence domain (Cronbach's α: 0.88–0.97; mean: 5.3 ± 1.4) and low internal consistency for the knowledge and understanding domain (Cronbach's α: 0.20–0.34; mean: 9.3 ± 0.98).

Furthermore, the results revealed that the CAPL-2 questionnaire exhibited highly predictive performance in identifying children active for at least 5 days (AUC: 0.95) compared to those active for at least 6 days (AUC: 0.89).

3.1. Psychometric Properties of the Questionnaire

Tables 2 and 3 provide an overview of the internal consistency, reliability, and systematic variations associated with the self-reported physical activity questions, motivation and confidence questions, and the knowledge and understanding questions from the CAPL-2 battery assessment.

Table 2. Reliability, test-retest and systematic differences in motivation and confidence questions from CAPL-2 battery assessment.

Motivation and Confidence	Mean (SD)	Item-Total Correlation (Test)	Item-Total Correlation (Retest)	Average Inter-Item Correlation	Cronbach's α
Item 1	2.19 (0.56)	0.97	0.92	0.79	0.88
Item 2	2.12 (0.63)	0.91	0.80	0.95	0.97
Item 3	2.15 (0.56)	0.96	0.92	0.79	0.89
Predilection	6.45 (1.67)	N/A	N/A	0.84	0.94
Item 1	1.96 (0.63)	0.91	0.79	0.87	0.93
Item 2	1.75 (0.64)	0.94	0.85	0.78	0.88
Item 3	1.87 (0.63)	0.95	0.88	0.75	0.85
Adequacy	5.59 (1.77)	N/A	N/A	0.80	0.92
Item 1	2.20 (0.43)	0.92	0.83	0.93	0.96
Item 2	2.04 (0.44)	0.97	0.93	0.93	0.96
Item 3	1.99 (0.42)	0.96	0.91	0.83	0.91
Intrinsic motivation	6.23 (1.22)	N/A	N/A	0.86	0.95
Item 1	1.89 (0.49)	0.97	0.93	0.82	0.90
Item 2	1.57 (0.52)	0.93	0.84	0.94	0.97
Item 3	1.83 (0.50)	0.96	0.92	0.83	0.91
Physical activity competence	5.30 (1.45)	N/A	N/A	0.86	0.95
Total domain score	23.51 (5.65)	N/A	N/A	0.74	0.97

Abbreviations: SD, standard deviation; N/A, not applicable. Item-total correlation refers to the magnitude of association between each item with its domain. Cronbach's a refers to the value when the item is removed.

Table 3. Reliability, test-retest and systematic differences in knowledge and understanding questions from CAPL-2 battery assessment.

Knowledge and Understanding	Mean (SD)	Item-Total Correlation (Test)	Item-Total Correlation (Retest)	Average Inter-Item Correlation	Cronbach's α
Physical activity (PA) guidelines	0.97 (0.19)	0.61	0.10	0.11	0.20
Cardiorespiratory fitness definition	1 (0)	N/A	N/A	N/A	N/A
Muscular endurance definition	1 (0)	N/A	N/A	N/A	N/A
Improve sport skills	0.53 (0.50)	0.70	0.23	0.21	0.34
PA comprehension	5.80 (0.60)	0.56	0.03	0.21	0.34
Total domain score	9.30 (0.86)	N/A	N/A	0.08	0.22

Abbreviations: SD, standard deviation; N/A, not applicable. Item-total correlation refers to the magnitude of association between each item with its domain. Cronbach's a refers to the value when the item is removed.

The Knowledge and Understanding domain exhibited low internal consistency (Cronbach's α: 0.20–0.34), likely due to limited variability and the relatively high baseline knowledge demonstrated by the sample, primarily composed of physically active children.

Correlation analysis of Pearson's r was performed for the first measurement of the tool (test). The results of these analyses are presented in Table 4.

Table 4. Correlations within the Motivation and Confidence domains.

	1	2	3	4
1. Predilection	-			
2. Adequacy	0.77 *	-		
3. Intrinsic Motivation	0.83 *	0.74 *	-	
4. PA competence	0.77 *	0.88 *	0.80 *	-
Motivation and Confidence	0.92 *	0.93 *	0.90 *	0.94 *

* $p < 0.05$.

Results showed that the analysis of the subscales of the Motivation and Confidence domain is nearly perfect, and associations were observed regarding the overall score of the Motivation and Confidence domain.

3.2. Predictiveness of the CAPL-2 Questionnaire Based on Physical Activity

As demonstrated from previous research [33], the questionnaire allows to check the overall diagnostic performance of the CAPL-2 questionnaire. For this purpose, the ROC curve analysis was performed, and the AUC was estimated. The analysis was made by setting two cut-points [9]: physically active for at least 60 min for 5 days a week; physically active for 6 days a week. The AUC values of the models were sufficient [42], indicating a good fit of the classification (Table 5). The highest predictive capability was found for the model based on the first cut-point.

Table 5. Results of ROC curve analysis for CAPL-2 Questionnaire total score based on children's physical activity.

MVPA Cut Point	Coefficient	St.Err.	z	p	[95% CI]		AUC (95% CI)	p
Active for at least 6 days	0.33	0.65	7.07	<0.001	0.20	0.46	0.89	<0.001
Active for at least 5 days	0.42	0.09	4.69	<0.001	0.24	0.59	0.95	<0.001

The ROC curve for the first physical activity cut-point (PA for 5 days and 60 min) is reported in Figure 1.

These results indicate that physical literacy scores are predictive of physical activity levels (engaging in at least 60 min of PA over at least 5 days).

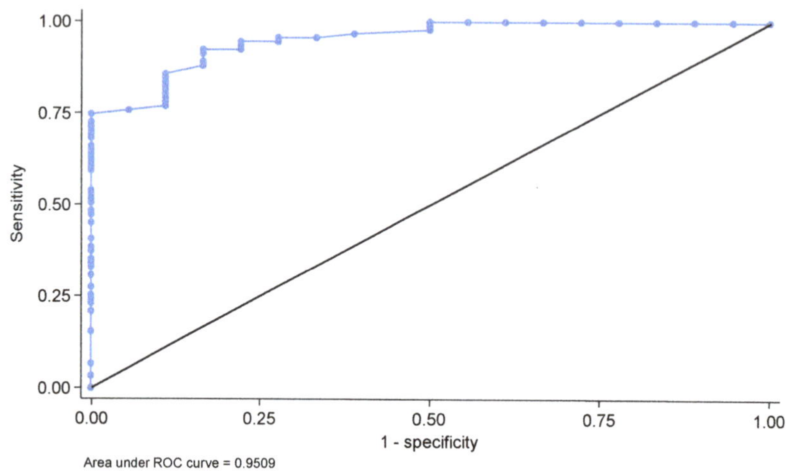

Figure 1. ROC curve for the physical activity cut-off point for 5 days and 60 min.

4. Discussion

The present study aimed to validate and culturally adapt the CAPL-2 questionnaire for Italian children aged 8 to 12 years. Our findings demonstrate that the Italian version of the CAPL-2 is a reliable and valid instrument for assessing PL in this population.

The Italian adaptation of the CAPL-2 questionnaire demonstrated excellent internal consistency within the Motivation and Confidence domain, with Cronbach's alpha values ranging from 0.88 to 0.97 across subscales (see Table 2). These findings align with previous validation studies in other cultural contexts. For instance, Elsborg et al. [32] reported high internal consistency in the Danish version of the CAPL-2, supporting the reliability of this domain across different populations. Similarly, Gunnell et al. [43] refined the Motivation and Confidence domain in the CAPL-2, resulting in a shorter, theoretically aligned questionnaire with strong psychometric properties. These consistent findings across studies suggest that the Motivation and Confidence domain is robust and effectively captures the intended constructs in diverse cultural settings [44]. The high item-total correlations underline the questionnaire's reliability and suggest that the translated and culturally adapted items effectively capture Italian children's motivational and self-perception dimensions associated with PA.

With respect to the Knowledge and Understanding domain, a low internal consistency was found, with Cronbach's alpha values ranging between 0.20 and 0.34 (see Table 3), hypothetically explained by the high homogeneity among answers, providing low variability. Nevertheless, results are consistent with previous international validation studies of the CAPL-2 questionnaire. For example, Pastor-Cisneros et al. [17] reported similar results in the Spanish version, suggesting potential challenges in measuring knowledge and understanding consistently across different populations. Similarly, in the Chinese version of CAPL-2, Li et al. [30] reported a Cronbach's α of 0.52 for the Knowledge and Understanding domain, whereas the Motivation and Confidence domain achieved a significantly higher α of 0.82, indicating that the cognitive domain consistently demonstrates lower internal consistency across cultural adaptations.

A Confirmatory Factor Analysis (CFA) was not performed in the present study due to the relatively small sample size, which would not meet the recommended criteria for stable estimation in a multi-item, multi-factor model [45,46]. Our primary aim was to translate, culturally adapt, and assess the internal consistency and test-retest reliability of the CAPL-2 questionnaire, in line with the methodological approach adopted by other cultural adaptation studies [17,32,33]. The consistently low Cronbach's α values reported internationally for the Knowledge and Understanding domain suggest that this is a recurring characteristic of the domain rather than a result of factorial misfit.

In our sample, the item "Physical activity guidelines" showed modest correlations (0.61 at test, significantly reduced to 0.10 at retest), while the "Improve sport skills" item also displayed low reliability (0.70 at test and 0.23 at retest). Moreover, the low average inter-item correlations (ranging from 0.11 to 0.34) suggest limited coherence among items. Given the consistently high mean scores (9.3 ± 0.98), the low variability among responses likely reduced internal consistency, suggesting a ceiling effect [47]. However, these findings do not necessarily indicate translation flaws or a lack of comprehension among Italian children. Rather, they may reflect both the characteristics of a well-informed and physically active sample, and the structural limitations of this domain across multiple contexts. In particular, the mixed item formats (multiple choice and gap-filling) and the limited number of items may not sufficiently capture the complexity of children's knowledge.

The inter-subscale correlations observed in Table 4 showed strong positive relationships among the four subscales of the Motivation and Confidence domain: Adequacy, Predilection, Intrinsic Motivation, and Perceived Physical Competence. These findings are consistent with previous studies that have validated the CAPL-2 in different cultural contexts. For instance, Gunnell et al. [43] conducted a factor analysis to refine the Motivation and Confidence domain, resulting in a model that included these four subscales, each demonstrating strong internal consistency and theoretical alignment with self-determination theory. Their study supports the structural coherence of these constructs within the CAPL-2 framework. Similarly, Elsborg et al. [32] reported high internal consistency within the Motivation and Confidence domain, further corroborating the robustness of these interrelated constructs across different populations. These consistent findings across studies reinforce the validity of the Motivation and Confidence domain in assessing PL among children.

Finally, the CAPL-2 demonstrated excellent predictive validity in identifying children meeting the World Health Organization's physical activity recommendations. The area under the curve (AUC) values were 0.95 for children active at least five days per week and 0.89 for those active six days per week, both statistically significant ($p < 0.001$). These findings are consistent with previous studies validating the CAPL-2 in various populations. For instance, Mendoza-Muñoz et al. [35] reported good fit indices in the Spanish version of the CAPL-2, supporting its validity in assessing physical literacy and predicting physical activity levels. In fact, the model showed better predictive capabilities for children meeting at least 5 days of physical activity, indicating the questionnaire's strong discriminative power, particularly among children closely adhering to minimum recommended activity levels. These findings confirm the CAPL-2's utility as a practical screening instrument in identifying physically inactive children and underscore its potential to guide targeted interventions.

Figure 1 visually supports the results, clearly displaying excellent sensitivity and specificity of the CAPL-2 questionnaire for predicting adherence to recommended activity levels, further reinforcing the quantitative evidence provided by Table 5. The curve's proximity to the top-left corner indicates optimal discriminatory performance, confirming the questionnaire's appropriateness for practical use in educational and health-related settings in Italy.

In the context of Italy's recent educational reforms in the PA and sport contexts, including the introduction of specialized physical education teachers in primary schools (Legge 234/2021) [36] the validation of CAPL-2 questionnaire could offer a valuable and culturally adapted instrument to trainers, teachers, educators and policymakers, enabling effective monitoring of PL and targeted interventions from an early age. By facilitating early identification of areas needing support, this instrument contributes to the establishment of active lifestyle trajectories that could persist throughout the lifespan [48,49]. In fact, motor illiteracy complicates motor development by reducing competence and confidence, often worsened by obesity [48]. This creates a barrier that negatively impacts emotional, behavioral, physical, and cognitive domains. Effective physical education strategies that promote autonomy, motivation, and confidence can increase enjoyment and perceived competence, encouraging long-term participation in physical activities [50,51].

The present study's purpose also aligns with broader European efforts promoting physical literacy, including the Erasmus+ project "Promoting Physical Literacy and Healthy Lifestyles through Digital Materials for University Students (ePhyLi)" (https://www.ephyliproject.eu/), involving Italian institutions. Furthermore, it aligns with global sustainability and health objectives, such as those outlined in the UN 2030 Agenda [52], fostering healthier lifestyles from childhood into adulthood and recognizing sport and physical activity as catalysts for health, education, inclusion, and equality. Our study supports this perspective by providing a validated tool to monitor and promote these outcomes through physical literacy.

Moreover, our study aligns with the Kazan Action Plan [53] that provides a relevant international framework emphasizing inclusive access for all to physical education, physical activity, and sport, with the specific aim to maximize contributions to sustainable development goals (SDGs). Among the Kazan priorities, our study specifically addresses objectives related to improving health and well-being (SDG 3), providing quality education and lifelong learning (SDG 4), fostering inclusive participation (SDG 10), and advancing gender equality (SDG 5). Furthermore, the Kazan Action Plan underscores the importance of using evidence-based tools, such as CAPL-2, for monitoring and evaluating policies and programs designed to enhance physical literacy, physical activity, and sport participation.

5. Limitations

While the present study provides a reliable and contextually adapted tool for assessing and promoting PL among Italian children, certain limitations should be considered when interpreting the findings. Although the sample size was sufficient to estimate internal consistency with confidence and is comparable to that used in other CAPL-2 questionnaire adaptations [17,32,33] it was not adequate to perform advanced factorial analyses such as Confirmatory Factor Analysis (CFA). Moreover, the use of a convenience sample from a national summer camp, while providing diversity in socio-cultural backgrounds, may limit the generalizability of the results to the broader pediatric population. In addition, the cross-sectional design did not allow for the assessment of long-term stability or predictive validity of the CAPL-2 questionnaire. Future research should involve larger, randomized, and demographically diverse samples to enhance external validity, and adopt longitudinal or intervention-based designs to examine how early PL levels influence sustained PA and sport participation across the lifespan.

6. Conclusions

To our knowledge, this is the first study adapting and validating the CAPL-2 questionnaire for Italian children aged 8 to 12 years, providing a reliable and contextually appropriate instrument to assess PL. It represents a significant advancement in aligning assessment tools with the holistic and inclusive conceptualization of PL [15], facilitating culturally tailored interventions aimed at lifelong engagement in physical activity.

The strong internal consistency observed in the Motivation and Confidence domain underscores the relevance of affective components in fostering sustained physical activity behaviors, supporting multicomponent interventions addressing these motivational dimensions [32,43]. Conversely, the lower reliability observed in the Knowledge and Understanding domain, likely due to limited variability among participants with high baseline knowledge, highlights the necessity for further refinement to ensure comprehensive assessment across all PL domains. These results suggest that future research should explore revised formulations or expanded item pools to enhance the psychometric performance of this domain.

Supplementary Materials: The following supporting information can be downloaded at: https://www.mdpi.com/article/10.3390/children12101290/s1. Figure S1: Graphical representation of the process of translation and cultural adaptation of the Italian version of the Canadian Physical Literacy Assessment-2 questionnaire; Supplementary Material S1: Italian version of the CAPL-2 questionnaire.

Author Contributions: Conceptualization, A.C., S.D. and V.A.; methodology, A.C., A.I. and V.A.; formal analysis, A.I. and B.F.; data collection, A.C., A.I., L.F. and V.A.; data analysis and curation, A.I. and B.F.; supporting analysis and data curation, L.F., M.C. and N.L.; writing—original draft preparation, A.C., A.I. and V.A.; writing—review and editing, M.C., N.L., S.D. and V.A.; S.D. and V.A. supervised the entire study. All authors have read and agreed to the published version of the manuscript.

Funding: The author(s) disclosed receipt of the following financial support for the research, authorship, and/or publication of this article: Project ECS 0000024 "Ecosistema dell'innovazione -Rome Technopole" financed by EU in NextGenerationEU plan through MUR Decree n. 1051 23.06.2022PNRR Missione 4Componente 2Investimento 1.5—CUPH33C22000420001.

Institutional Review Board Statement: This study was conducted in accordance with the Declaration of Helsinki and approved by the Ethics Committee of University of Cassino and Southern Lazio—IRB Department of Human Sciences, Society and Health (Approval number: 4R.2024.09.11).

Informed Consent Statement: Informed consent was obtained prior to any procedure by the parents or their legal guardians.

Data Availability Statement: The data are available from the corresponding author on reasonable request.

Acknowledgments: Authors would like to thank all participants and the master student Alessandra Genovese for their contribution to this project.

Conflicts of Interest: The authors declare no conflicts of interest.

References

1. Boer, M.; van den Eijnden, R.J.J.M.; Boniel-Nissim, M.; Wong, S.L.; Inchley, J.C.; Badura, P.; Craig, W.M.; Gobina, I.; Kleszczewska, D.; Klanšček, H.J.; et al. Adolescents' Intense and Problematic Social Media Use and Their Well-Being in 29 Countries. *J. Adolesc. Health* **2020**, *66*, S89–S99. [CrossRef]
2. Galeotti, T.; Canale, N.; Charrier, L.; Bacigalupo, I.; Lazzeri, G.; Vieno, A. *La Sorveglianza HBSC-Italia 2022 Health Behaviour in School-Aged Children: I Comportamenti Di Dipendenza*; Italian Institute of Public Health: Rome, Italy, 2024.
3. Kern, M.R.; Duinhof, E.L.; Walsh, S.D.; Cosma, A.; Moreno-Maldonado, C.; Molcho, M.; Currie, C.; Stevens, G.W.J.M. Intersectionality and Adolescent Mental Well-Being: A Cross-Nationally Comparative Analysis of the Interplay Between Immigration Background, Socioeconomic Status and Gender. *J. Adolesc. Health* **2020**, *66*, S12–S20. [CrossRef] [PubMed]
4. Digennaro, S.; Iannaccone, A. Imagining Another Self: The Use of Social Media Among Preadolescents and Its Body-Related Consequences. An Exploratory Study. *Sage Open* **2025**, *15*, 21582440251321364. [CrossRef]
5. Digennaro, S.; Iannaccone, A. Check Your Likes but Move Your Body! How the Use of Social Media Is Influencing Pre-Teens Body and the Role of Active Lifestyles. *Sustainability* **2023**, *15*, 3046. [CrossRef]
6. Piccerillo, L.; Tescione, A.; Iannaccone, A.; Digennaro, S. Alpha Generation's Social Media Use: Sociocultural Influences and Emotional Intelligence. *Int. J. Adolesc. Youth* **2025**, *30*, 2454992. [CrossRef]
7. Guthold, R.; Stevens, G.A.; Riley, L.M.; Bull, F.C. Global Trends in Insufficient Physical Activity among Adolescents: A Pooled Analysis of 298 Population-Based Surveys with 1·6 Million Participants. *Lancet Child. Adolesc. Health* **2020**, *4*, 23–35. [CrossRef] [PubMed]

8. Wilhite, K.; Booker, B.; Huang, B.-H.; Antczak, D.; Corbett, L.; Parker, P.; Noetel, M.; Rissel, C.; Lonsdale, C.; del Pozo Cruz, B.; et al. Combinations of Physical Activity, Sedentary Behavior, and Sleep Duration and Their Associations With Physical, Psychological, and Educational Outcomes in Children and Adolescents: A Systematic Review. *Am. J. Epidemiol.* **2023**, *192*, 665–679. [CrossRef]
9. Bull, F.C.; Al-Ansari, S.S.; Biddle, S.; Borodulin, K.; Buman, M.P.; Cardon, G.; Carty, C.; Chaput, J.-P.; Chastin, S.; Chou, R.; et al. World Health Organization 2020 Guidelines on Physical Activity and Sedentary Behaviour. *Br. J. Sports Med.* **2020**, *54*, 1451–1462. [CrossRef]
10. Carl, J.; Barratt, J.; Arbour-Nicitopoulos, K.P.; Barnett, L.M.; Dudley, D.A.; Holler, P.; Keegan, R.; Kwan, M.; Scurati, R.; Sum, R.K.-W.; et al. Development, Explanation, and Presentation of the Physical Literacy Interventions Reporting Template (PLIRT). *Int. J. Behav. Nutr. Phys. Act.* **2023**, *20*, 21. [CrossRef]
11. Dlugonski, D.; Gadd, N.; McKay, C.; Kleis, R.R.; Hoch, J.M. Physical Literacy and Physical Activity Across the Life Span: A Systematic Review. *Transl. J. Am. Coll. Sports Med.* **2022**, *7*, e000201. [CrossRef]
12. Agosti, V.; Sirico, M. Motor Imagery as a Tool for Motor Learning and Improving Sports Performance: A Mini Review on the State of the Art. *Sport Sci.* **2020**, *13*, 13–17.
13. Neil-Sztramko, S.E.; Caldwell, H.; Dobbins, M. School-Based Physical Activity Programs for Promoting Physical Activity and Fitness in Children and Adolescents Aged 6 to 18. *Cochrane Database Syst. Rev.* **2009**, *1*, 1452. [CrossRef]
14. Farias, C.; Wallhead, T.; Mesquita, I. "The Project Changed My Life": Sport Education's Transformative Potential on Student Physical Literacy. *Res. Q. Exerc. Sport* **2020**, *91*, 263–278. [CrossRef]
15. Whitehead, M. Definition of Physical Literacy: Development and Issues. In *Physical Literacy Across the World*; Routledge: London, UK, 2019.
16. Whitehead, M. *Physical Literacy: Throughout the Lifecourse*; Routledge: London, UK, 2010.
17. Pastor-Cisneros, R.; Carlos-Vivas, J.; Adsuar, J.C.; Barrios-Fernández, S.; Rojo-Ramos, J.; Vega-Muñoz, A.; Contreras-Barraza, N.; Mendoza-Muñoz, M. Spanish Translation and Cultural Adaptation of the Canadian Assessment of Physical Literacy-2 (CAPL-2) Questionnaires. *Int. J. Environ. Res. Public Health* **2022**, *19*, 8850. [CrossRef]
18. Rudd, J.R.; Pesce, C.; Strafford, B.W.; Davids, K. Physical Literacy—A Journey of Individual Enrichment: An Ecological Dynamics Rationale for Enhancing Performance and Physical Activity in All. *Front. Psychol.* **2020**, *11*, 1904. [CrossRef]
19. Carl, J.; Jaunig, J.; Schnith, L.; Mayer, J.; O'Connor, J.; Young, L. Mapping the 'Lifelong Journey' of Physical Literacy: A Biographical Assessment Method for the Physical Activity and Health Context. *Sport Educ. Soc.* **2024**, 1–15. [CrossRef]
20. Hadier, S.G.; Liu, Y.; Long, L.; Hamdani, S.M.Z.H.; Khurram, H.; Hamdani, S.D.; Danish, S.S.; Fatima, S.U. Assessment of Physical Literacy in 8- to 12-Year-Old Pakistani School Children: Reliability and Cross-Validation of the Canadian Assessment of Physical Literacy-2 (CAPL-2) in South Punjab, Pakistan. *BMC Public Health* **2024**, *24*, 1726. [CrossRef]
21. Dania, A.; Kaioglou, V.; Venetsanou, F. Validation of the Canadian Assessment of Physical Literacy for Greek Children: Understanding Assessment in Response to Culture and Pedagogy. *Eur. Phys. Educ. Rev.* **2020**, *26*, 903–919. [CrossRef]
22. Barnett, L.M.; Jerebine, A.; Keegan, R.; Watson-Mackie, K.; Arundell, L.; Ridgers, N.D.; Salmon, J.; Dudley, D. Validity, Reliability, and Feasibility of Physical Literacy Assessments Designed for School Children: A Systematic Review. *Sports Med.* **2023**, *53*, 1905–1929. [CrossRef]
23. Boldovskaia, A.; Dias, N.M.G.; Silva, M.N.; Carraça, E.V. Physical Literacy Assessment in Adults: A Systematic Review. *PLoS ONE* **2023**, *18*, e0288541. [CrossRef] [PubMed]
24. Carl, J.; Barratt, J.; Wanner, P.; Töpfer, C.; Cairney, J.; Pfeifer, K. The Effectiveness of Physical Literacy Interventions: A Systematic Review with Meta-Analysis. *Sports Med.* **2022**, *52*, 2965–2999. [CrossRef] [PubMed]
25. Pascali, G.; Colella, D. Physical Literacy Assessment. A Literature Review. *Eur. J. Phys. Educ. Sport Sci.* **2025**, *12*. [CrossRef]
26. Edwards, L.C.; Bryant, A.S.; Keegan, R.J.; Morgan, K.; Jones, A.M. Definitions, Foundations and Associations of Physical Literacy: A Systematic Review. *Sports Med.* **2017**, *47*, 113–126. [CrossRef] [PubMed]
27. World Health Organization. *Global Action Plan on Physical Activity 2018–2030: More Active People for a Healthier World*; World Health Organization: Geneva, Switzerland, 2018.
28. Carl, J.; Mazzoli, E.; Mouton, A.; Sum, R.K.-W.; Singh, A.; Niederberger, M.; Martins, J.; Kriellaars, D.; Green, N.; Elsborg, P.; et al. Development of a Global Physical Literacy (GloPL) Action Framework: Study Protocol for a Consensus Process. *PLoS ONE* **2024**, *19*, e0307000. [CrossRef]
29. Longmuir, P.E.; Gunnell, K.E.; Barnes, J.D.; Belanger, K.; Leduc, G.; Woodruff, S.J.; Tremblay, M.S. Canadian Assessment of Physical Literacy Second Edition: A Streamlined Assessment of the Capacity for Physical Activity among Children 8 to 12 Years of Age. *BMC Public Health* **2018**, *18*, 1047. [CrossRef]
30. Li, M.H.; Sum, R.K.W.; Tremblay, M.; Sit, C.H.P.; Ha, A.S.C.; Wong, S.H.S. Cross-Validation of the Canadian Assessment of Physical Literacy Second Edition (CAPL-2): The Case of a Chinese Population. *J. Sports Sci.* **2020**, *38*, 2850–2857. [CrossRef]

31. Vuletic, P.R.; Kesic, M.G.; Gilic, B.; Pehar, M.; Uzicanin, E.; Idrizovic, K.; Sekulic, D. Evaluation of Physical Literacy in 9- to 11-Year-Old Children: Reliability and Validity of Two Measurement Tools in Three Southeastern European Countries. *Children* **2023**, *10*, 1722. [CrossRef]
32. Elsborg, P.; Melby, P.S.; Kurtzhals, M.; Tremblay, M.S.; Nielsen, G.; Bentsen, P. Translation and Validation of the Canadian Assessment of Physical Literacy-2 in a Danish Sample. *BMC Public Health* **2021**, *21*, 2236. [CrossRef]
33. Knisel, E.; Bremer, M.; Nałęcz, H.; Wascher, L.; Laudańska-Krzemińska, I. Validation of The Canadian Assessment of Physical Literacy—CAPL-2 Questionnaire for German and Polish School Children. *Phys. Cult. Sport* **2024**, *104*, 1–14. [CrossRef]
34. Mendoza-Muñoz, M.; Carlos-Vivas, J.; Castillo-Paredes, A.; Parraca, J.A.; Raimundo, A.; Alegrete, J.; Pastor-Cisneros, R.; Gomez-Galan, R. Portuguese Translation and Validation of the Questionnaires from the Canadian Physical Literacy Assessment-2: A Pilot Study. *Front. Psychol.* **2023**, *14*, 1244566. [CrossRef]
35. Mendoza Muñoz, M.; López-Gil, J.F.; Pastor-Cisneros, R.; Castillo Paredes, A.; Urbano Mairena, J.; Tremblay, M.; Carlos Vivas, J. Cross-Validation of the Canadian Assessment of Physical Literacy Second Edition (CAPL-2) for Spanish Children. *BMJ Open Sport Exerc. Med.* **2024**, *10*, e001971. [CrossRef] [PubMed]
36. Ministero Dell'Istruzione. Dipartimento per Il Sistema Educativo Di Istruzione e Formazione. Gazzetta Ufficiale Della Repubblica. Legge 30 Dicembre 2021, n. 234, Bilancio Di Previsione Dello Stato per l'anno Finanziario 2022 e Bilancio Pluriennale per Il Triennio 2022-2024, Art. 1, Co. 332, in G.U., Serie Generale, n. 310 Del 31.12.2021, S.O. n. 49. Available online: https://www.gazzettaufficiale.it/eli/id/2021/12/31/21G00256/s (accessed on 15 July 2025).
37. Longmuir, P.E.; Woodruff, S.J.; Boyer, C.; Lloyd, M.; Tremblay, M.S. Physical Literacy Knowledge Questionnaire: Feasibility, Validity, and Reliability for Canadian Children Aged 8 to 12 Years. *BMC Public Health* **2018**, *18*, 1035. [CrossRef]
38. Walde, P.; Völlm, B.A. The TRAPD Approach as a Method for Questionnaire Translation. *Front. Psychiatry* **2023**, *14*, 1199989. [CrossRef]
39. Nunnally, J.C. Psychometric Theory (2nd...—Google Scholar). 1978. Available online: https://scholar.google.com/scholar?hl=it&as_sdt=0%2C5&q=Nunnally%2C+J.+C.+%281978%29.+Psychometric+theory+%282nd+ed.%29.+McGraw-Hill.&btnG= (accessed on 21 August 2025).
40. George, D. *SPSS for Windows Step by Step: A Simple Study Guide and Reference, 17.0 Update, 10/e.*; Pearson Education India: Bangalore, India, 2011.
41. Landis, J.R.; Koch, G.G. The Measurement of Observer Agreement for Categorical Data. *Biometrics* **1977**, *33*, 159. [CrossRef]
42. Polo, T.C.F.; Miot, H.A. Use of ROC Curves in Clinical and Experimental Studies. *J. Vasc. Bras.* **2020**, *19*, e20200186. [CrossRef]
43. Gunnell, K.E.; Longmuir, P.E.; Woodruff, S.J.; Barnes, J.D.; Belanger, K.; Tremblay, M.S. Revising the Motivation and Confidence Domain of the Canadian Assessment of Physical Literacy. *BMC Public Health* **2018**, *18*, 1045. [CrossRef] [PubMed]
44. Cudicio, A.; Agosti, V. Beyond Belief: Exploring the Alignment of Self-Efficacy, Self-Prediction, Self-Perception, and Actual Performance Measurement in a Squat Jump Performance—A Pilot Study. *J. Funct. Morphol. Kinesiol.* **2024**, *9*, 16. [CrossRef]
45. Kyriazos, T.A. Applied Psychometrics: Sample Size and Sample Power Considerations in Factor Analysis (EFA, CFA) and SEM in General. *Psychology* **2018**, *9*, 2207–2230. [CrossRef]
46. Worthington, R.L.; Whittaker, T.A. Scale Development Research. *Couns. Psychol.* **2006**, *34*, 806–838. [CrossRef]
47. Terwee, C.B.; Bot, S.D.M.; de Boer, M.R.; van der Windt, D.A.W.M.; Knol, D.L.; Dekker, J.; Bouter, L.M.; de Vet, H.C.W. Quality Criteria Were Proposed for Measurement Properties of Health Status Questionnaires. *J. Clin. Epidemiol.* **2007**, *60*, 34–42. [CrossRef] [PubMed]
48. Colella, D. Physical Literacy e Stili d'insegnamento. Ri-Orientare l'educazione Fisica a Scuola Physical Literacy and Teaching Styles. Re-Orienting Physical Education at School. *Form. Insegn.* **2018**, *16* (Suppl. S1), 33–42.
49. Monacis, D.; Sannicandro, I.; Colella, D. Exploring Self-Reported Physical Activity Levels and Physical Fitness in Italian Children: A Mediation and Moderation Analysis. *Children* **2025**, *12*, 204. [CrossRef] [PubMed]
50. Trecroci, A.; Invernizzi, P.L.; Monacis, D.; Colella, D. Physical Illiteracy and Obesity Barrier: How Physical Education Can Overpass Potential Adverse Effects? A Narrative Review. *Sustainability* **2021**, *14*, 419. [CrossRef]
51. Faella, P.; Digennaro, S.; Iannaccone, A. Educational Practices in Motion: A Scoping Review of Embodied Learning Approaches in School. *Front. Educ.* **2025**, *10*, 1568744. [CrossRef]
52. United Nation Agenda Sustainable Development 2030. Available online: https://www.un.org/sustainabledevelopment/ (accessed on 30 July 2025).
53. UNESCO. UNESCO Kazan Action Plan. In Proceedings of the International Conference of Ministers and Senior Officials Responsible for Physical Education and Sport, 6th, Kazan, Russia, 3–15 July 2017; pp. 1–26.

children

MDPI

Systematic Review

Cluttering in Children and Adolescents: Speech Motor Development, Neurocognitive Mechanisms, and Allied Health Implications

Weifeng Han *, Lin Zhou, Juan Lu and Shane Pill

College of Education, Psychology and Social Work, Flinders University, Bedford Park, SA 5042, Australia
* Correspondence: weifeng.han@flinders.edu.au

Highlights

What are the main findings?

- Cluttering in childhood and adolescence reflects a developmental vulnerability in motor–cognitive integration, rather than a purely rate-based fluency disturbance.
- Symptoms emerge most clearly under high linguistic and cognitive load, demonstrating the central role of task demands and contextual variability in the expression of cluttering.

What are the implications of the main findings?

- Assessment should prioritise connected speech tasks that reveal timing instability, articulatory blurring and reduced monitoring, with attention to discourse and cognitive load.
- Intervention and future research should adopt developmentally informed, motor–cognitive frameworks capable of guiding more precise diagnosis, treatment and theoretical refinement.

Abstract

Background/Objectives: Cluttering in childhood and adolescence is characterised by unstable speech timing, excessive coarticulation, irregular rate and reduced intelligibility, yet the developmental mechanisms underpinning these behaviours remain partially understood. This review synthesises empirical and conceptual evidence to examine cluttering through the lenses of speech motor development, neurocognitive mechanisms, task demands and allied-health practice. Four research questions guided the review, focusing on motor characteristics, developmental and neurocognitive mechanisms, task dependence and clinical implications. **Methods:** Following the PRISMA guidelines, a comprehensive search across seven databases identified studies examining cluttering in children and adolescents. Screening and full-text review were conducted in Covidence by two reviewers, with disagreements resolved by the first author. Twelve studies met the inclusion criteria. Data were extracted into a structured evidence table, and findings were synthesised. **Results:** Across studies, cluttering emerged as a developmental motor–cognitive integration disorder. Speech motor systems, linguistic formulation and executive control showed difficulty aligning under real-world communicative demands, leading to timing instability, articulatory blurring and reduced intelligibility. Symptoms were strongly influenced by task complexity, with spontaneous and extended discourse eliciting the most pronounced breakdowns. **Conclusions:** Cluttering reflects a developmental vulnerability in coordinating speech motor, linguistic and executive processes. Understanding cluttering in this way challenges narrow rate-based definitions and supports more nuanced approaches to assessment and intervention. Significant evidence gaps remain, particularly in longitudinal, mechanistic, multilingual and ecologically valid research. This developmental motor–cognitive framework strengthens the conceptual foundations of cluttering and clarifies its relevance to children's motor development.

Keywords: cluttering; speech motor development; motor–cognitive integration; neurodevelopment; speech timing; developmental communication disorders

1. Introduction

Cluttering is a fluency disorder characterised by an abnormally rapid or irregular speech rate, excessive coarticulation, reduced intelligibility, atypical pausing, and deficits in self-monitoring [1]. Although traditionally discussed alongside stuttering, contemporary perspectives increasingly emphasise that cluttering reflects a distinct pattern of impaired speech motor control and cognitive-linguistic regulation, with symptoms often emerging during late childhood and adolescence [2]. The Limited Consensus Definition (LCD) [3] identifies three core features, i.e., perceived rapid or irregular speech rate, atypical fluency, and reduced intelligibility resulting from over-coarticulation or collapsing syllables, all supported by additional characteristics such as deficits in pragmatic, linguistic, and executive functioning.

Understanding cluttering from a developmental perspective is of importance for two reasons. First, speech is a highly specialised motor skill that undergoes maturation throughout childhood and adolescence. Motor development frameworks [4] emphasise the progressive stabilisation of timing, sequencing, coordination, and automatization, i.e., domains directly implicated in cluttering. Dynamic systems models (e.g., [5]), describe speech as the coordinated integration of multiple subsystems (respiratory, phonatory, articulatory, prosodic), each sensitive to cognitive load and task demands. When system demands exceed developmental capacity, instability, variability, and breakdowns occur. This motor-development lens highlights the interplay between perceptual, cognitive, linguistic, and motor processes across maturation. Cluttering, when viewed as an emerging speech motor coordination disorder with neurodevelopmental roots [6], aligns naturally with this focus.

Assessment represents a central challenge in the study of cluttering, particularly in children and adolescents [7]. Unlike more narrowly defined fluency disorders, cluttering is typically identified through patterns observed in connected speech, including variable speech rate, reduced intelligibility, excessive coarticulation, and limited self-monitoring, rather than through discrete, task-independent markers [8,9]. As a result, assessment practices often rely on extended discourse tasks and clinical judgement, and may vary substantially across settings. These challenges highlight the importance of understanding how speech motor development, linguistic and cognitive load, and task demands interact to shape the manifestation of cluttering and underscore the need for a clearer developmental framework to inform assessment decisions.

However, emerging evidence indicates that cluttering rarely exists in isolation. Its behavioural presentation often reflects the combined influence of speech motor control, linguistic planning, executive functioning, and broader neurodevelopmental profiles. For example, Bangert, Scott [10] identified cluttering-like features in children with fragile X syndrome, and suggested that atypical timing and working memory may contribute to fluency breakdowns. Fidan and Sarıyer [7] reported that children with cluttering show weaknesses in attention, working memory, and motor planning abilities, particularly in those with co-

https://doi.org/10.3390/children13010097

occurring attention-deficit/hyperactivity disorder (ADHD). Scott [11], Scott [12] provided developmental insights into rapid speech, over-coarticulation, and contextual variability across tasks, while Kelkar [1] and Duchan and Felsenfeld [13] emphasised the need for integrated motor, linguistic, and pragmatic assessment frameworks. Collectively, current evidence underscores the importance of examining cluttering as a multidimensional, developmentally sensitive, and context-dependent phenomenon.

Despite these advances, major gaps remain. Most studies addressing speech motor control in cluttering have been conducted with adults (e.g., [14]), therefore limiting their applicability to childhood development. Paediatric research is scarce and heterogeneous, with few studies exploring underlying motor or neurocognitive mechanisms directly. Few studies used kinematic, neuroimaging, or physiological measures to examine motor coordination or timing processes. Instead, existing paediatric literature relies largely on behavioural description, or indirect indices of cognitive load and motor planning (e.g., [15]). This gap limits our understanding of how speech motor control, linguistic formulation, and executive processes interact during critical periods of motor and cognitive growth.

Given these limitations, there is a need for a comprehensive synthesis and analysis of what is currently known about the speech motor, neurocognitive, and neurodevelopmental mechanisms underpinning cluttering in children and adolescents, and that situates these mechanisms within contemporary motor development frameworks. Such a review is essential for informing allied health practice, refining assessment, and guiding future intervention research grounded in motor-learning principles. Moreover, an integrative perspective is essential for improving early identification, particularly for children whose cluttering co-occurs with ADHD, fragile X syndrome, developmental language disorder, or other neurodevelopmental conditions (see, for example, [7,10,16,17]). A developmental motor–cognitive model may also inform school-based practice and educational participation that will ensure young people with cluttering receive support that aligns with their communication needs and developmental profile.

This review is intended as a systematic synthesis with a structured narrative and developmental focus, aiming to clarify patterns, constraints, and gaps in an emerging literature rather than to establish empirically validated causal models. It was guided by four interrelated research questions that together form the conceptual framework of the manuscript. Specifically, we asked: how speech motor characteristics are described in children and adolescents who clutter (RQ1); what developmental and neurocognitive mechanisms are proposed to underpin these characteristics (RQ2); how task demands and contextual factors shape the expression of cluttering (RQ3); and what implications these findings have for allied-health assessment and intervention (RQ4). Each section of the review is explicitly aligned with one or more of these questions, enabling a structured synthesis of a heterogeneous evidence base and a clear argumentative progression from description to interpretation and application.

2. Methods

This review employed a systematic search strategy combined with a structured narrative synthesis to examine cluttering in children and adolescents. While systematic procedures were used to identify, screen, and select relevant studies, a meta-analytic approach was not appropriate due to substantial heterogeneity in study designs, participant characteristics, outcome measures, and theoretical orientations. Instead, findings were synthesised narratively using a domain-based framework aligned to the four research questions, allowing integration of empirical, developmental, and clinically informative evidence while preserving conceptual coherence. Our procedures followed PRISMA guide-

https://doi.org/10.3390/children13010097

lines [18,19], and the screening process was facilitated using Covidence [20] to ensure consistency and reproducibility.

2.1. Search Strategy

We conducted a comprehensive search of four major databases commonly used in communication sciences and allied health research: Scopus, PsycINFO, PubMed, and CINAHL. Our search terms combined cluttering-related descriptors (such as "cluttering", "fluency disorder", "rapid rate", "irregular rate", "over-coarticulation"), motor and neurocognitive terminology (including "motor planning", "speech motor", "timing", "coarticulation", "executive function", "working memory", "attention", etc.), and developmental descriptors (e.g., "child", "children", "adolescent", "school-aged", "developmental"). Boolean operators and truncation ensured high sensitivity across databases. We supplemented database searching with manual screening of reference lists of key cluttering publications and forward citation tracking of foundational cluttering papers to ensure full coverage of relevant empirical studies. Tables 1 and 2 outline the PICO framework, key concepts and terms that facilitated the search.

Table 1. PICO framework.

Element	Description
Population	Children and adolescents (0–18 years) with cluttering
Intervention	Speech motor control, motor learning, neuromotor development, or neurological correlates
Comparison	Typically developing peers, or other fluency/motor disorders (e.g., stuttering, CAS, dysarthria)
Outcomes	Speech fluency, intelligibility, prosody, motor timing/coordination, neurological or genetic findings, intervention outcomes

Table 2. Concepts and search terms. Asterisks (*) are used as a truncation or wildcard symbol to broaden the search by retrieving various forms and spellings of a word from a single root term, which is a standard/default practice in systematic searches of literature.

Concept	Key Terms
Cluttering/Fluency Disorder	"clutter*", "fluency disorder", "disfluency", "rate disorder", "tachylalia", "rapid speech", "stutter*"
Motor control/Motor speech	"motor control", "motor timing", "motor coordination", "motor learning", "speech motor control", "speech movement", "articulatory control", "neuromotor"
Neurodevelopment	"neurodevelopment", "developmental disorder", "neural correlates", "neurological", "cerebellar", "basal ganglia", "executive function", "genetic"
Comparative disorders	"stutter*", "childhood apraxia of speech", "CAS", "dysarthria", "speech sound disorder"
Allied health/intervention	"speech pathology*", "speech therap*", "occupational therap*", "physiotherapy*", "interven*", "motor learning", "rehab*", "communica*"
Population	"child*", "adolescen*", "youth", "p?ediatric", "school-age*"

2.2. Inclusion and Exclusion Criteria

To ensure that the final corpus addressed RQ1–RQ4 directly and reflected contemporary definitions of cluttering, we applied the inclusion and exclusion criteria summarised in Table 3. These criteria were developed prior to screening and applied consistently

 https://doi.org/10.3390/children13010097

throughout. These criteria ensured that each included study contributed directly to at least one of the four research questions.

Table 3. Inclusion and exclusion criteria.

Inclusion Criteria	Exclusion Criteria
Research examining cluttering in children or adolescents (≤18 years), or mixed-age samples with extractable paediatric data	Studies involving adults only
Cluttering is defined using behavioural indicators (e.g., rapid or irregular rate, excessive coarticulation, reduced intelligibility, atypical fluency)	Studies describing fluency or motor speech disorders unrelated to cluttering (e.g., isolated stuttering, dysarthria, or CAS)
Evidence relevant to speech motor development, neurocognition, neurodevelopmental mechanisms, contextual task effects or allied-health clinical practice	Studies using the term cluttering without describing cluttering-consistent behaviours
Peer-reviewed studies published after 1 January 2000	Non-peer-reviewed studies; or studies published before 2000
Published in English	Non-English studies
No geographical restrictions	

Importantly, studies published from the year 2000 onwards were included to ensure alignment with contemporary diagnostic frameworks, assessment practices, and developmental models of speech motor and neurocognitive functioning. Earlier literature, while foundational in defining cluttering as a clinical construct, often predates greater consensus regarding diagnostic criteria and task-based assessment approaches, limiting its direct comparability with more recent developmental research.

Studies were also excluded if the term "cluttering" was used without accompanying descriptions consistent with established behavioural characteristics of cluttering, such as irregular or rapid speech rate, reduced intelligibility in connected speech, excessive coarticulation, or limited self-monitoring. This criterion was applied to ensure conceptual consistency across included studies. Decisions regarding exclusion on this basis were made through independent screening by two reviewers, with discrepancies discussed and resolved through consensus, and final determinations made by the first author.

Given the limited number of empirical paediatric studies directly examining cluttering, the review included multiple types of scholarly sources, including theoretical, conceptual, and clinically grounded papers, provided they addressed at least one of the research questions. These sources were not treated as equivalent to empirical studies; rather, they were used to inform the interpretation of developmental mechanisms, contextualise empirical findings, and articulate implications for assessment and intervention. This approach reflects established practice in integrative developmental reviews where empirical evidence is sparse or methodologically heterogeneous.

2.3. *Study Screening and Selection*

All search results were imported into Covidence for automated deduplication. The screening process followed the PRISMA framework [18,19]. Title and abstract screening was conducted independently by the second and third authors, who applied the eligibility criteria to each record. Full-text screening followed the same procedure. When disagreements occurred, the first author resolved conflicts through discussion and final decision-making. Twelve studies were included in the final synthesis and analysis, which provided the evidence foundation for addressing RQ1, RQ2, RQ3 and RQ4. The PRISMA

 https://doi.org/10.3390/children13010097

flow diagram (Figure 1) provides a detailed account of the number of records identified, screened, excluded and retained.

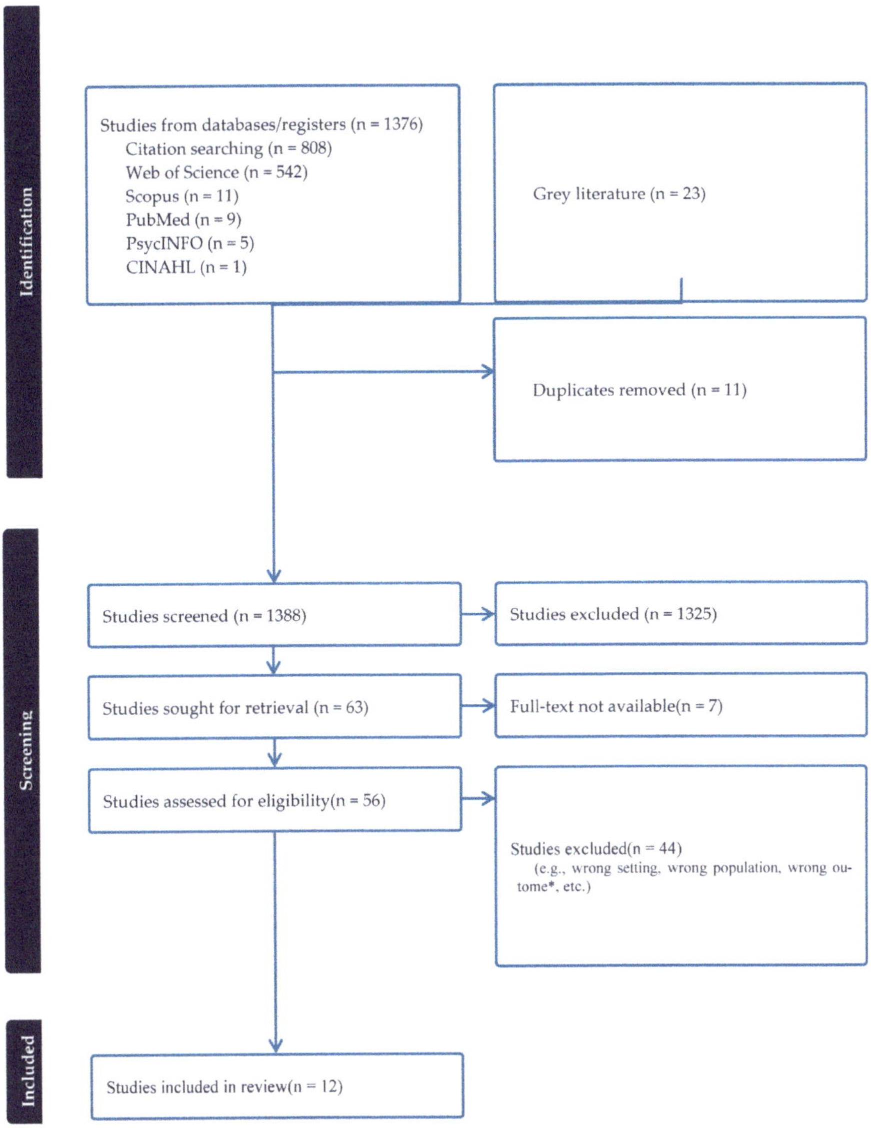

Figure 1. PRISMA chart. * Note. Research of wrong outcomes denotes those that did not report motor, neurocognitive, or task/context outcomes relevant to RQ1–RQ4, including Adult-only sample; that did not examine cluttering (term used without cluttering-consistent behaviours); or that did not report outcomes relevant to motor/neurocognitive/task-demand aims (RQ1–RQ4).

2.4. Data Extraction and Synthesis

Once the final corpus was established, the first author extracted all data into a structured template that captured study design, participant characteristics, definitions of cluttering, speech motor, neurocognitive or contextual features addressed, and primary findings. Each study was also mapped to the research questions it informed. Our synthesis proceeded

https://doi.org/10.3390/children13010097

by grouping extracted findings according to the four research questions: RQ1 (speech motor development), RQ2 (neurocognitive and neurodevelopmental mechanisms), RQ3 (task and contextual influences) and RQ4 (allied-health assessment and intervention implications).

Given the heterogeneity of the cluttering literature, synthesis was guided by explicit differentiation criteria rather than statistical aggregation. Studies were interpreted according to their primary analytic focus and developmental relevance, including empirical investigations of paediatric speech motor and cognitive characteristics, developmentally informative mechanistic studies, and clinically grounded conceptual or assessment-oriented work. This distinction informed a structured narrative synthesis aligned to the research questions, enabling identification of converging patterns, areas of divergence, and levels of evidential support across domains while avoiding inappropriate homogenisation of clinically and methodologically diverse sources.

Notably, the included literature reflects an emerging evidence base with substantial methodological diversity. To support transparent synthesis, we interpreted findings using an evidence-tier approach. Empirical paediatric studies were treated as direct evidence for observable speech motor and task-related characteristics. Mechanistic or developmentally informative work was used to propose functional interpretations, without being treated as causal evidence for paediatric mechanisms. Conceptual and clinical literature were used to clarify definitions, assessment considerations, and plausible pathways linking speech motor and cognitive demands, with inferences explicitly identified as interpretive rather than empirically established. This approach allowed integration across domains while keeping claims aligned with the strength and type of evidence available.

To support transparency and provide a clear overview of the evidence base, Table 4 summarises the twelve included studies. For each study, we summarise study design, participant characteristics, focal domains and their contribution to RQ1–RQ4. The table provides a point of reference for the subsequent synthesis and highlights the methodological diversity of the existing literature on cluttering in children and adolescents.

Table 4. Summary of included studies.

Study	Type/Design	Age Range	Focus	Motor/Neurodevelopmental Emphasis	Allied-Health Relevance	Relevance to RQs
Alm [21]	Theoretical paper	Lifespan (developmentally relevant)	Neurobiological mechanisms	Speech motor timing; cortico-basal ganglia circuits	Rate/timing assessment considerations	RQ1, RQ2
Bakker, Myers [22]	Empirical (cross-sectional)	Adults with developmental relevance	Motor performance under rate demands	Capacity-based motor control	Rate control; monitoring	RQ1, RQ3, RQ4
Bangert, Scott [10]	Empirical (cross-sectional phenotype study)	Young adults with FXS	Neurodevelopmental phenotype	FXS-related timing, cognition, and disfluency	Complex-needs assessment	RQ2, RQ4
Drayna [17]	Evidence synthesis	Lifespan	Genetic and heritable factors	Neural circuitry; familial aggregation	Family history; referrals	RQ2
Duchan [6]	Conceptual paper	Lifespan	Multilayered clinical construct	Motor-language-pragmatics interaction	Contextualised assessment	RQ1, RQ3, RQ4
Duchan and Felsenfeld [13]	Theoretical paper	Lifespan	Historical evolution of cluttering	Motor + cognitive shifts over time	Diagnostic implications	RQ1, RQ4
Fidan and Sarıyer [7]	Empirical (comparative)	Children/adolescents with ADHD	EF, WM, reading, cluttering	ADHD-linked executive and motor-planning difficulties	Integrated cognitive-motor assessment	RQ2, RQ4

 https://doi.org/10.3390/children13010097

Table 4. *Cont.*

Study	Type/Design	Age Range	Focus	Motor/Neurodevelopmental Emphasis	Allied-Health Relevance	Relevance to RQs
Kelkar, Sanghi [23]	Instrument validation	SLPs (Speech Language Pathologists)/consumer samples	Impact of cluttering	Participation-level impacts	Outcome measurement in practice	RQ4
Scott [12]	Empirical (child speech study)	School-aged children	Contextual variability in cluttering	Motor timing + discourse load	Task-based assessment	RQ1, RQ3
Scott [11]	Clinical/ educational discussion	School-aged children	Symptomatology and management	Motor, cognitive, and linguistic features	Assessment, differential diagnosis	RQ1, RQ3, RQ4
Ward [24]	Theoretical paper	Lifespan	Motor speech mechanisms	Timing, articulation, prosody	Motor-focused intervention	RQ1, RQ3, RQ4
Ward [25]	Clinical practice paper	Lifespan	Motor-focused treatment	Rate control, over-articulation	Clinically actionable strategies	RQ3, RQ4

3. Developmental and Theoretical Foundations of Cluttering

Cluttering during childhood and adolescence unfolds within a developmental period marked by ongoing refinement of speech motor control, linguistic organisation and executive functioning. These systems mature at different rates, and their interaction forms the foundation for understanding the speech characteristics and the contextual influences addressed in RQ1 and RQ3. By situating cluttering within a developmental motor framework, we can interpret the varied behaviours observed in children who clutter and understand why symptoms fluctuate across tasks and contexts.

Speech production is among the most temporally complex motor behaviours acquired in childhood [26]. Throughout the school years, children continue to refine articulatory timing, coarticulation and prosodic control as their speech motor patterns stabilise. Developmental research (e.g., [27,28]), shows that children's articulatory gestures are more variable, their segmental timing is less consistent, and their prosodic patterns are more easily disrupted than those of adults. These patterns reflect a motor system still consolidating automatization [29].

This developmental context is essential for understanding cluttering. Paediatric research shows that children who clutter exhibit timing variability, imprecise articulation and instability in rhythm, particularly during spontaneous or complex speech [11,12]. Such findings align with developmental speech literature (e.g., [30,31]), that when linguistic formulation demands increase, a less stable motor system becomes more vulnerable to irregular timing and articulatory "blurring". Cluttering becomes especially salient during the school years, when communicative and cognitive expectations increase, and children are required to produce longer, more complex verbal output.

Although rapid or irregular speech rate is often emphasised clinically, cluttering is widely understood as a multidimensional phenomenon involving the interaction of motoric, linguistic and pragmatic processes [1]. Historical analyses outline cluttering as encompassing imprecise articulation, disorganised verbal output and reduced self-monitoring [13], while more recent descriptions highlight excessive coarticulation, unstable prosody and difficulty coordinating extended discourse [11]. Consensus work underscores that no single feature defines cluttering; rather, individuals present with different constellations of symptoms that shift across contexts [2,6,21,24,25].

This multidimensionality is reflected across the included studies. Children who clutter not only speak rapidly or irregularly but often show reduced monitoring, challenges with discourse organisation and difficulty maintaining intelligibility across tasks [11,12].

 https://doi.org/10.3390/children13010097

Evidence from neurocognitive comparisons indicates that weaknesses in executive functioning or working memory can compound motor difficulties [7], therefore reinforcing the need to understand cluttering as the outcome of interacting systems rather than a purely motoric disorder.

Speech timing and sequencing are also central to the motor profile of cluttering. Empirical work shows that individuals who push speech beyond their capacity limits experience timing breakdowns and decreased intelligibility [22]. In children who clutter, timing instability is especially evident during connected speech production, where the motor system must coordinate rapid sequences while managing linguistic formulation demands. Rapid bursts, uneven rhythm and variable segment durations have been documented in school-aged children [12], particularly during tasks requiring spontaneous or extended speech.

Theoretical accounts also support these observations. Models of speech motor control describe cluttering as involving vulnerabilities in systems responsible for temporal regulation and articulatory coordination [24] and potential inefficiencies in neural circuits associated with rhythm and sequencing [21]. Together, these models and empirical findings suggest that cluttering reflects a developmental weakness in achieving stable, well-regulated timing, especially when cognitive or linguistic load increases.

In general, fluency disorders arise from the interplay between speech motor control, linguistic organisation and executive functioning [32]. Weaknesses in any of these domains can, therefore, amplify demands on the others. For example, rapid linguistic formulation may exceed the motor system's capacity to execute articulatory sequences with precision, leading to excessive coarticulation or syllable collapse [33]. Similarly, unstable motor execution may increase the cognitive load required to monitor speech, reducing efficiency in discourse organisation [34].

The included studies provide evidence of these cross-domain interactions. Children with ADHD who clutter show greater difficulty with executive functioning and working memory than their non-cluttering peers [7], evidencing how neurocognitive load can intensify motor variability. Studies also show that cluttering behaviours often increase during narrative or expository tasks that require sustained planning and monitoring [11,12]. These findings are consistent with developmental research and demonstrate that fluent speech in complex tasks depends on well-coordinated cognitive, linguistic and motor systems.

When cluttering is viewed through a developmental motor lens, a coherent interpretation emerges, i.e., cluttering reflects an imbalance in the synchronisation of speech motor, linguistic and cognitive subsystems. Dynamic systems theories emphasise that motor output becomes less stable under increased cognitive load or rapid transitions [5], precisely the conditions under which cluttering features are most prominent. Structured tasks that reduce linguistic demands often minimise cluttering behaviours, while spontaneous discourse and complex communicative activities reveal the system's vulnerabilities. Understanding cluttering as a dynamic coordination disorder, therefore, clarifies why symptoms fluctuate across tasks and contexts and prepares the ground for examining the neurocognitive mechanisms that underpin these patterns.

Taken together, findings across these studies converge on the presence of instability in speech timing and articulatory coordination, particularly during connected speech, despite variability in study design and measurement approaches. While empirical paediatric studies provide direct evidence of these features, clinically oriented and mechanistic accounts offer complementary insights into how such motor instability may emerge under increased linguistic and cognitive load. Differences across studies appear to reflect task demands and analytic focus rather than contradictory findings, supporting a coherent interpretation of speech motor disruption as a central feature of cluttering.

 https://doi.org/10.3390/children13010097

4. Speech Motor Characteristics of Cluttering in Childhood and Adolescence

The empirical studies included in this review offer converging evidence on the speech motor characteristics of cluttering in children and adolescents and directly inform RQ1 and RQ3. Although the evidence base is modest and varied in scope, clear patterns emerge across studies: children who clutter demonstrate instability in speech timing and rhythm, variability in rate regulation, reduced articulatory precision and pronounced task-dependent fluctuations. These findings complement the conceptual foundations established in Section 3 and illustrate how developmental vulnerabilities across motor, linguistic and cognitive systems manifest in observable speech behaviours.

Timing instability is one of the most consistent findings across the included studies. Research has demonstrated that when speakers exceed their speech motor capacity, timing becomes irregular and intelligibility declines [22]. Although the study involved clients across the life span, its capacity-demand framework is directly applicable to developmental populations. In school-aged children, research found that cluttering symptoms were marked by variable syllable durations, abrupt shifts in tempo and irregular rhythmic patterns [12]. These timing disruptions were especially evident during spontaneous and linguistically complex tasks and were less prominent in structured activities. Descriptive synthesis [11] reinforces this pattern, noting that inconsistent rhythm and uneven timing frequently co-occur with reduced intelligibility in children who clutter. Together, these findings show that timing instability is not a superficial feature of cluttering but a core indicator of underlying vulnerability in temporal regulation systems. These instabilities also form a bridge to RQ2, where timing-related mechanisms are examined more directly from a neurocognitive and neurodevelopmental perspective.

Irregular or excessively rapid speech rate is another key behavioural marker of cluttering, and the included studies emphasise difficulties regulating rate rather than deliberate speaking fast. Children who clutter often accelerate unintentionally, which suggests limited capacity to modulate output in real time. For example, children who clutter were found to produce rapid bursts of speech during narrative and expository tasks, even when explicitly cued to reduce rate [12]. These uncontrolled accelerations were accompanied by reductions in intelligibility and increased articulatory imprecision. Speech, therefore, deteriorates when speakers operate beyond their individual capacity thresholds [22]. Rate regulation difficulties in cluttering thus reflect disruptions in the dynamic balance between linguistic formulation and motor execution. These findings support the developmental motor framework outlined previously and illustrate how regulation demands increase as communicative complexity grows.

Further, reduced intelligibility in cluttering primarily arises from excessive coarticulation and imprecise or incomplete articulatory gestures. Paediatric data (e.g., [11,12]), show that children who clutter produced blurred articulatory transitions and collapsed syllables, particularly during longer, less structured speech tasks. These articulatory patterns were less evident in word-level responses, therefore indicating that cluttering becomes more salient as linguistic and cognitive demands increase. Similarly, the motor speech framework [24] describes cluttering as involving excessive anticipatory coarticulation and reduced segmental precision. Although not focused exclusively on children, this framework is consistent with empirical observations in paediatric samples and aligns with developmental research showing that coarticulation patterns continue maturing through adolescence. When combined with irregular timing and inadequate monitoring, excessive coarticulation contributes significantly to intelligibility breakdowns in children who clutter.

One of the clearest findings across the included studies is that cluttering symptoms vary substantially across speaking tasks. For example, cluttering behaviours tend to inten-

 https://doi.org/10.3390/children13010097

sify during spontaneous and cognitively demanding contexts, whereas more structured tasks yield fewer or milder symptoms [12]. It is, therefore, important to sample connected speech across a range of communicative contexts to capture the full breadth of cluttering behaviours in school-aged children. That means task-dependent variability is not diagnostic noise; it is a defining characteristic of cluttering. This aligns with developmental models of motor coordination, which show that stability decreases as cognitive or linguistic load increases. The evidence, therefore, indicates that cluttering cannot be fully understood without considering the interaction between motor capacity and communicative context.

Several included studies also highlight the relevance of cognitive and neurodevelopmental factors in amplifying motor instability. For example, children with ADHD who clutter are found to exhibit greater weaknesses in executive functioning and working memory than peers with ADHD who did not clutter [7]. These findings suggest that cluttering in some children may arise from combined motor and executive vulnerabilities, which can influence rate regulation, timing consistency and self-monitoring.

Further insights come from research on neurodevelopmental conditions that present with cluttering-like characteristics. Rapid speech, timing irregularities and segmental imprecision were also documented in individuals with fragile X syndrome [10]. The evidence supports the possibility that cluttering shares characteristics with broader timing and sequencing difficulties observed in neurodevelopmental disorders. These findings lay the groundwork for understanding the neurobiological mechanisms.

5. Neurocognitive and Neurodevelopmental Mechanisms Underpinning Cluttering

Cluttering emerges during a developmental period characterised not only by the refinement of speech motor control but also by substantial growth in executive functioning, working memory, linguistic integration and neural efficiency. RQ2 seeks to clarify how neurocognitive and neurodevelopmental factors interact with motor control to shape cluttering behaviours in children and adolescents. While empirical paediatric studies provide direct evidence of observable speech motor and task-related features, conceptual and clinically oriented work offers complementary perspectives on how these features may arise developmentally and how they manifest in practice. Although the included studies provide limited direct neurological data, they collectively point to a set of convergent mechanisms involving timing, sequencing, executive control, processing speed and self-regulation. These mechanisms help explain why cluttering varies across tasks and why symptoms often intensify during spontaneous or cognitively demanding communication.

Timing and sequencing processes underpin fluent speech and rely on the coordinated activity of cortical and subcortical neural pathways. Theoretical models highlight the involvement of cortico-basal ganglia-cerebellar circuits in rate control and temporal precision [21], and disruptions in these systems have long been proposed as contributors to cluttering. Although the included studies do not provide direct neurophysiological evidence, their behavioural findings strongly suggest underlying timing vulnerabilities. Observations of inconsistent rhythm, variable segment durations and rapid bursts, for example, indicate reduced temporal stability in children who clutter [12]. The evidence suggests that cluttering-like features may emerge when neural timing mechanisms are compromised. Collectively, these findings align with the developmental motor perspective outlined earlier, i.e., children with cluttering may have a narrower margin of temporal stability, causing motor coordination to break down when cognitive or linguistic load increases.

Fluent speech also requires continuous coordination of linguistic formulation, monitoring and real-time motor sequencing. Executive functions, and working memory in particular, play a key role in managing these processes. Evidence from the included studies

 https://doi.org/10.3390/children13010097

demonstrates that children who clutter may present with executive function vulnerabilities that intensify speech motor instability. For example, research found that children with ADHD who cluttered showed weaker working memory and executive control than children with ADHD who did not clutter [7]. Because working memory supports planning, sequencing and linguistic coherence, reduced capacity can lead to rapid, poorly monitored speech and disorganised utterances. Furthermore, executive control assists in regulating rate, inhibiting premature articulatory gestures and adjusting output based on listener feedback. When these capacities are compromised, rate regulation becomes difficult, monitoring is inconsistent, and cluttering emerges more readily, particularly with complex communication needs [35]. This neurocognitive interpretation fits well with observations that individuals who clutter may outpace their planning during speech [36]. Rather than attributing cluttering solely to a fast rate, as a result, our findings support that cognitive-linguistic processes and motor planning become misaligned when executive resources are insufficient to manage the load.

Evidence from children's speech supports that in cluttering, linguistic planning outpaces the motor system's ability to execute articulatory sequences with stability. For example, documented cases where children appeared to generate linguistic content rapidly, leading to compressed syllables, excessive coarticulation and reduced intelligibility [12] are consistent with a planning-execution mismatch, i.e., when linguistic content is generated more quickly than motor commands can be precisely implemented, speech becomes blurred and irregular. Such a mismatch may be further compounded by children's developing neural systems. For example, neural efficiency increases throughout childhood and adolescence [37], and processing speed in both linguistic and motor domains improves with age [38]. Therefore, when these systems do not develop synchronously, timing conflicts can arise [39]. The evidence reviewed suggests that cluttering manifests when linguistic formulation is rapid but motor control is insufficiently stabilised, which results in an unstable output pattern.

Another critical component of fluent communication is self-monitoring, the ability to attend to one's speech in real time and adjust output accordingly. Multiple studies and clinical descriptions note that individuals who clutter often show reduced self-monitoring or limited awareness of speech breakdowns [6,11]. This reduced monitoring may reflect limitations in attention allocation or in the integration of auditory and proprioceptive feedback. Self-monitoring demands increase substantially during extended discourse, where children must maintain coherence, adjust rate and attend to listener needs simultaneously. When monitoring systems are taxed, children may fail to detect rapid rate increases or articulatory imprecision until the breakdown is already perceptible to the listener. Executive vulnerabilities may, therefore, limit not only planning but also retrospective awareness, creating a cycle in which cluttering behaviours persist without timely self-correction.

Although cluttering can occur independently, several neurodevelopmental conditions present with cluttering-like speech characteristics. For example, rapid rate, irregular timing and imprecise articulation are found in individuals with conditions associated with atypical neural connectivity and developmental timing differences [10]. Such findings suggest that cluttering behaviours may arise when underlying neural systems involved in sequencing and rhythm are affected. Studies examining cluttering in the context of ADHD provide similar insights. Similarly, executive function weaknesses were also found to contribute to increased cluttering behaviours [7]. These results suggest that cluttering may, in some children, reflect broader neurodevelopmental vulnerabilities rather than isolated speech motor disruption. These observations, however, do not imply that cluttering is secondary to other developmental conditions; rather, they highlight shared mechanisms, such as

https://doi.org/10.3390/children13010097

timing instability, working memory load, and reduced monitoring, that may manifest across different neurodevelopmental profiles.

In interpreting these findings, it is important to distinguish between observed behavioural characteristics and the mechanisms proposed to account for them. While disruptions in speech timing and articulatory coordination are directly observed, for example, associations with linguistic formulation, attentional control, and executive functioning are inferred from task effects and developmental patterns rather than demonstrated as causal relationships. These associations are therefore best understood as functionally linked dimensions within a broader developmental system rather than as isolated or hierarchically ordered deficits.

The mechanisms described above, therefore, converge to support an integrated account of cluttering in childhood and adolescence. Cluttering appears to arise from the interaction of (a) timing and sequencing vulnerabilities, which reflect inefficiencies in neural circuits responsible for temporal regulation; (b) executive function and working memory limitations, which impair planning, attention shifting and monitoring; (c) processing speed mismatches, which cause linguistic formulation to outpace motor stability; and (d) reduced self-monitoring, which limit the ability to regulate rate and correct breakdowns. These interacting vulnerabilities provide a coherent explanation for the speech motor patterns and the contextual sensitivity observed across studies. They also align with developmental models emphasising that speech fluency depends on synchronised contributions from cognitive, linguistic and motor systems. A pattern we found from the synthesis is that when these systems develop asynchronously or operate under increased load, the risk of cluttering behaviours increases.

6. Assessment and Intervention Implications for Allied Health Practice

The empirical and conceptual evidence in earlier sections has clear implications for how cluttering should be assessed and managed within allied-health practice. RQ4 focuses on identifying elements of assessment and intervention that are supported by the existing evidence base and are appropriate for children and adolescents, whose speech motor, cognitive and linguistic systems are still developing. Although the twelve included studies vary in design and purpose, they converge on a set of clinically meaningful insights that can guide practice.

Our findings have implications for assessment. Across multiple included studies, cluttering symptoms were most evident during spontaneous or extended speech [11,12]. Rapid rate, timing instability, excessive coarticulation and reduced intelligibility often diminished in structured tasks but returned during longer monologic or narrative speech. For assessment, this underscores the need to obtain samples across a range of contexts, including conversation, narrative and expository tasks. Reliance on single-word or heavily scaffolded tasks is likely to under-identify cluttering behaviours.

Rate variability and unintentional acceleration are prominent in children who clutter. Findings that speech deteriorates when speakers exceed their capacity limits [22] suggest that assessment should examine not only habitual rate but also rate flexibility and behaviours under increased load. This may involve having the child shift between speaking rates, sustain a slower rate during complex tasks or demonstrate rate control while simultaneously organising linguistic content.

Children who clutter also often present with reduced intelligibility caused by blurred articulatory transitions and excessive coarticulation [12,24]. Assessment should therefore include careful analysis of articulatory precision, segmental clarity and syllable integrity within naturalistic speech. Because intelligibility breakdowns frequently emerge only under

 https://doi.org/10.3390/children13010097

specific conditions, clinicians must attend to task-based variability rather than relying solely on averaged scores or structured elicitation.

Evidence (e.g., [7]), shows that children who clutter may have weaknesses in working memory and executive control. Although SLPs do not formally diagnose executive function disorders, they can observe behaviours such as difficulty sustaining attention, rapid shifts between ideas, limited awareness of communication breakdowns and challenges organising multi-clause discourse. These behaviours provide essential contextual information when forming a differential diagnosis and determining whether cluttering emerges primarily from motor, cognitive-linguistic or combined vulnerabilities.

Cluttering often co-occurs with other communication or developmental conditions, including stuttering, ADHD and, in some cases, broader neurodevelopmental differences [10,11]. Assessment procedures should therefore incorporate differential diagnosis protocols that consider shared symptoms (such as rapid rate or disfluencies) while distinguishing cluttering from related disorders based on timing instability, coarticulatory excess, monitoring behaviours and task-dependent variability. Interviews with families and teachers can provide insights into when cluttering behaviours are most noticeable and how they affect functional communication in school and social settings.

The findings also share implications for intervention. Current evidence shows that because rate instability is a core feature of childhood cluttering, rate control remains a central therapeutic focus. However, the evidence also suggests that therapy should not aim merely to "slow speech," but rather to support children in developing regulation of rate across tasks and contexts. For example, research notes that children often accelerate unintentionally even when aware of the need to slow down, which indicates limited self-regulation rather than a preference for fast speech [12]. Intervention should therefore integrate strategies such as pausing cues, pacing boards, rhythmic supports, metronomic guidance and visual counters, used flexibly to promote internalised tempo regulation.

Excessive coarticulation and imprecise articulation contribute significantly to reduced intelligibility in cluttering. Motor-based strategies such as over-articulation practice, syllable stretching, targeted contrast drills and explicit focus on articulatory gestures may help strengthen clarity. For example, research highlights the value of combining rate control with articulatory cueing, which allows children to allocate sufficient time for complete gestural execution [24,25].

Many children who clutter have reduced awareness of breakdowns. Intervention should include activities that enhance the child's ability to monitor their speech in real time, evaluate intelligibility and adjust output. Approaches may involve video or audio playback, supported self-rating scales, and guided reflection activities. The ultimate importance is to help children recognise when their speech accelerates or becomes disorganised and develop strategies for re-establishing control [11].

Given the evidence linking cluttering to working memory and executive function challenges [7], therapy may be strengthened by incorporating supports that reduce cognitive load or increase predictability. These may include organising frameworks for narrative tasks, visual planning for longer utterances, chunking strategies and scaffolds that promote sustained attention. While not executive-function training per se, these supports may improve fluency by aligning linguistic planning with motor execution.

The clinical implications outlined here are grounded primarily in converging behavioural evidence and established developmental principles, rather than in direct experimental manipulation of underlying mechanisms, and should be interpreted accordingly. Furthermore, because cluttering behaviours shift across tasks, intervention should be delivered across a variety of communicative contexts. Structured tasks may help children develop foundational skills, but therapy must eventually extend into spontaneous dis-

https://doi.org/10.3390/children13010097

course, functional classroom activities and real-life conversational contexts. This approach helps ensure that improvements generalise to settings where cluttering is most pronounced.

When cluttering co-occurs with other communication or developmental conditions, intervention may require adaptation. For example, when ADHD is present, therapy may integrate brief, highly engaging activities, predictable routines and external cues to support sustained attention. For young people with broader neurodevelopmental differences, intervention may need to address sensory, attentional or pragmatic challenges that influence speech motor stability. Cross-disciplinary research (e.g., [10]), suggests that cluttering-like behaviours in some populations may reflect underlying neurobiological timing vulnerabilities, underscoring the importance of interdisciplinary collaboration.

Finally, viewing cluttering through a developmental lens highlights the importance of synchronising assessment and intervention with a child's evolving motor, cognitive and linguistic capacities. The combined evidence suggests that cluttering is best supported through approaches that capture variability across contexts, focus on rate regulation and articulatory stability, build self-monitoring, scaffold executive functioning demands, and accommodate co-occurring conditions when present.

7. General Discussion

This review set out to examine cluttering in children and adolescents from four interrelated angles: speech motor development (RQ1), neurocognitive and neurodevelopmental mechanisms (RQ2), task and contextual influences (RQ3), and implications for allied-health assessment and intervention (RQ4). Across the twelve included studies, a coherent picture emerges. Cluttering in childhood and adolescence is best understood as a developmental disorder of motor–cognitive integration, in which speech motor systems, executive processes and linguistic planning fail to synchronise efficiently under real-world communicative demands. Importantly, the synthesis presented here distinguishes between types of evidence and their respective contributions, integrating empirical paediatric findings with developmentally informative mechanistic and clinical literature to build a coherent account of cluttering without conflating distinct levels of analysis. In what follows, we integrate findings across Sections 3–6 to articulate this developmental account, highlight the central role of task demands, and consider implications for theory, classification and practice. Where explanatory mechanisms are discussed, these are framed as integrative, developmentally informed interpretations that organise existing evidence and generate testable hypotheses, rather than as definitive accounts of causality.

Rather than treating heterogeneity as noise, therefore, we operationalised variability in cluttering along analytically relevant dimensions that are consistently implicated across studies: developmental stage, diagnostic practice, task demands (structured speech vs. spontaneous discourse), and cognitive–linguistic load. This typology supports the interpretation of why cluttering features vary across contexts and explains why connected speech tasks are most informative for identifying timing instability, coarticulatory blurring, and reduced self-monitoring. Importantly, this framework does not assume discrete subtypes on current evidence; instead, it provides a structured way to interpret variation while highlighting priorities for future mechanistic and longitudinal research.

7.1. Cluttering as a Developmental Motor–Cognitive Disorder

The evidence reviewed across Sections 3–5 indicates that cluttering cannot be reduced to a single domain of impairment. Rather than a purely motor speech disorder or a purely cognitive-linguistic difficulty, cluttering in childhood appears where developing systems for motor timing, linguistic formulation, and executive regulation intersect and occasionally misalign. Children who clutter are navigating the same maturational processes as their

https://doi.org/10.3390/children13010097

peers: refinement of speech motor patterns, growth in linguistic complexity and increasing demands on planning and self-regulation. What distinguishes them is the fragility of the coordination among these systems when communicative demands are high.

From a developmental perspective, this coordination problem is unsurprising. Speech requires fine-grained temporal control while simultaneously accommodating lexical retrieval, syntactic assembly, discourse organisation and monitoring of listener needs. The studies reviewed suggest that in children who clutter, temporal and articulatory systems are more vulnerable to disruption when executive resources are stretched, working memory is taxed or linguistic formulation becomes rapid and dense. The characteristic "blurring" of segments, irregular bursts of speech and fluctuating intelligibility are thus not isolated symptoms but the surface expression of a deeper integration difficulty.

This account also helps clarify how cluttering is similar to, and distinct from, other fluency and motor speech disorders. Like stuttering, cluttering appears to involve vulnerabilities in timing and sequencing [2]; like some dysarthrias or developmental coordination disorders, it reflects challenges in achieving stable motor patterns [29]. Unlike these conditions, however, cluttering is defined by its close coupling to discourse-level formulation and monitoring. The speech motor system does not fail in isolation; rather, it fails when asked to keep pace with the child's linguistic and cognitive tempo. This motor–cognitive integration view, therefore, offers a unifying framework that honours the multidimensional descriptions of cluttering without fragmenting it into unrelated symptom clusters.

Importantly, conceptualising cluttering as a developmental integration disorder also aligns with work in motor development [40], which emphasises that complex motor behaviours emerge from the interaction of multiple subsystems rather than from a single locus of control. In this sense, cluttering offers a valuable case study for motor development research as it shows how high-level cognitive and linguistic processes can destabilise a maturing motor system, and how motor constraints can, in turn, shape the expression of language and discourse.

7.2. The Central Role of Task Demands and Environmental Load

A second major insight from this review is the centrality of task demands and environmental load in shaping how cluttering is expressed. Section 4 documented that cluttering behaviours are most evident during spontaneous, extended and linguistically rich speech, and attenuated in highly structured or constrained tasks. Section 5 linked this task sensitivity to the limited capacity of developing executive systems to manage planning, sequencing and monitoring under pressure. Taken together, these findings suggest that cluttering is not simply a property of the individual. It is rather equally a property of the interaction between the child and the communicative environment. The implications outlined below are therefore presented as practice relevant inferences grounded in converging behavioural evidence and developmental theory, while acknowledging that direct mechanistic validation in paediatric samples remains a priority for future research.

This interactional view has important conceptual implications. If cluttering emerges most reliably when children must generate ideas, structure discourse, monitor their listener and regulate their rate simultaneously, then variability across tasks is not a nuisance variable but a defining feature of the condition. It follows that "inconsistency" in cluttering across contexts should not be interpreted as diagnostic unreliability, but as evidence that the underlying vulnerability is highly sensitive to load. This perspective reframes longstanding clinical frustrations, such as children who "do not clutter" during a short structured assessment but clutter extensively in the classroom, as predictable outcomes of the capacity-demand balance.

 https://doi.org/10.3390/children13010097

The role of environmental load extends beyond task structure. Classroom expectations, assessment practices and interactional norms can either mask or reveal cluttering. For example, tightly scaffolded question-answer formats may fail to elicit cluttering behaviours, whereas open-ended show-and-tell, oral presentations and narrative tasks are much more likely to expose the limits of motor–cognitive coordination. Similarly, noisy environments, rapid turn-taking, or time pressure may all increase the risk of cluttering behaviours in children whose systems are already working near capacity.

Recognising this dependence on task and context has methodological implications for research as well. Studies relying solely on reading tasks or brief picture descriptions will underestimate the presence and severity of cluttering, especially in younger speakers. Research designs that incorporate ecologically valid tasks, such as curriculum-based oral activities or semi-structured peer interactions, are more likely to capture the phenomena that concern children, families and teachers. In this way, the cluttering literature highlights a broader lesson for motor development research, i.e., understanding a developing system requires studying it under the kinds of loads it routinely experiences, not just under idealised clinical conditions.

7.3. Implications for Theory, Classification and Clinical Practice

A third contribution of this review lies in its implications for how cluttering is conceptualised and classified, and how these conceptual choices shape clinical practice. Traditional definitions anchored in rapid or irregular rates are increasingly at odds with the multi-component picture emerging from empirical and clinical work. Rate instability remains central, but on its own it is insufficient to differentiate cluttering from other fluency disturbances or from typical developmental variability in fast-talking children.

The integrated account developed here suggests that cluttering is better characterised by a constellation of features, including vulnerability in temporal regulation of speech, a tendency for linguistic formulation to outpace stable motor execution, reduced effectiveness of monitoring under high load and marked contextual variability, etc. Such a profile does not map neatly onto existing diagnostic categories, which often separate "motor" and "language" disorders as if they were independent. A developmental motor–cognitive integration framework provides a more accurate description and encourages classification systems to recognise cluttering as a disorder that sits at the interface of motor speech and developmental neurocognition.

Clinically, this shift has several consequences. For assessment, it supports the use of multi-context, discourse-level tasks, explicit attention to timing and coarticulation and targeted observation of monitoring and executive behaviours. It also justifies integrating information from teachers and families, who observe the child in precisely the high-load settings where cluttering is most evident. For intervention, it encourages programmes that go beyond rate control drills to encompass self-monitoring, discourse planning and management of cognitive load.

There are also implications for team-based practice. Because cluttering often co-occurs with broader developmental differences, such as ADHD or neurogenetic conditions, SLPs may need to work closely with psychologists, paediatricians, educators and, where appropriate, neurologists. A shared understanding of cluttering as a motor–cognitive integration difficulty allows these professionals to situate cluttering within the child's overall developmental profile rather than treating it as a discrete symptom to be "fixed" in isolation. This, in turn, supports more coherent planning of supports across home, school and clinic.

Finally, this integrated perspective has consequences for how cluttering is communicated to children and families. Framing cluttering as a difficulty in coordinating fast-moving

 https://doi.org/10.3390/children13010097

systems, rather than as a flaw in character or effort, can reduce stigma and support more collaborative goal-setting. It also provides a rationale for why certain situations feel particularly challenging and why therapy may focus on building skills for managing complex communicative demands rather than simply "slowing down.". It should also be pointed out that the integrative account advanced in this review does not assume direct causal relationships between linguistic, cognitive, attentional, and neurodevelopmental dimensions. Instead, cluttering is conceptualised as emerging from the dynamic interaction of these processes during speech production, particularly under conditions of increased communicative load. Empirical studies provide evidence for observable speech motor instability and task sensitivity, while developmental and neurocognitive accounts offer plausible explanatory frameworks for these patterns. Explicitly distinguishing observed phenomena from proposed mechanisms allows a coherent synthesis without overstating the strength of causal inference.

7.4. Gaps and Future Directions

The integrated account presented here reveals several gaps and opportunities in the current evidence base. It was necessary for this review to exclude studies that used the term "cluttering" without describing cluttering-consistent behaviours, which highlights a broader issue within the literature. Inconsistent or imprecise use of terminology complicates comparison across studies and contributes to uncertainty in prevalence estimates, assessment practices, and research synthesis. This lack of terminological consistency represents an important gap in the field and underscores the need for clearer operational definitions and reporting standards in future research on cluttering, particularly in paediatric populations.

Another striking limitation is the scarcity of longitudinal work. Most studies offer snapshots of cluttering at a single point in time, leaving open questions about how motor–cognitive integration evolves across development, why some children appear to "grow out of" cluttering and how intervention influences trajectories. Longitudinal studies following children from early school years into adolescence would allow researchers to examine whether cluttering reflects a transient delay in integration, a persistent vulnerability or multiple developmental pathways. Nevertheless, it is worth pointing out that the small number of empirical paediatric studies underscores the limited state of mechanistic research on cluttering in childhood, rather than a weakness of the present review. Accordingly, this synthesis integrates empirical findings with developmentally informative theoretical and clinical literature to construct a coherent account of cluttering as a motor–cognitive integration difficulty. Empirical evidence anchors the description of observable phenomena, while non-empirical sources contribute to theory-building and clinical interpretation, allowing conclusions to be calibrated to the available evidence.

Methodologically, there is a need for studies that combine detailed behavioural observations with more fine-grained measures of timing, sequencing and neural function. Acoustic and kinematic techniques could elucidate how temporal patterns in cluttering differ from those in other speech motor disorders. Neuroimaging or electrophysiological methods, used judiciously, therefore, could begin to map the neural correlates of motor–cognitive coordination difficulties. At present, mechanistic accounts remain largely inferential; more direct evidence would allow the field to refine or revise current models.

There is also a notable gap in cross-linguistic and multilingual research. Given that cluttering involves interactions between motor control and linguistic structure, languages with different phonological, prosodic or morphosyntactic profiles may shape its expression in distinct ways [41]. Studies in non-English languages, particularly those that are typologically different from English [42], and in children acquiring more than one language [43], would not only broaden the empirical base but also test the generalisability of the motor–

https://doi.org/10.3390/children13010097

cognitive integration model proposed here. Such work would be particularly valuable in contexts where multilingualism is the norm and where cluttering may be under-recognised or misattributed to second-language learning difficulties.

Variability in diagnostic practices, sample sizes, and task paradigms across studies, therefore, necessarily constrains the generalisability of individual findings, which underscores the importance of interpreting convergence across domains rather than relying on any single study or methodological approach.

A further underdeveloped area concerns real-world participation and quality of life. For example, there is limited research on how cluttering affects children's academic engagement, peer relationships and self-concept, or how these outcomes change with intervention. Integrating participation-level outcomes into research designs would align cluttering research more closely with contemporary frameworks in speech-language pathology and with the priorities of the clients, their families and care teams [44], as well as the integration of modern technologies [45].

Finally, future work would benefit from closer integration with the broader motor development literature. The challenges of coordinating speech under high cognitive load are mirrored in other motor domains, such as complex limb movements [46] or bimanual tasks [47]. Collaborative research across speech science, motor control and developmental psychology could yield richer models of how motor–cognitive integration develops and why it sometimes falters. Future reviews may also build on this work by examining the historical evolution of cluttering concepts in earlier literature, particularly to trace how definitional and diagnostic shifts have shaped contemporary research and practice. In this way, cluttering research can both draw from and contribute to a wider understanding of children's motor development.

8. Conclusions

In this review, we synthesised developmental, motor, cognitive, and clinical evidence to examine cluttering in children and adolescents. Across the twelve included studies, a consistent picture emerged, i.e., cluttering reflects a developmental vulnerability in the coordination of speech motor timing, linguistic formulation, and executive control. These findings address all four research questions by clarifying the speech motor characteristics of cluttering (RQ1), identifying the developmental and neurocognitive mechanisms that underpin them (RQ2), demonstrating the central role of task and contextual demands in symptom expression (RQ3), and outlining the implications for allied-health assessment and intervention (RQ4).

By framing cluttering as a motor–cognitive integration disorder, we strengthened its alignment with contemporary theories of children's motor development. Cluttering arises most clearly when linguistic, cognitive, and motor systems must operate simultaneously under load, revealing the limits of an integration process that is still maturing. This perspective challenges rate-based definitions and supports a more coherent model in which temporal instability, articulatory blurring, reduced monitoring, and contextual variability are understood as interdependent manifestations of a single developmental mechanism.

While the available empirical literature remains limited, the synthesis presented here integrates behavioural findings with developmentally informative theoretical and clinical work to advance a coherent framework for understanding cluttering in childhood and adolescence. In the meantime, the evidence base remains limited, particularly in relation to paediatric samples, longitudinal trajectories, mechanistic studies, and multilingual contexts. Addressing these gaps will be essential for refining theoretical models, informing classification systems, and improving clinical practice. Even with these constraints, the developmental motor–cognitive account advanced here provides a foundation for

https://doi.org/10.3390/children13010097

future research and a clearer rationale for assessment and intervention in both clinical and educational settings.

Cluttering is often under-recognised, misunderstood, or misclassified. By articulating cluttering as a developmental motor–cognitive integration difficulty, this review advances conceptual clarity in the field and provides a foundation for more precise assessment, intervention, and future research in children's motor development.

Author Contributions: Conceptualization, W.H.; methodology, W.H., L.Z. and J.L.; validation, W.H., L.Z. and J.L.; formal analysis, W.H.; writing—original draft preparation, W.H.; writing—review and editing, W.H. and S.P. All authors have read and agreed to the published version of the manuscript.

Funding: This research received no external funding.

Institutional Review Board Statement: Not applicable.

Informed Consent Statement: Not applicable.

Data Availability Statement: No new data were created or analyzed in this study. Data sharing is not applicable to this article.

Conflicts of Interest: The authors declare no conflicts of interest.

Abbreviations

The following abbreviations are used in this manuscript:

ADHD	Attention-Deficit/Hyperactivity Disorder
LCD	Limited Consensus Definition
SLP	Speech-Language Pathologist

References

1. Kelkar, P. Cluttering. In *Understanding and Managing Fluency Disorders*; Maruthy, S., Kelkar, P., Eds.; Routledge: London, UK, 2023; pp. 186–210.
2. Scott, K.S. Stuttering and Cluttering. In *Research in Clinical Pragmatics*; Cummings, L., Ed.; Springer International Publishing: Cham, Switzerland, 2017; pp. 471–490.
3. St. Louis, K.O.; Schulte, K. Defining cluttering: The lowest common denominator. In *Cluttering: Research, Intervention and Education*; Ward, D., Scott, K.S., Eds.; Routledge: London, UK, 2011; pp. 233–253.
4. Cech, D.J.; Martin, S.T. Chapter 3—Motor Development. In *Functional Movement Development Across the Life Span*, 3rd ed.; Cech, D.J., Martin, S.T., Eds.; W.B. Saunders: Saint Louis, MI, USA, 2012; pp. 45–67.
5. Van Lieshout, P.H.H.M. Dynamical Systems Theory and Its Application in Speech. In *Speech Motor Control in Normaland Disordered Speech*; Oxford University Press: Oxford, UK, 2004.
6. Duchan, J.F. Frameworks used in cluttering treatments: Past, present, and future. *Adv. Commun. Swallowing* **2021**, *24*, 87–97. [CrossRef]
7. Fidan, S.T.; Sarıyer, M.N. Cluttering and Working Memory in Attention Deficit and Hyperactivity Disorder. *Psychiatry Clin. Psychopharmacol.* **2025**, *35*, 234–244. [CrossRef] [PubMed]
8. Neumann, K.; Euler, H.A.; Bosshardt, H.-G.; Cook, S.; Sandrieser, P.; Sommer, M. The Pathogenesis, Assessment and Treatment of Speech Fluency Disorders. *Dtsch. Aerzteblatt Online* **2017**, *114*, 383–390. [CrossRef]
9. Icht, M.; Zukerman, G.; Zigdon, A.; Korn, L. There is more to cluttering than meets the eye: The prevalence of cluttering and association with psychological well-being indices in an undergraduate sample. *Int. J. Lang. Commun. Disord.* **2023**, *58*, 2022–2032. [CrossRef] [PubMed]
10. Bangert, K.; Scott, K.S.; Adams, C.; Kisenwether, J.S.; Giuffre, L.; Reed, J.; Thurman, A.J.; Abbeduto, L.; Klusek, J. Cluttering in the Speech of Young Men with Fragile X Syndrome. *J. Speech Lang. Hear. Res.* **2022**, *65*, 954–969. [CrossRef]
11. Scott, K.S. Cluttering in a School-Aged Child: Tackling the Challenges Step by Step. *Semin. Speech Lang.* **2022**, *43*, 130–146. [CrossRef]
12. Scott, K.S. Cluttering symptoms in school-age children by communicative context: A preliminary investigation. *Int. J. Speech-Lang. Pathol.* **2020**, *22*, 174–183. [CrossRef] [PubMed]
13. Duchan, J.F.; Felsenfeld, S. Cluttering framed: An historical overview. *Adv. Commun. Swallowing* **2021**, *24*, 75–85. [CrossRef]

 https://doi.org/10.3390/children13010097

14. Ward, D.; Connally, E.L.; Pliatsikas, C.; Bretherton-Furness, J.; Watkins, K.E. The neurological underpinnings of cluttering: Some initial findings. *J. Fluen. Disord.* **2015**, *43*, 1–16. [CrossRef]
15. LaSalle, L.R.; Wolk, L. Stuttering, cluttering, and phonological complexity: Case studies. *J. Fluen. Disord.* **2011**, *36*, 285–289. [CrossRef]
16. Blood, G.W.; Blood, I.M.; Tellis, G. Auditory Processing and Cluttering in Young Children. *Percept. Mot. Ski.* **2000**, *90*, 631–639. [CrossRef]
17. Drayna, D. Possible Genetic Factors in Cluttering. In *Cluttering: A Handbook of Research, Intervention and Education*; Ward, D., Scott, K.S., Eds.; Routledge: London, UK, 2011; pp. 51–56.
18. Page, M.J.; Moher, D.; Bossuyt, P.M.; Boutron, I.; Hoffmann, T.C.; Mulrow, C.D.; Shamseer, L.; Tetzlaff, J.M.; Akl, E.A.; Brennan, S.E.; et al. PRISMA 2020 explanation and elaboration: Updated guidance and exemplars for reporting systematic reviews. *BMJ* **2021**, *372*, n160. [CrossRef] [PubMed]
19. Page, M.J.; McKenzie, J.E.; Bossuyt, P.M.; Boutron, I.; Hoffmann, T.C.; Mulrow, C.D.; Shamseer, L.; Tetzlaff, J.M.; Akl, E.A.; Brennan, S.E.; et al. The PRISMA 2020 statement: An updated guideline for reporting systematic reviews. *BMJ* **2021**, *372*, 71. [CrossRef]
20. Covidence Systematic Review Software, Veritas Health Innovation. 2023. Available online: https://www.covidence.org/ (accessed on 7 January 2026).
21. Alm, P.A. Cluttering: A Neurological Perspective. In *Cluttering: A Handbook of Research, Intervention and Education*; Ward, D., Scott, K.S., Eds.; Routledge: London, UK, 2011; pp. 22–50.
22. Bakker, K.; Myers, F.L.; Raphael, L.J.; Louis, K.O.S. A Preliminary Comparison of Speech Rate, Self-Evaluation, and Disfluency of People Who Speak Exceptionally Fast, Clutter, or Speak Normally. In *Cluttering: A Handbook of Research, Intervention and Education*; Ward, D., Scott, K.S., Eds.; Routledge: London, UK, 2011; pp. 69–91.
23. Kelkar, P.; Sanghi, M.; Chaudhari, S. The Impact Scale for Assessment of Cluttering and Stuttering (ISACS): Preliminary analyses. *Evid.-Based Commun. Assess. Interv.* **2025**, *18*, 160–182. [CrossRef]
24. Ward, D. Motor Speech Control and Cluttering. In *Cluttering: A Handbook of Research, Intervention and Education*; Ward, D., Scott, K.S., Eds.; Routledge: London, UK, 2011; pp. 57–68.
25. Ward, D. The Nature of Cluttering. In *Stuttering and Cluttering*; Ward, D., Ed.; Psychology Press: London, UK, 2017; pp. 143–170.
26. Perkell, J.; Guenther, F.; Lane, H.; Matthies, M.; Payan, Y.; Perrier, P.; Vick, J.; Wilhelms-Tricarico, R.; Zandipour, M. The sensorimotor control of speech production. In Proceedings of the International Symposium of Measurement, Analysis and Modeling of Human Function, Sapporo, Japan, 21–23 September 2001.
27. Lau, J.C.; Losh, M.; Speights, M. Differences in speech articulatory timing and associations with pragmatic language ability in autism. *Res. Autism Spectr. Disord.* **2023**, *102*, 102118. [CrossRef] [PubMed]
28. Redford, M.A. Speech Production from a Developmental Perspective. *J. Speech Lang. Hear. Res.* **2019**, *62*, 2946–2962. [CrossRef] [PubMed]
29. Iuzzini-Seigel, J. Motor Performance in Children with Childhood Apraxia of Speech and Speech Sound Disorders. *J. Speech Lang. Hear. Res.* **2019**, *62*, 3220–3233. [CrossRef]
30. Jiang, J.; Benhamou, E.; Waters, S.; Johnson, J.C.S.; Volkmer, A.; Weil, R.S.; Marshall, C.R.; Warren, J.D.; Hardy, C.J.D. Processing of Degraded Speech in Brain Disorders. *Brain Sci.* **2021**, *11*, 394. [CrossRef]
31. Sommer, M.; Koch, M.A.; Paulus, W.; Weiller, C.; Büchel, C. Disconnection of speech-relevant brain areas in persistent developmental stuttering. *Lancet* **2002**, *360*, 380–383. [CrossRef]
32. Anderson, J.D.; Ofoe, L.C. The Role of Executive Function in Developmental Stuttering. *Semin. Speech Lang.* **2019**, *40*, 305–319. [CrossRef]
33. Walsh, B.; Mettel, K.M.; Smith, A. Speech motor planning and execution deficits in early childhood stuttering. *J. Neurodev. Disord.* **2015**, *7*, 1–12. [CrossRef]
34. MacPherson, M.K. Cognitive Load Affects Speech Motor Performance Differently in Older and Younger Adults. *J. Speech Lang. Hear. Res.* **2019**, *62*, 1258–1277. [CrossRef]
35. Han, W.; Wang, T. From Motor Skills to Digital Solutions: Developmental Dysgraphia Interventions over Two Decades. *Children* **2025**, *12*, 542. [CrossRef]
36. Louis, K.O.S.; Myers, F.L.; Faragasso, K.; Townsend, P.S.; Gallaher, A.J. Perceptual aspects of cluttered speech. *J. Fluen. Disord.* **2004**, *29*, 213–235. [CrossRef]
37. Baker, A.E.; Galván, A.; Fuligni, A.J. The connecting brain in context: How adolescent plasticity supports learning and development. *Dev. Cogn. Neurosci.* **2025**, *71*, 101486. [CrossRef] [PubMed]
38. Eckert, M.A.; Keren, N.I.; Roberts, D.R.; Calhoun, V.D.; Harris, K.C. Age-related changes in processing speed: Unique contributions of cerebellar and prefrontal cortex. *Front. Hum. Neurosci.* **2010**, *4*, 1178. [CrossRef]

39. Yoo, H.; McNeil, M.R.; Dickey, M.W.; Terhorst, L. Linguistic and nonlinguistic processing speed across age-matched normal healthy controls and individuals with left-hemisphere damage, with and without aphasia. *Aphasiology* **2022**, *36*, 147–169. [CrossRef]
40. Adolph, K.E.; Franchak, J.M. The development of motor behavior. *Wiley Interdiscip Rev. Cogn. Sci.* **2017**, *8*, e1430. [CrossRef] [PubMed]
41. Han, W. Chapter 7: "Grammar, I hate" or "I grammar hate"? L1 and L2 word order differences and bilingual DLD assessment. In *Multifaceted Multilingualism*; Grohmann, K.K., Ed.; John Benjamins: Amsterdam, The Netherlands; Philadelphia, PA, USA, 2024; pp. 186–205.
42. Han, W.; Shi, D. Topic and Left Periphery in Shanghainese. *J. Chin. Linguist.* **2016**, *44*, 29–60.
43. Han, W. *Universal Grammar and the Initial State of Second Language Learning: Evidence of Chinese Multidialectal Children's Acquisition of English at the Syntax-Semantics Interface*; Springer: Singapore, 2020.
44. Xiao, L.D.; Chen, L.; Han, W.; Meyer, C.; Müller, A.; Low, L.; Brijnath, B.; Mohammadi, L. Optimising social conditions to improve autonomy in communication and care for ethnic minority residents in nursing homes: A meta-synthesis of qualitative research. *Nurs. Inq.* **2022**, *29*, e12469. [CrossRef] [PubMed]
45. Liang, Y.; Han, W. Source text pre-editing versus target text post-editing in using Google Translate to provide health services to culturally and linguistically diverse clients. *Sci. Eng. Health Stud.* **2022**, *16*, 22050009.
46. Van Hove, O.; Pichon, R.; Pallanca, P.; Cebolla, A.M.; Noel, S.; Feipel, V.; Deboeck, G.; Bonnechère, B. Influence of Speech and Cognitive Load on Balance and Timed up and Go. *Brain Sci.* **2022**, *12*, 1018. [CrossRef] [PubMed]
47. Devillers-Réolon, L.; Temprado, J.-J.; Sleimen-Malkoun, R. Mindfulness meditation and bimanual coordination control: Study of acute effects and the mediating role of cognition. *Front. Psychol.* **2023**, *14*, 1162390. [CrossRef] [PubMed]

 https://doi.org/10.3390/children13010097

children

MDPI

Article

Effects of the SmartACT Intervention on Motor and Psychological Variables in Adolescent Athletes: A Controlled Trial Using BlazePod and Microgate

Barabási Madár Timea [1], Costea-Bărluţiu Carmen [2], Ordean Mircea Nicolae [3,*], Mancini Nicola [4,*], Grosu Vlad Teodor [5], Sabău Anca Maria [6], Popovici Cornelia [7], Carlos Hervás-Gómez [8], Grosu Emilia Florina [1] and Monea Dan [1]

1 Faculty of Physical Education and Sport, "Babes-Bolyai" University, Mihail Kogălniceanu 1, 400347 Cluj-Napoca, Romania; timea.barabasi@ubbcluj.ro (B.M.T.); emilia.grosu@ubbcluj.ro (G.E.F.); dan.monea@ubbcluj.ro (M.D.)

2 Faculty of Psychology and Educational Sciences, "Babes-Bolyai" University, Sindicatelor 7, 400347 Cluj-Napoca, Romania; carmen.costea@ubbcluj.ro

3 Department of Physical Education and Sports, "December 1, 1918" University, Gabriel Bethlen 5, 510009 Alba Iulia, Romania

4 Department of Science of Education and Sport, Pegaso Telematic University, 80143 Naples, Italy

5 Faculty of Industrial Engineering, Robotics, and Production Management, Technical University of Cluj-Napoca, Muncii 103-105, 400461 Cluj-Napoca, Romania; vlad.grosu@mdm.utcluj.ro or vtgrosu@gmail.com

6 Departament of Physical Education and Sport and Kinetotherapy, Faculty of Geography, Turism and Sport, University of Oradea, 410087 Oradea, Romania; sabauancamaria@yahoo.com

7 Physical Education Discipline, University of Medicine and Pharmacy "Iuliu Haţieganu", Pasteur 6, 400347 Cluj-Napoca, Romania; popovicicornelia@yahoo.com or cornelia.popovici@umfcluj.ro

8 Department of Teaching and Educational Organization, University of Sevilla, 41013 Sevilla, Spain; hervas@us.es

* Correspondence: mircea.ordean@uab.ro (O.M.N.); nicola.mancini@unipegaso.it (M.N.)

Abstract: Background/Objectives: Agility and reaction speed are critical components of sports performance and are influenced by both physical conditioning and psychological state. Interventions such as SmartACT, which integrate mindfulness, acceptance, and commitment, guided imagery and hypnosis techniques are still underexplored in high-performance sport, despite their potential to affect both psychological and motor dimensions. **Methods**: This 7-week controlled trial investigated the effectiveness of SmartACT in reducing psychological and somatic symptoms and enhancing motor performance in adolescent athletes. A total of 193 athletes aged 15–18 years were assigned to three groups: SmartACT (n = 69), MAC (*Mindfulness–Acceptance–Commitment*, the standardized Gardner & Moore protocol; n = 65), and a control group (n = 59). Agility was measured using the T-Drill Agility Test with Microgate electronic timing, and reaction speed was assessed using BlazePod devices. Psychological and somatic symptoms were evaluated using the Depression, Anxiety, and Stress Scale (DASS-21) and the Ghent Multidimensional Somatic Complaints Scale (GMSCS). **Results**: The SmartACT group showed significantly improved agility ($MD = -1.07$ s, $p < 0.001$, $d = 2.50$, 95% CI [1.79, 3.35]), faster reaction times ($MD = -643.75$ ms, $p < 0.001$, $d = 0.85$, 95% CI [0.35, 1.41]), and a higher number of BlazePod touches ($MD = +2.53$, $p < 0.001$, $d = 1.43$, 95% CI [0.87, 2.07]). Psychological symptoms (DASS-21) and somatic complaints (GMSCS) decreased significantly more than in the MAC and control groups. **Conclusions**: SmartACT appears to be an effective hybrid psychological intervention to simultaneously improve physical performance and reduce psychological and psychosomatic distress in adolescent athletes.

Keywords: SmartACT; adolescent athletes; agility; reaction time; DASS-21; GMSCS; ACT; hypnosis; performance psychology

1. Introduction

Early participation in organized sport contributes to psychophysical development and long-term well-being in youth [1,2]. Agility is a complex skill that integrates coordination, speed, and rapid decision-making with perceptual–cognitive processes such as visual scanning and anticipation; it is a key determinant of performance in open-skill team sports where athletes must respond to unpredictable stimuli [3–13]. Contemporary accounts emphasize reactive agility—changes in direction in response to sport-specific cues—because it better captures real game demands and predicts talent more accurately than pre-planned agility [5,7,14], with implications for identification and development pathways [4,6,7,15].

Across ball and racket sports, rapid reactions and efficient visual processing underpin success under tactical pressure [4,15–17]. Accordingly, reaction time (RT) is not only a marker of performance potential but is tightly coupled with reactive-agility outcomes and decision speed in ecologically valid tasks [4–7,15]. Considering this linkage, the present study treats RT as a core motor outcome alongside agility, as both reflect the integration of perceptual, cognitive, and motor processes that our intervention seeks to influence.

Beyond motor performance, adolescent sport participation is associated with psychological benefits—including improved self-esteem and lower symptoms of depression and anxiety—whereas stress and anxiety can contribute to somatic complaints (e.g., fatigue, pain, gastrointestinal discomfort) that interfere with training and competition [18–39]. In applied settings where maximal testing is not always feasible, combining quick motor tests with validated questionnaires such as the Ghent Multidimensional Somatic Complaints Scale (GMSCS) provides a practical screen for psychophysiological imbalance [40,41].

Interest in psychological methods that target attention, emotion regulation, and imagery has grown in performance sport. Mindfulness- and acceptance-based approaches, guided imagery, and hypnosis have been linked to reduced psychosomatic symptoms and improved execution under pressure [42–62]. However, the SmartACT protocol—integrating mindfulness, acceptance, commitment, guided imagery, and hypnosis—has not been systematically tested in adolescent athletes on both motor and psychological outcomes simultaneously, leaving a relevant gap in the literature.

Aims and Hypotheses

This study aims to evaluate the effects of a 7-week SmartACT intervention on both motor performance (agility, reaction time) and psychological well-being (anxiety, depression, somatic symptoms) in adolescent athletes. Based on prior literature, we hypothesize that SmartACT will produce greater improvements than the MAC and control conditions across all measured outcomes.

2. Materials and Methods

This study followed a quasi-experimental, controlled, repeated-measures design with pretest and posttest assessments over seven weeks. A total of 193 student athletes (age 15–18 years, M = 16.34; SD = 0.64) were recruited from sports-focused high schools in Transylvania (Romania) and educational centers in Hungary (Table 1). Participants were assigned to the three groups (SmartACT, MAC, Control) using cluster allocation at the school or training-group level, rather than individual randomization, which justifies the quasi-experimental design. Inclusion criteria were: (i) age between 15 and 18 years, (ii) participation in structured sports training at least twice per week, and (iii) informed consent from both athletes and their guardians. Exclusion criteria included: (i) current musculoskeletal or neurological injuries, (ii) ongoing psychological treatment, or (iii) incomplete participation in pre- or post-assessments.

Table 1. Participant characteristics at baseline (N = 193).

Characteristic	Category	*n* (%)
Age (years), mean ± SD	—	16.34 ± 0.64
Primary sport	Volleyball 46 (23.9%); Basketball 45 (23.4%); Football 42 (21.8%); Handball 20 (10.2%); Athletics 13 (6.6%); Wrestling 12 (6.1%); Others ≤ 2% each	
Sports experience	>4 years 107 (55.3%); 3–4 years 26 (13.7%); 1–2 years 44 (22.8%); 1st year 16 (8.1%)	
Training frequency	≥5×/week 105 (54.3%); 4×/week 43 (22.3%); 2–3×/week 43 (22.3%); 1×/week 2 (1.0%)	
Additional sports	Yes 66 (34.0%); No 127 (66.0%)	
Diet pattern	Balanced 89 (46.0%); High-protein 58 (29.9%); Carbohydrate-dominant 28 (14.7%); Sugar-rich 6 (3.3%); Not reported 12 (6.2%)	

Note. *n* = number of participants; % = percentage; *SD* = standard deviation.

Participants completed an assessment that addressed both motor and psychological components. From a motor perspective, agility was tested using the T-Drill agility task using the Microgate electronic timing system, and reaction speed was assessed using BlazePod devices, which involve rapid responses to visual stimuli. Psychologically, participants completed two validated instruments: the Depression, Anxiety, and Stress Scale (DASS-21) [63], which measures depression, anxiety, and distress, and the Ghent Multidimensional Somatic Complaints Scale (GMSCS) [64], which assesses the presence and intensity of psychosomatic symptoms.

2.1. Motor Assessment: Agility and Reaction Speed

Before testing, all participants completed a 10 min standardized warm-up under supervision, including dynamic stretches, joint rotations, and functional drills designed to activate major muscle groups [65]. The T-Drill agility protocol was demonstrated and explained to ensure consistent execution.

A total of 168 participants performed the T-Drill Agility Test (Figure 1), applied both in the pre-test and post-test stages. This test assesses movement speed, the ability to quickly change direction and motor coordination, in conditions that require quick reactions and precision. The T-Drill agility has been shown to have high test–retest reliability and validity in athletic populations [66]. The execution time was recorded using a Microgate Racetime Light Radio electronic timing system (Microgate, Bolzano, Italy; Figure 2), installed at the start–finish line to ensure the objectivity of the measurements. The route was visually delimited by colored cones, which indicated the directions of movement and the mandatory touch points, according to the sequence provided by the standard T-Drill agility protocol.

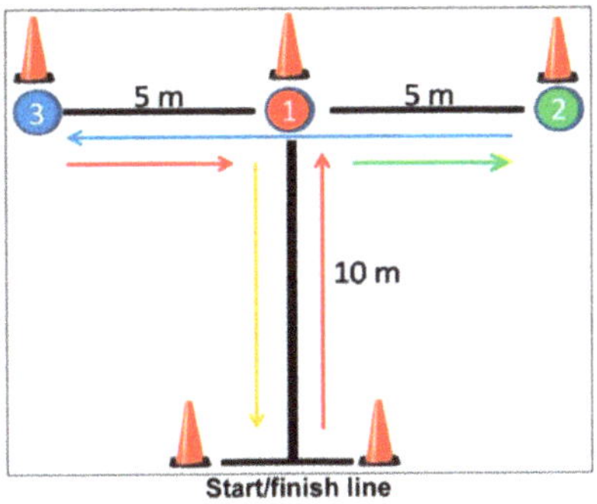

Figure 1. T-Drill Agility Test.

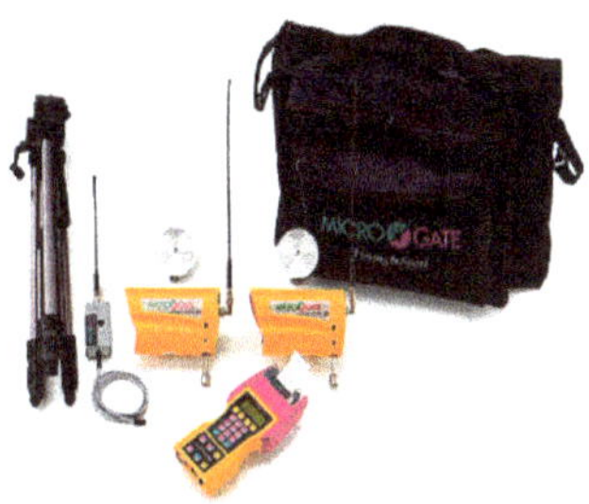

Figure 2. Microgate equipment kit Racetime Light Radio.

A total of 185 participants were assessed in terms of reaction speed and total number of touches using the BlazePod training and testing system (BlazePod Ltd., Tel Aviv, Israel; Figure 3), both in the pretest and posttest stages. BlazePod is a modern motor assessment and training system (BlazePod Ltd., Tel Aviv, Israel), designed to develop and measure psychomotor functions through visual light stimuli, emitted by portable LED modules. In this study, a set of 12 modules was used, controlled via the BlazePod mobile application (www.blazepod.eu, accessed on 5 April 2025), installed on a phone compatible with the iOS operating system. The reliability and validity of this system in assessing reactive agility have already been confirmed in the specialized literature, being frequently used in sports testing contexts [67,68]. The devices were configured to allow simultaneous testing of six participants. Each athlete was assigned a personal code entered in the application, allowing individual monitoring of performance. The motor exercise used, called "Color Catch", involved the rapid reaction of the participants by touching visually activated color modules. The 12 pods were placed on adjustable tripods at a height of 90–120 cm, arranged in a semicircle of ~3 m in front of the participant to allow multidirectional reaching. Pods were spaced 50–70 cm apart to require lateral and forward movements. The testing was carried out in two consecutive rounds of 60 s each, separated by a 30 s break. Instructions were clearly communicated before the start of the test, and the activity was standardized. Performance was monitored in real time by the application, which automatically recorded parameters such as the total number of touches and the average reaction speed.

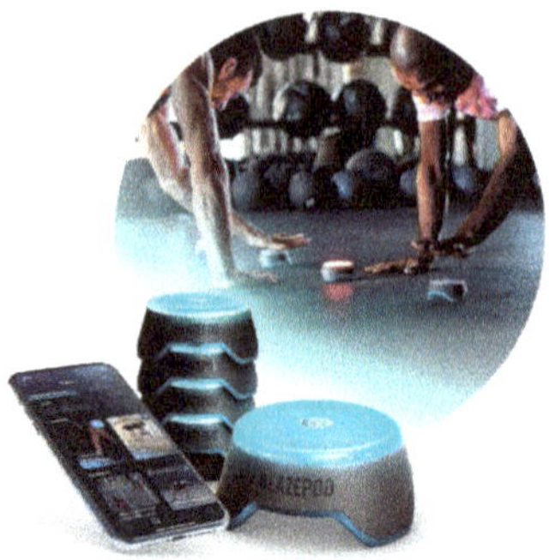

Figure 3. BlazePod Ltd. (www.blazepod.eu).

2.2. *Psychological and Psychosomatic Assessment*

A total of 193 participants completed the Depression, Anxiety, and Stress Scales (DASS-21) [63] and the Ghent Multidimensional Somatic Complaints Scale (GMSCS) [64] at both pre- and post-test assessments. The Depression, Anxiety and Stress Scale (DASS-21) is a quantitative instrument used to assess depression, anxiety and stress. Based on the scores obtained, individuals can be classified into five severity categories for each subscale: normal, mild, moderate, severe and extremely severe.

The questionnaire consists of 21 items, and respondents rate the frequency with which they have experienced certain states in the past week, using a scale from 0 ("not at all") to 3 ("very much or most of the time") [63].

The Ghent Multidimensional Somatic Complaints Scale (GMSCS) was used to assess symptoms in experimental subjects. They rated 18 somatic symptoms that had occurred in the past four weeks, in terms of frequency and intensity, using a scale from 0 to 7. Frequency was rated as follows: 0 = never, 7 = constantly; and intensity: 0 = not at all, 7 = unbearable.

The scale includes five subscales: pain localized to the head, shoulders and stomach, sensations of cold or heat, cardiac manifestations and fatigue [64]. Both scales were linguistically adapted in Romanian [69–71] and Hungarian [69–71] languages.

2.3. *Participant Flow and Outcome Completion*

Of the 193 athletes initially enrolled, completion rates differed across outcome measures due to occasional absences or missing data. A total of 168 completed the T-Drill agility, 185 completed the BlazePod tests, and all 193 completed the DASS-21 and GMSCS questionnaires (Table 2). No adverse events or intervention-related withdrawals were reported.

Table 2. Participant flow by outcome (pre–post analyzed).

Outcome	Baseline Enrolled (N)	Completed Pre–Post (n)	Missing (n)	Reason for Missing
T-Drill agility	193	168	25	Absence or incomplete timing data
BlazePod tests	193	185	8	Device availability/missed session
DASS-21	193	193	0	—
GMSCS	193	193	0	—

Note. Reasons for non-completion were administrative or logistical (e.g., absence, missing data, device unavailability). No adverse events or intervention-related withdrawals were reported. N = total number of participants enrolled at baseline; n = number of participants; — = not applicable.

2.4. Blinding

Outcome assessors were not blinded to group assignment. However, motor outcomes were recorded using automated and objective systems (Microgate electronic timing, BlazePod application), and standardized procedures were applied across groups to minimize detection bias.

The study was built on a repeated measures design, including an initial assessment (pretest) and a subsequent assessment (posttest), conducted at an interval of seven weeks. Participants were divided into three experimental groups. The first group, SmartACT ($n = 69$, 35.8%), benefited from a structured psychological program, carried out over seven weeks, which integrated principles of acceptance and commitment therapy (ACT) with hypnosis and guided imagery techniques, adapted to the specifics of sports activity. The second group, MAC (Mindfulness–Acceptance–Commitment), consisting of 65 participants (33.7%), followed the standardized protocol proposed by Gardner and Moore (2007) [72], focused on developing full awareness of internal experiences, their acceptance and orientation towards action in accordance with one's own values. The control group ($n = 59$, 30.6%) continued their usual sports and educational activity, without participating in any specific psychological intervention during the study.

It is assumed that there are significant relationships between motor performance and psychological indicators, such that a more balanced level of emotional state and a more functional body perception correlate with superior motor efficiency. In this context, it is considered that the general psychological state and somatic perceptions of adolescent athletes significantly influence motor performance and psychomotor reactivity. It is also anticipated that the SmartACT psychological intervention, which combines mindfulness, acceptance and commitment techniques, guided imagery and hypnotherapy, will lead to significant improvements in both physical (agility, reaction speed) and psychological aspects, by reducing symptoms of depression, anxiety, stress and psychosomatic symptoms. The SmartACT group is expected to obtain significantly higher scores in the posttest stage, compared to the MAC group and the control group, which would support the effectiveness of a hybrid intervention in simultaneously optimizing psychological functioning and motor performance in a sports context.

2.5. Statistical Analysis

Data were analyzed using SPSS Statistics v25 (IBM, Armonk, NY, USA). Descriptive statistics are reported as mean ± SD (with 95% confidence intervals where relevant). Pearson's r quantified bivariate associations. Within-group changes were tested with paired-samples t-tests; time × group effects were examined with a mixed repeated-measures ANOVA (within-subject factor: time [pre, post]; between-subject factor: group [SmartACT, MAC, Control]). When appropriate, between-group pairwise comparisons at posttest used Tukey–Kramer HSD. All tests were two-tailed with $\alpha = 0.05$.

Effect sizes were calculated as Cohen's d for t-tests and partial eta squared (η^2p) for ANOVAs, each with 95% confidence intervals. Benchmarks were: Cohen's d small = 0.20, medium = 0.50, large = 0.80; Pearson's r small = 0.10, medium = 0.30, large = 0.50; η^2p small = 0.01, medium = 0.06, large = 0.14. Assumptions of normality and homogeneity of variances were checked with Shapiro–Wilk (and Q–Q plots) and Levene's tests; with two time points, sphericity is not applicable. Analyses were performed per outcome using all available paired observations (pairwise deletion).

3. Results

3.1. Analysis of Correlations Between Motor Variables, Perception of Somatic Symptoms and Indicators of Psychological Distress

Table 3 reports significant correlations between motor performance (T-Drill agility, BlazePod Hits, and Reaction Time) and scores from the DASS-21 and GMSCS, which assess psychological distress and psychosomatic symptoms.

Table 3. Correlations between motor, psychological and psychosomatic variables.

	1	2	3	4	5	6	7	8	9	10	11	12
1.T-Drill agility												
2.BlazePod Hits	−0.400 **											
3.BlazePod React. Time	0.371 **	−0.894 **										
4.GMSCS Head Should	0.214 **	−0.075	0.112									
5.GMSCS Heart Chest	0.172 *	−0.049	0.140	0.670 **								
6.GMSCS Stom Abd	0.313 **	−0.106	0.114	0.471 **	0.502 **							
7.GMSCS Warm Cold	0.223 **	−0.030	0.038	0.500 **	0.531 **	0.607 **						
8.GMSCS Fatigue	0.283 **	−0.052	0.085	0.592 **	0.602 **	0.565 **	0.658 **					
9.GMSCS TOTAL	0.295 **	−0.074	0.118	0.780 **	0.810 **	0.764 **	0.806 **	0.879 **				
10.DASS-21 Depression	0.391 **	−0.172 *	0.189 *	0.492 **	0.529 **	0.450 **	0.431 **	0.623 **	0.635 **			
11.DASS-21 Anxiety	0.307 **	−0.147 *	0.151 *	0.574 **	0.674 **	0.452 **	0.568 **	0.650 **	0.726 **	0.715 **		
12.DASS-21 Stress	0.368 **	−0.189 *	0.213 **	0.548 **	0.549 **	0.444 **	0.519 **	0.677 **	0.688 **	0.766 **	0.767 **	
13.DASS-21 TOTAL	0.386 **	−0.186 *	0.203 **	0.588 **	0.637 **	0.491 **	0.552 **	0.712 **	0.747 **	0.909 **	0.902 **	0.927 **

**. Correlation is significant at the 0.01 level (2-tailed); *. Correlation is significant at the 0.05 level (2-tailed).

T-Drill agility times were negatively correlated with BlazePod Hits ($r = -0.400$, $p < 0.01$), indicating a moderate-to-strong association whereby faster agility was linked to more effective visual–motor responses. BlazePod Hits and Reaction Time were strongly and inversely related ($r = -0.894$, $p < 0.01$), confirming that increased reactivity corresponds to shorter response times. T-Drill agility times were also positively associated with several GMSCS subscales, especially fatigue ($r = 0.283$, $p < 0.01$), warm–cold sensations ($r = 0.223$, $p < 0.01$), and abdominal symptoms ($r = 0.313$, $p < 0.01$), suggesting that slower agility is linked to greater perceived somatic discomfort. Significant positive correlations were further observed between DASS-21 scores and T-Drill agility times (r range = 0.307−0.391, $p < 0.01$), indicating that higher emotional distress is associated with slower agility. BlazePod Hits showed weak but significant negative correlations with DASS-21 subscales (e.g., Depression $r = -0.172$, $p < 0.05$), suggesting that better reaction performance is associated with lower emotional distress. Conversely, Reaction Time positively correlated with DASS-21 Total ($r = 0.203$, $p < 0.01$) and GMSCS Total ($r = 0.118$, $p < 0.01$), indicating that slower responses are linked to greater psychological and somatic symptoms.

3.2. Analysis of Pretest–Posttest Differences in the SmartACT Group for Motor Variables (T-Drill Agility, BlazePod Hits and Reaction Time)

Paired-sample t-tests were used to assess within-group changes in agility (T-Drill agility), BlazePod Hits, and Reaction Time for the SmartACT group. Results are presented in Table 4 and demonstrate significant pre–post improvements across all motor outcomes.

- T-Drill agility improved significantly from pretest (M = 11.80 s) to posttest (M = 10.78 s), MD = −1.07 s, t(68) = 10.29, $p < 0.001$, with a large effect size (d = 2.50, 95% CI [1.79–3.35]).
- BlazePod Hits increased from 16.34 to 19.01, MD = +2.53, t(68) = −5.90, $p < 0.001$, also with a large effect size (d = 1.43, 95% CI [0.87–2.07]).
- BlazePod Reaction Time decreased from 3770.84 ms to 3108.10 ms, MD = −643.75 ms, t(68) = 3.52, $p < 0.001$, with a large effect size (d = 0.85, 95% CI [0.35–1.41]).

These results confirm that SmartACT produced strong and practically meaningful improvements in both agility and visual-motor reactivity.

Table 4. Significant pretest–posttest differences in the SmartACT group for the analyzed motor variables (T-Drill agility, BlazePod Hits, BlazePod Reaction Time).

Variable	Time	M	MD	*T* (df)	*p*	Cohen's *d* [95% CI]
T-Drill agility (s)	Pretest Posttest	11.80 10.78	−1.07	10.29 (68)	<0.001	2.50 [1.79, 3.35]
BlazePod Hits	Pretest Posttest	16.34 19.01	+2.53	−5.90 (68)	<0.001	1.43 [0.87, 2.07]
BlazePod Reaction Time (ms)	Pretest Posttest	3770.84 3108.10	−643.75	3.52 (68)	<0.001	0.85 [0.35, 1.41]

Note. MD = mean difference; *t* = t statistic; *p* = probability value; *d* = Cohen's d; CI = confidence interval.

3.2.1. Motor Agility—T-Drill

T-Drill agility times in the SmartACT group improved significantly from pretest (M = 11.80 s) to posttest (M = 10.78 s), with a mean difference of −1.07 s, $t(68) = 10.29$, $p < 0.001$. This change corresponds to a large effect size (d = 2.50, 95% CI [1.79–3.35]), confirming the strong impact of the intervention on agility. The MAC and Control groups showed minimal or no change.

3.2.2. Visual Response—BlazePod Hits

BlazePod Hits increased significantly in the SmartACT group from 16.34 to 19.01 ($MD = +2.53$, $t(68) = -5.90$, $p < 0.001$). This improvement reflects a large effect size ($d = 1.43$, 95% CI [0.87–2.07]), indicating substantial gains in visual reactivity. No comparable improvements were observed in the MAC or Control groups.

3.2.3. Reaction Time—BlazePod Reaction Time (RT)

Reaction Time significantly decreased in the SmartACT group from 3770.84 ms to 3108.10 ms ($MD = -643.75$ ms, $t(68) = 3.52$, $p < 0.001$). This corresponds to a large effect size ($d = 0.85$, 95% CI [0.35–1.41]), demonstrating faster psychomotor responses following the intervention. No meaningful changes occurred in the MAC or Control groups.

3.3. Repeated Measures ANOVA: Pretest–Posttest Evolution in the Three Groups for Motor Variables and Psychological Indicators

To further investigate the differential effects of the interventions, repeated-measures ANOVAs were conducted for each outcome, followed by Tukey's post hoc tests where appropriate. The results are presented below for motor variables (T-Drill agility, BlazePod Hits, Reaction Time) and psychological indicators (DASS-21, GMSCS).

3.3.1. Group Comparison Regarding T-Drill Agility Test

A repeated-measures ANOVA was conducted on T-Drill agility scores ($n = 168$) to assess changes in agility across time and between groups, followed by Tukey's post hoc comparisons. Results showed a significant main effect of time, $F(1,165) = 13.14$, $p < 0.001$, and a significant time × group interaction, $F(2,165) = 20.29$, $p < 0.001$, indicating that agility improvements varied across groups. Tukey's post hoc test (Table 5) revealed that the SmartACT group outperformed both the MAC group (MD = −1.11, $p < 0.001$, $\eta^2 p = 0.19$, 95% CI [0.09–0.29]) and the Control group (MD = −1.07, $p < 0.001$, $\eta^2 p = 0.18$, 95% CI [0.08–0.28]). No significant difference emerged between MAC and Control (MD = 0.04, $p = 0.987$, $\eta^2 p = 0.00$).

Table 5. Results of the Tukey post hoc test for comparing T-Drill Agility scores (sec) between groups.

Compare Groups	MD	SE	*p*	η^2p (95% CI)
SmartACT vs. MAC	−1.11	0.226	0.000	0.19 [0.09–0.29]
SmartACT vs. Control	−1.07	0.232	0.000	0.18 [0.08–0.28]
MAC vs. Control	0.04	0.246	0.987	0.00 [0.00–0.04]

Note. MD = mean difference; SE = standard error; *p* = probability value; η^2p = partial eta squared; CI = confidence interval.

The graphical representation of the execution times in the T-Drill Agility Test for the three groups, at the pre- and post-test assessments, is illustrated in Figure 4.

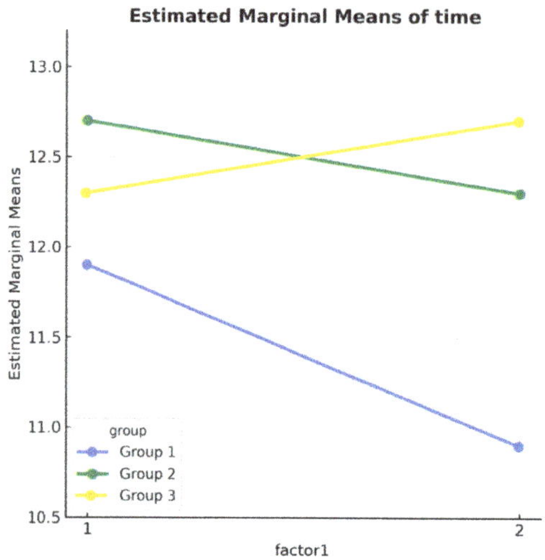

Figure 4. Mean T-Drill agility execution time (seconds) at pretest and posttest across the three groups (SmartACT, MAC, Control). Group 1—SMARTACT—is marked in blue, group 2—MAC—is represented in green, and group 3—control—is indicated in yellow.

3.3.2. Group Comparison Regarding DASS-21 Total

DASS-21 and GMSCS data were collected from all 193 participants at both pretest and posttest time points. Tukey's post hoc analysis (Table 6) showed that posttest DASS-21 scores were significantly lower in the SmartACT group compared to both the MAC group (*MD* = −6.43, $p = 0.002$, $\eta^2p = 0.11$, 95% CI [0.03–0.21]) and the Control group (*MD* = −4.87, $p = 0.029$, $\eta^2p = 0.07$, 95% CI [0.01–0.16]). No significant difference was observed between the MAC and Control groups ($p = 0.697$, $\eta^2p = 0.01$).

Table 6. Results of the Tukey post hoc test for comparing DASS-21 Total between groups.

Compare Groups	MD	SE	*p*	η^2p (95% CI)
SmartACT vs. MAC	−6.43	1.844	0.002	0.11 [0.03–0.21]
SmartACT vs. Control	−4.87	1.891	0.029	0.07 [0.01–0.16]
MAC vs. Control	1.56	1.918	0.697	0.01 [0.00–0.06]

Note. MD = mean difference; SE = standard error; *p* = probability value; η^2p = partial eta squared; CI = confidence interval.

These differences confirm that the intervention applied to the SmartACT group had a superior impact compared to the other groups regarding the Depression, Anxiety and Stress Scale (DASS-21), as illustrated in Figure 5. The magnitude of these differences was moderate-to-large (η^2p = 0.07−0.11), indicating not only statistical significance but also practical relevance.

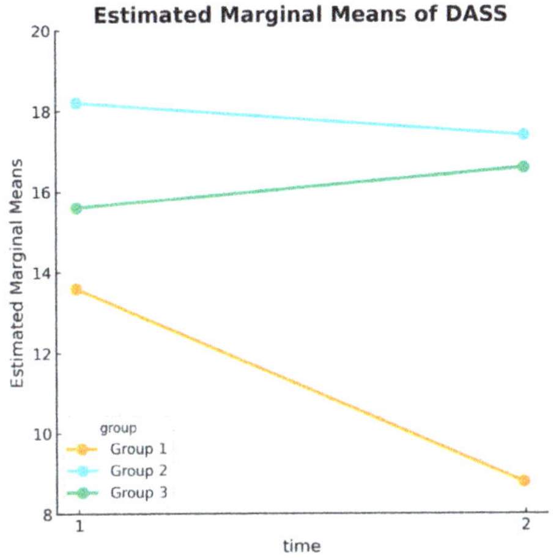

Figure 5. Mean DASS-21 Total scores at pretest and posttest across groups. A larger reduction is evident in the SmartACT group.

3.3.3. Group Comparison Regarding GMSCS Total

Somatic symptoms (GMSCS Total) decreased significantly in the SmartACT group (from 38.91 to 30.54), with smaller reductions in the MAC group (49.69 to 45.00) and negligible changes in the Control group (42.85 to 40.98). The Tukey post hoc test (Table 7) revealed significant differences between groups. Specifically, SmartACT showed greater efficacy than MAC (MD = −12.62, $p < 0.001$, η^2p = 0.15, 95% CI [0.07–0.25]) in reducing somatic symptoms. The difference between SmartACT and Control was also significant (MD = −7.19, p = 0.050, η^2p = 0.08, 95% CI [0.01–0.17]), suggesting a relevant benefit compared to the absence of intervention.

Table 7. Results of the Tukey post hoc test for comparing GMSCS Total scores between groups.

Compare Groups	MD	SE	p	η^2p (95% CI)
SmartACT vs. MAC	−12.62	2.968	0.000	0.15 [0.07–0.25]
SmartACT vs. Control	−7.19	3.045	0.050	0.08 [0.01–0.17]
MAC vs. Control	5.43	3.088	0.186	0.03 [0.00–0.09]

Note. MD = mean difference; SE = standard error; p = probability value; η^2p = partial eta squared; CI = confidence interval.

In contrast, no significant differences were identified between the MAC and Control groups (p = 0.186, η^2p = 0.03), indicating that the MAC intervention did not substantially impact somatic symptoms in this context.

GMSCS scores decreased significantly over time, suggesting an overall improvement in somatic symptomatology among participants. Group 1 (SmartACT) experienced significantly fewer symptoms compared to Group 2 (MAC) and marginally fewer than Group 3 (Control), as also highlighted in Figure 6. Although the interaction between time and group did not reach statistical significance (p = 0.080), post hoc analysis confirmed that Group 1 benefited most from the intervention, with effect sizes in the moderate-to-large range (η^2p = 0.08–0.15). This indicates that SmartACT produced not only statistically significant but also practically relevant reductions in somatic complaints.

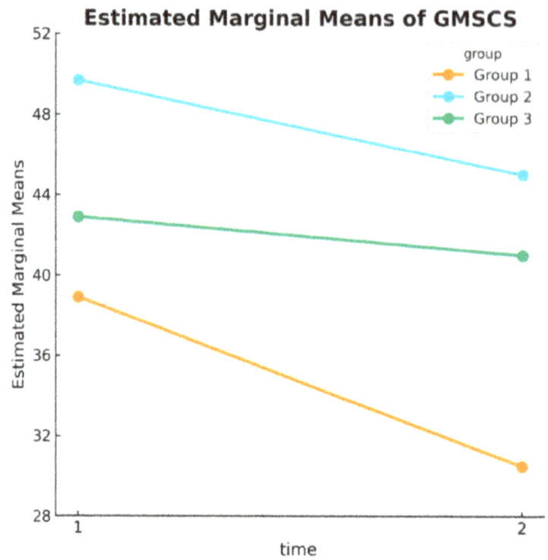

Figure 6. GMSCS Total scores at pretest and posttest across groups. The SmartACT group exhibited the greatest reduction in somatic symptoms.

3.3.4. Group Comparison Regarding GMSCS Fatigue

Fatigue scores significantly declined over time in all groups ($p < 0.001$), though post hoc analysis revealed that SmartACT led to significantly greater reductions than the other conditions. The mean difference between SmartACT and MAC was −4.88 ($p < 0.001$), and between SmartACT and Control was −2.91 ($p = 0.014$), confirming the superior effectiveness of SmartACT.

No significant differences were observed between MAC and Control ($p = 0.143$). Table 8 presents in detail the results of the Tukey post hoc test for the comparison of perceived fatigue scores (GMSCS) between groups.

Table 8. Results of the Tukey post hoc test for comparing GMSCS fatigue scores between groups.

Compare Groups	MD	SE	p	η^2p (95% CI)
SmartACT vs. MAC	−4.88	.998	0.000	0.17 [0.08–0.27]
SmartACT vs. Control	−2.91	1.024	0.014	0.09 [0.01–0.18]
MAC vs. Control	1.97	1.038	0.143	0.04 [0.00–0.11]

Note. MD = mean difference; SE = standard error; p = probability value; η^2p = partial eta squared; CI = confidence interval.

3.3.5. Group Comparison Regarding GMSCS Stomach/Abdominal Symptoms

The Tukey post hoc test showed a significant difference between SmartACT and MAC ($MD = -1.84$, $p = 0.014$), indicating fewer stomach/abdominal symptoms in the SmartACT group. The comparison between SmartACT and Control did not reach significance ($p = 0.272$), and no difference was found between MAC and Control ($p = 0.449$) (Table 9).

Table 9. Results of the Tukey post hoc test for comparing GMSCS Stomach/Abdominal scores between groups.

Compare Groups	MD	SE	p	η^2p (95% CI)
SmartACT vs. MAC	−1.84	0.647	0.014	0.08 [0.01–0.17]
SmartACT vs. Control	−1.03	0.664	0.272	0.03 [0.00–0.09]
MAC vs. Control	0.81	0.673	0.449	0.02 [0.00–0.07]

Note. MD = mean difference; SE = standard error; p = probability value; η^2p = partial eta squared; CI = confidence interval.

3.3.6. Group Comparison Regarding GMSCS Head/Shoulder Symptoms

Tukey's post hoc test (Table 10) showed a statistically significant difference between SmartACT and MAC ($MD = -2.36$, $p < 0.001$, $\eta^2p = 0.13$, 95% CI [0.05–0.23]), indicating that participants in the SmartACT group reported fewer head/shoulder symptoms. Differences between SmartACT and Control were not significant ($MD = -1.02$, $p = 0.194$, $\eta^2p = 0.04$), nor were differences between MAC and Control ($MD = 1.34$, $p = 0.067$, $\eta^2p = 0.05$). These findings confirm that SmartACT was significantly more effective than MAC in reducing head/shoulder pain.

Table 10. Results of the Tukey post hoc test for comparing GMSCS Head/Shoulder scores between groups.

Compare Groups	MD	SE	p	η^2p (95% CI)
SmartACT vs. MAC	−2.36	0.574	0.000	0.13 [0.05–0.23]
SmartACT vs. Control	−1.02	0.588	0.194	0.04 [0.00–0.11]
MAC vs. Control	1.34	0.597	0.067	0.05 [0.00–0.12]

Note. MD = mean difference; SE = standard error; p = probability value; η^2p = partial eta squared; CI = confidence interval.

3.3.7. Group Comparison Regarding GMSCS Warm–Cold Symptoms

All three groups experienced decreases in scores between pretest and posttest, suggesting an overall reduction in somatic Warm–Cold symptoms, although the differences between groups were not statistically significant. The most pronounced reduction was observed in the SmartACT group, where the score decreased from approximately 7.7 to 6.0.

This indicates a clear effect of the intervention in this group, contributing to the reduction in perceived thermal discomfort at the body level. The MAC and Control groups experienced smaller decreases of approximately one point.

3.3.8. Group Comparison Regarding GMSCS Heart/Chest Symptoms

Although the SmartACT group showed the greatest reductions in scores on the Heart/Chest subscale, the differences between groups were not statistically significant. This suggests a general tendency toward improvement across all groups, without evidence of a specific intervention effect.

4. Discussion

The present findings indicate that psychological well-being and somatic symptomatology are closely linked to motor performance in adolescent athletes. SmartACT produced meaningful gains in agility and visual–motor reactivity—evidenced by shorter T-Drill agility times and better BlazePod performance—together with larger reductions on DASS-21 and GMSCS than both the MAC and Control conditions. This pattern suggests that an integrated, performance-oriented psychological program can enhance athletic readiness by acting simultaneously on attentional control, emotion regulation, and perceived somatic discomfort. Given the magnitude of the pre–post changes observed in the SmartACT group, these effects are likely to be practically relevant for youth athletes and their coaches. These outcomes align with contemporary models that conceptualize agility as primarily reactive, with changes in direction triggered by sport-specific stimuli and constrained by perceptual–cognitive demands [3–7,9–13,15]. Faster reaction to external cues is a hallmark of higher competitive levels in open-skill sports, and measures that capture stimulus–response speed are considered informative for talent identification and training monitoring [4–7,15,68]. The improvements on BlazePod indices therefore fit within this framework, adding experimental evidence that targeted psychological work can translate into better reactive behavior on the field.

A plausible mechanism for SmartACT's superiority over MAC is its hybrid structure, which combines ACT processes with guided imagery and hypnosis. Prior work shows that these techniques can strengthen attentional focus, emotion regulation, and self-efficacy, and can facilitate access to optimal performance states such as relaxation and flow [43–46,49–51,58–62,72]. Imagery and hypnosis have also been associated with improvements in technical execution and competitive precision across several sports, including cycling, shooting, golf, football, basketball, and volleyball [50,53–57,73]. In parallel, reductions in GMSCS scores observed here are consistent with evidence that mindfulness/ACT-based methods and imagery can attenuate psychophysiological stress responses and improve interoceptive awareness, thereby lowering the salience of somatic complaints [44,58–62,74,75].

By contrast, the smaller changes in the MAC group may reflect dose and age-fit issues. Seven weeks may be insufficient for adolescents to consolidate mindfulness and acceptance skills, which often require longer daily practice to yield robust transfer to performance contexts [58,72]. In addition, adolescents may engage more readily with techniques that feel directly sport-embedded (imagery, hypnosis, performance routines) than with introspective exercises, leading to stronger motivation and adherence in SmartACT [58,60,61]. These considerations, together with the current data, support the utility of hybrid, performance-linked mental training for youth athletes.

4.1. Literature Context and Theoretical Framing

The present study extends literature that ties agility and reaction time to perceptual–cognitive factors and sport-specific stimuli [3–7,9–13,15,68] by showing that a brief, structured psychological intervention can enhance these motor outcomes alongside mental-health indicators. It also integrates strands of evidence on ACT/mindfulness and on imagery/hypnosis in sport: ACT-based approaches reduce emotional symptoms and improve regulation under stress [58–62,72], while imagery and hypnosis improve focus, confidence, and flow, with demonstrated benefits for performance execution [49–51,53–57,73]. Taken together, these findings align with models of cognitive–motor integration in which attentional control and affective regulation act as proximal drivers of skilled action under time pressure [44,45,75]. Within this framework, SmartACT likely operates through complementary pathways—top-down regulation (ACT), sensorimotor simulation (imagery), and autonomic/attentional tuning (hypnosis)—to yield concurrent gains in motor efficiency and reductions in psychosomatic distress [44,49–51,58–62,74–76].

4.2. Practical Implications

From an applied perspective, these findings support integrating brief, structured mental training alongside routine physical preparation in youth sport. Coach-delivered micro-sessions that combine ACT-consistent skills (present-moment attention, acceptance, values-guided actions) with sport-specific imagery, concise hypnosis scripts, and competition routines can help athletes translate psychological regulation into faster, more efficient responses in open-skill contexts—i.e., improved T-Drill agility and stimulus–response speed consistent with agility and perceptual–cognitive models [14,15], and with device-based reactivity work [4,68]. Evidence that ACT/mindfulness improves regulation under stress [58–62], and that imagery/hypnosis can enhance focus, flow, self-efficacy, and execution across sports, provides a mechanistic rationale for this hybrid approach in adolescents [49–51,54,57,73]. For implementation, sessions can be embedded twice weekly for ~10–15 min during warm-ups or cooldowns over 7 weeks, using simple scripts aligned with technical goals (e.g., cue-based focusing, brief imagery of sport-specific decision points, and short relaxation/hypnosis inductions appropriate for minors and delivered or overseen by trained staff) [49–51,54,57–62,73]. Programs should be integrated with existing load- and recovery-monitoring to address perceived fatigue and somatic complaints—domains linked to performance and injury risk—using low-burden tools (e.g., DASS-21, GMSCS) alongside standard fatigue practices [40,41,77–81]. Motor tracking can rely on field-friendly tests already used here (T-Drill, BlazePod "Color Catch") to ensure that psychological skills training remains performance-embedded and ecologically valid [4,15,66,68].

4.3. Limitations and Future Directions

Several limitations should be acknowledged. The lack of random assignment limits internal validity, and although baseline equivalence was partly ensured, unmeasured confounders may have influenced the results. Moreover, the absence of a long-term follow-up prevents conclusions about durability, and reliance on self-report for psychological variables introduces potential response bias. Future research should prioritize randomized controlled designs, incorporate objective physiological markers (e.g., HRV, cortisol), and include follow-ups to assess maintenance of change. It will also be valuable to stratify by sport type (team vs. individual; endurance vs. power-based) to account for differing cognitive-motor and emotional demands, and to test dose–response relations to identify the minimal effective dose for adolescent athletes.

5. Conclusions

Agility and visual reaction speed are decisive components of sport performance in open-skill disciplines that demand rapid responses to unpredictable stimuli. In this controlled trial, the SmartACT program produced greater gains in T-Drill agility and BlazePod performance than both MAC and Control, together with larger reductions in DASS-21 and GMSCS. For somatic symptoms, all groups improved over time, but the decreases were consistently greatest in SmartACT, indicating added value beyond usual practice and a mindfulness-only approach. While the quasi-experimental design and lack of follow-up limit causal and durability inferences, the magnitude and consistency of effects support the utility of SmartACT as a complement to standard training. Future studies should test SmartACT in randomized designs, include longer follow-ups, and examine differential responses across sport types and competitive levels.

Author Contributions: Conceptualization, B.M.T., O.M.N. and M.D.; methodology M.N., G.E.F. and P.C.; software, C.-B.C. and B.M.T.; validation, C.H.-G., P.C. and M.N.; formal analysis, B.M.T. and G.V.T.; investigation, G.E.F., C.-B.C., G.V.T. and S.A.M.; resources, B.M.T., M.D. and G.V.T.; data curation, C.-B.C., G.V.T. and S.A.M.; writing—original draft preparation, B.M.T. and M.N.; writing—review and editing, P.C., B.M.T. and M.N.; visualization, G.E.F.; supervision, C.H.-G. and M.N.; project administration, G.E.F., C.H.-G. and B.M.T.; funding acquisition O.M.N. All authors have read and agreed to the published version of the manuscript.

Funding: This research received no external funding.

Institutional Review Board Statement: The study was conducted in accordance with the Declaration of Helsinki and approved by the Institutional Review Board (or Ethics Committee) of The Scientific Council of the Babeș-Bolyai University of Cluj-Napoca (7355/4/7 June 2023).

Informed Consent Statement: Informed consent was obtained from all subjects involved in the study. This article is part of the first author's doctoral thesis Barabási Madár Timea.

Data Availability Statement: The data presented in this study are available on request from the corresponding author due to privacy and ethical restrictions.

Acknowledgments: This article is part of the first author's doctoral thesis. We thank Barabási Madár Timea for her collaboration. The authors have reviewed and edited the output and take full responsibility for the content of this publication.

Conflicts of Interest: The authors declare no conflicts of interest.

Abbreviations

The following abbreviations are used in this manuscript:

MAC	Mindfulness Acceptance Commitment
SmartACT	Smart Acceptance and Commitment Therapies
DASS-21	Depression, Anxiety and Stress Scales (21-item)
GMSCS	Ghent Multidimensional Somatic Complaints Scale
RT	Reaction Time
CI	Confidence Interval
ANOVA	Analysis of Variance
η^2p	partial eta squared
MD	Mean Difference
SD	Standard Deviation

References

1. Vella, S.A.; Cliff, D.P.; Magee, C.A.; Okely, A.D. Sports participation and parent-reported health-related quality of life in children: Longitudinal associations. *J. Pediatr.* **2014**, *164*, 1469–1474. [CrossRef] [PubMed]
2. Hoffmann, M.D.; Barnes, J.D.; Tremblay, M.S.; Guerrero, M.D. Associations between organized sport participation and mental health difficulties: Data from over 11,000 US children and adolescents. *PLoS ONE* **2022**, *17*, e0268583. [CrossRef] [PubMed]
3. Sheppard, J.M.; Young, W.B. Agility literature review: Classifications, training and testing. *J. Sports Sci.* **2006**, *24*, 919–932. [CrossRef]
4. Mancini, N.; Di Padova, M.; Polito, R.; Mancini, S.; Dipace, A.; Basta, A.; Colella, D.; Limone, P.; Messina, G.; Monda, M.; et al. The Impact of Perception–Action Training Devices on Quickness and Reaction Time in Female Volleyball Players. *J. Funct. Morphol. Kinesiol.* **2024**, *9*, 147. [CrossRef]
5. Zemková, E.; Vilman, T.; Kováciková, Z.; Hamar, D. Reaction time in the Agility Test under simulated competitive and noncompetitive conditions. *J. Strength Cond. Res.* **2013**, *27*, 3445–3449. [CrossRef]
6. Trajković, N.; Sporiš, G.; Krističević, T.; Madić, D.M.; Bogataj, Š. The Importance of Reactive Agility Tests in Differentiating Adolescent Soccer Players. *Int. J. Environ. Res. Public Health* **2020**, *17*, 3839. [CrossRef]
7. Young, W.; Farrow, D. The importance of a sport-specific stimulus for training agility. *Strength Cond. J.* **2013**, *35*, 39–43. [CrossRef]
8. Chow, C.G.; Kong, Y.H.; Wong, C.L. Reactive-Agility in Touch Plays an Important Role in Elite Playing Level: Reliability and Validity of a Newly Developed Repeated Up-and-Down Agility Test. *J. Sports Sci. Med.* **2022**, *21*, 413–418. [CrossRef] [PubMed]
9. Young, W.; Farrow, D. A review of agility: Practical applications for strength and conditioning. *Strength Cond. J.* **2006**, *28*, 24–29. [CrossRef]
10. Sporiš, G.; Milanović, Z.; Trajković, N.; Joksimović, A. Correlation between speed, agility and quickness (SAQ) in elite young soccer players. *Acta Kinesiol.* **2011**, *5*, 36–41.
11. Wang, P.; Shi, C.; Chen, J.; Gao, X.; Wang, Z.; Fan, Y.; Mao, Y. Training methods and evaluation of basketball players' agility quality: A systematic review. *Heliyon* **2024**, *10*, e24296. [CrossRef] [PubMed]
12. Delextrat, A.; Grosgeorge, B.; Bieuzen, F. Determinants of performance in a new test of planned agility for young elite basketball players. *Int. J. Sports Physiol. Perform.* **2015**, *10*, 160–165. [CrossRef] [PubMed]
13. Yilmaz, G. The effects of Power, Speed, Skill and Anaerobic Capacity of different training models in young male basketball players. *Anthropologist* **2014**, *18*, 877–883. [CrossRef]
14. Forster, J.W.D.; Uthoff, A.M.; Rumpf, M.C.; Cronin, J.B. Training to Improve Pro-Agility Performance: A Systematic Review. *J. Hum. Kinet.* **2023**, *85*, 35–51. [CrossRef]
15. Paul, D.J.; Gabbett, T.J.; Nassis, G.P. Agility in Team Sports: Testing, Training and Factors Affecting Performance. *Sports Med.* **2016**, *46*, 421–442. [CrossRef]
16. Baker, D.G.; Newton, R.U. Comparison of lower body strength, power, acceleration, speed, agility, and sprint momentum to describe and compare playing rank among professional rugby league players. *J. Strength Cond. Res.* **2008**, *22*, 153–158. [CrossRef]
17. Shedge, S.S.; Ramteke, S.U.; Jaiswal, P.R. Optimizing Agility and Athletic Proficiency in Badminton Athletes Through Plyometric Training: A Review. *Cureus* **2024**, *16*, e52596. [CrossRef]
18. Sabiston, C.M.; Jewett, R.; Ashdown-Franks, G.; Belanger, M.; Brunet, J.; O'Loughlin, E.; O'Loughlin, J. Number of Years of Team and Individual Sport Participation During Adolescence and Depressive Symptoms in Early Adulthood. *J. Sport Exerc. Psychol.* **2016**, *38*, 105–110. [CrossRef]

19. Eime, R.M.; Young, J.A.; Harvey, J.T.; Charity, M.J.; Payne, W.R. A systematic review of the psychological and social benefits of participation in sport for children and adolescents: Informing development of a conceptual model of health through sport. *Int. J. Behav. Nutr. Phys. Act.* **2013**, *10*, 98. [CrossRef]
20. Panza, M.J.; Graupensperger, S.; Agans, J.P.; Doré, I.; Vella, S.A.; Evans, M.B. Adolescent Sport Participation and Symptoms of Anxiety and Depression: A Systematic Review and Meta-Analysis. *J. Sport Exerc. Psychol.* **2020**, *42*, 201–218. [CrossRef]
21. He, J.P.; Paksarian, D.; Merikangas, K.R. Physical Activity and Mental Disorder Among Adolescents in the United States. *J. Adolesc. Health* **2018**, *63*, 628–635. [CrossRef]
22. Murray, R.M.; Sabiston, C.M.; Doré, I.; Bélanger, M.; O'Loughlin, J.L. Association between pattern of team sport participation from adolescence to young adulthood and mental health. *Scand. J. Med. Sci. Sports* **2021**, *31*, 1481–1488. [CrossRef] [PubMed]
23. Ashdown-Franks, G.; Sabiston, C.M.; Solomon-Krakus, S.; O'Loughlin, J.L. Sport participation in high school and anxiety symptoms in young adulthood. *Ment. Health Phys. Act.* **2017**, *12*, 19–24. [CrossRef]
24. Merikangas, K.R.; Nakamura, E.F.; Kessler, R.C. Epidemiology of mental disorders in children and adolescents. *Dialogues Clin. Neurosci.* **2009**, *11*, 7–20. [CrossRef] [PubMed]
25. Serido, J.; Almeida, D.M.; Wethington, E. Chronic stressors and daily hassles: Unique and interactive relationships with psychological distress. *J. Health Soc. Behav.* **2004**, *45*, 17–33. [CrossRef]
26. Kovács, I.K.; Borcsa, M. The relationship between anxiety, somatic symptoms and hardiness in adolescence. *Rom. J. Appl. Psychol.* **2017**, *19*, 42–49. [CrossRef]
27. Demuthova, S. The school environment as a source of somatic problems in adolescents. *Rev. Românească Educ. Multidimens.* **2019**, *11*, 59–71. [CrossRef]
28. Vulić-Prtorić, A. Somatic complaints in adolescence: Prevalence patterns across gender and age. *Psihologijske Teme* **2016**, *25*, 75–105. Available online: https://hrcak.srce.hr/file/230450 (accessed on 1 April 2025).
29. Gallant, S. Assessing adverse neural tension in athletes. *J. Sport Rehabil.* **1998**, *7*, 128–139. [CrossRef]
30. Barroso, G.C.; Thiele, E.S. Muscle injuries in athletes. *Rev. Bras. Ortop.* **2015**, *46*, 354–358. [CrossRef]
31. Roșioară, A.I.; Năsui, B.A.; Ciuciuc, N.; Sîrbu, D.M.; Curșeu, D.; Vesa, Ș.C.; Popescu, C.A.; Bleza, A.; Popa, M. Beyond BMI: Exploring Adolescent Lifestyle and Health Behaviours in Transylvania, Romania. *Nutrients* **2025**, *17*, 268. [CrossRef]
32. Diduch, B.K. Gastrointestinal Conditions in the Female Athlete. *Clin. Sports Med.* **2017**, *36*, 655–669. [CrossRef]
33. de Oliveira, E.P.; Burini, R.C.; Jeukendrup, A. Gastrointestinal complaints during exercise: Prevalence, etiology, and nutritional recommendations. *Sports Med.* **2014**, *44* (Suppl. 1), S79–S85. [CrossRef]
34. Waterman, J.J.; Kapur, R. Upper gastrointestinal issues in athletes. *Curr. Sports Med. Rep.* **2012**, *11*, 99–104. [CrossRef]
35. Wright, H.; Collins, M.; Schwellnus, M.P. Gastrointestinal (GIT) symptoms in athletes: A review of risk factors associated with the development of GIT symptoms during exercise. *Int. SportMed J.* **2009**, *10*, 116–123. Available online: https://hdl.handle.net/10520/EJC48379 (accessed on 1 April 2025).
36. Wilson, P.B. The Psychobiological Etiology of Gastrointestinal Distress in Sport: A Review. *J. Clin. Gastroenterol.* **2020**, *54*, 297–304. [CrossRef]
37. Cronin, O.; Molloy, M.G.; Shanahan, F. Exercise, fitness, and the gut. *Curr. Opin. Gastroenterol.* **2016**, *32*, 67–73. [CrossRef]
38. Coleman, N. Gastrointestinal Issues in Athletes. *Curr. Sports Med. Rep.* **2019**, *18*, 185–187. [CrossRef] [PubMed]
39. Poucher, Z.A.; Tamminen, K.A.; Sabiston, C.M.; Cairney, J.; Kerr, G. Prevalence of symptoms of common mental disorders among elite Canadian athletes. *Psychol. Sport Exerc.* **2021**, *57*, 102018. [CrossRef]
40. Robson-Ansley, P.J.; Gleeson, M.; Ansley, L. Fatigue management in the preparation of Olympic athletes. *J. Sports Sci.* **2009**, *27*, 1409–1420. [CrossRef]
41. Halson, S.L. Monitoring training load to understand fatigue in athletes. *Sports Med.* **2014**, *44* (Suppl. 2), S139–S147. [CrossRef] [PubMed]
42. Budgett, R. Fatigue and underperformance in athletes: The overtraining syndrome. *Br. J. Sports Med.* **1998**, *32*, 107–110. [CrossRef]
43. Hasyim, A.H.; Muhammad, A.; Sujarwo, H. The impact of sport hypnosis on volleyball athlete performance: An empirical study. *J. Sport Area* **2023**, *8*, 360–370. [CrossRef] [PubMed]
44. Rosendahl, J.; Alldredge, C.T.; Haddenhorst, A. Meta-analytic evidence on the efficacy of hypnosis for mental and somatic health issues: A 20-year perspective. *Front. Psychol.* **2024**, *14*, 1330238. [CrossRef]
45. Li, Z.; Li, S.X. The Application of Hypnosis in Sports. *Front. Psychol.* **2022**, *12*, 771162. [CrossRef]
46. Di Corrado, D.; Guarnera, M.; Vitali, F.; Quartiroli, A.; Coco, M. Imagery ability of elite level athletes from individual vs. *team and contact vs. no-contact sports. PeerJ* **2019**, *7*, e6940. [CrossRef]
47. Khoury, B.; Sharma, M.; Rush, S.E.; Fournier, C. Mindfulness-based stress reduction for healthy individuals: A meta-analysis. *J. Psychosom. Res.* **2015**, *78*, 519–528. [CrossRef] [PubMed]
48. Shearer, A.; Hunt, M.; Chowdhury, M.; Nicol, L. Effects of a brief mindfulness meditation intervention on student stress and heart rate variability. *Int. J. Stress Manag.* **2016**, *23*, 232. [CrossRef]
49. Pates, J.; Palmi, J. The effects of hypnosis on flow states and performance. *J. Excell.* **2002**, *6*, 48–62.

50. Milling, L.S.; Randazzo, E.S. Enhancing sports performance with hypnosis: An ode for Tiger Woods. *Psychol. Conscious. Theory Res. Pract.* **2016**, *3*, 45. [CrossRef]
51. Straub, W.F.; Bowman, J.J. A review of the development of sport hypnosis as a performance enhancement method for athletes. *J. Psychol. Clin. Psychiatry* **2016**, *6*, 00378. [CrossRef]
52. Lindsay, P.; Maynard, I.; Thomas, O. Effects of hypnosis on flow states and cycling performance. *Sport Psychol.* **2005**, *19*, 164–177. [CrossRef]
53. Pates, J.; Maynard, I. Effects of hypnosis on flow states and golf performance. *Percept. Mot. Skills* **2000**, *91 Pt 2*, 1057–1075. [CrossRef]
54. Mattle, S.; Birrer, D.; Elfering, A. Feasibility of Hypnosis on Performance in Air Rifle Shooting Competition. *Int. J. Clin. Exp. Hypn.* **2020**, *68*, 521–529. [CrossRef]
55. Hamid, N.; Abdoli, R.; Shahroie, A. Efficacy of cognitive behavior therapy with positive imagination of success during hypnotism on athletic performance. *Hormozgan Med. J.* **2018**, *22*, e86481. [CrossRef]
56. Sahabuddin, S.; Sofyan, D.; Fadillah, A. Integrating Self-Hypnotherapy Techniques into Physical Conditioning Programs for Volleyball Performance Enhancement. *Compet. J. Pendidik. Kepelatihan Olahraga* **2025**, *17*, 503–518. [CrossRef]
57. Barker, J.B.; Jones, M.; Greenlees, I. Using Hypnosis to Enhance Self-Efficacy in Sport Performers. *J. Clin. Sport Psychol.* **2013**, *7*, 228–247. [CrossRef]
58. Noetel, M.; Ciarrochi, J.; Van Zanden, B.; Lonsdale, C. Mindfulness and acceptance approaches to sporting performance enhancement: A systematic review. *Int. Rev. Sport Exerc. Psychol.* **2019**, *12*, 139–175. [CrossRef]
59. González-García, M.; Álvarez, J.C.; Pérez, E.Z.; Fernandez-Carriba, S.; López, J.G. Feasibility of a Brief Online Mindfulness and Compassion-Based Intervention to Promote Mental Health Among University Students During the COVID-19 Pandemic. *Mindfulness* **2021**, *12*, 1685–1695. [CrossRef] [PubMed]
60. Johles, L.; Gustafsson, H.; Jansson-Fröjmark, M.; Classon, C.; Hasselqvist, J.; Lundgren, T. Psychological Flexibility Among Competitive Athletes: A Psychometric Investigation of a New Scale. *Front. Sports Act. Living* **2020**, *2*, 110. [CrossRef]
61. Petterson, H.; Olson, B.L. Effects of mindfulness-based interventions in high school and college athletes for reducing stress and injury, and improving quality of life. *J. Sport Rehabil.* **2017**, *26*, 578–587. [CrossRef]
62. Tang, Y.Y.; Hölzel, B.K.; Posner, M.I. The neuroscience of mindfulness meditation. *Nat. Rev. Neurosci.* **2015**, *16*, 213–225. [CrossRef]
63. Henry, J.D.; Crawford, J.R. The short-form version of the Depression Anxiety Stress Scales (DASS-21): Construct validity and normative data in a large non-clinical sample. *Br. J. Clin. Psychol.* **2005**, *44 Pt 2*, 227–239. [CrossRef] [PubMed]
64. Beirens, K.; Fontaine, J.R. Development of the Ghent Multidimensional Somatic Complaints Scale. *Assessment* **2010**, *17*, 70–80. [CrossRef] [PubMed]
65. Aguilar, A.J.; DiStefano, L.J.; Brown, C.N.; Herman, D.C.; Guskiewicz, K.M.; Padua, D.A. A dynamic warm-up model increases quadriceps strength and hamstring flexibility. *J. Strength Cond. Res.* **2012**, *26*, 1130–1141. [CrossRef]
66. Pauole, K.; Madole, K.; Garhammer, J.; Lacourse, M.; Rozenek, R. Reliability and validity of the T-test as a measure of agility, leg power, and leg speed in college-aged men and women. *J. Strength Cond. Res.* **2000**, *14*, 443–450. [CrossRef]
67. Polechoński, J.; Pilch, J.; Langer, A.; Prończuk, M.; Markowski, J.; Maszczyk, A. Assessment of the reliability and validity of simple and complex reaction speed tests in mixed martial arts athletes using the BlazePod system. *Baltic J. Health Phys. Act.* **2025**, *17*, 2. [CrossRef]
68. Hoffman, J.R. Evaluation of a Reactive Agility Assessment Device in Youth Football Players. *J. Strength Cond. Res.* **2020**, *34*, 3311–3315. [CrossRef]
69. Barabási-Madár, T.; Monea, D.; Costea-Bărluţiu, C. Effects of a Mindfulness-Based Intervention on the Physical and Psychological Well-Being in Teenagers. *Educ. Health Perform.* **2023**, 25–37. [CrossRef]
70. Barabási-Madár, T.; Costea-Bărluţiu, C.; Vargha, J.L. Preliminary data on the effectiveness of in This Moment program: Investigation of its impact on Romanian high school students' stress management abilities. In Proceedings of the Poster Presentation, ACBS World Conference 17, Dublin, Ireland, 25–30 June 2019.
71. Barabási-Madár, T.; Costea-Bărluţiu, C.; Vargha, J.L. Studiul utilizării smartphone-ului de către elevii de liceu. In *Punţi Între Teorii, Cercetări, Studii de Caz. Abordări Multidisciplinare*; Jardan, V.A., Ed.; Editura APAR: Braşov, Romania, 2019.
72. Gardner, F.L.; Moore, Z.E. *The Psychology of Enhancing Human Performance: The Mindfulness-Acceptance-Commitment (MAC) Approach*; Springer Publ. Co.: New York, NY, USA, 2007.
73. Miró, A.; Mesperuza, M.; Jensen, M.P.; Day, M.A.; García, F.; Miró, J. Therapeutic hypnosis and sports performance: A systematic review. *Int. Rev. Sport Exerc. Psychol.* **2025**, 1–21. [CrossRef]
74. Volgemute, K.; Vazne, Z.; Malinauskas, R. The benefits of guided imagery on athletic performance: A mixed-methods approach. *Front. Psychol.* **2025**, *16*, 1500194. [CrossRef]
75. Gutman, T.; Gottlieb, A. Performance mindfulness: Integrating ACT matrix, imagery and mindfulness for performance enhancement. *J. Sport Psychol.* **2024**, 1–17. [CrossRef]

76. Jovanovic, M.; Sporis, G.; Omrcen, D.; Fiorentini, F. Effects of speed, agility, quickness training method on power performance in elite soccer players. *J. Strength Cond. Res.* **2011**, *25*, 1285–1292. [CrossRef] [PubMed]
77. Thorpe, R.T.; Atkinson, G.; Drust, B.; Gregson, W. Monitoring Fatigue Status in Elite Team-Sport Athletes: Implications for Practice. *Int. J. Sports Physiol. Perform.* **2017**, *12* (Suppl. 2), S227–S234. [CrossRef] [PubMed]
78. Almonroeder, T.G.; Tighe, S.M.; Miller, T.M.; Lanning, C.R. The influence of fatigue on decision-making in athletes: A systematic review. *Sports Biomech.* **2020**, *19*, 76–89. [CrossRef]
79. Radin, E.L. Role of muscles in protecting athletes from injury. *Acta Med. Scand.* **1986**, *220* (Suppl. 711), 143–147. [CrossRef]
80. Sikora, M.; Mikołajczyk, R.; Łakomy, O.; Karpiński, J.; Żebrowska, A.; Kostorz-Nosal, S.; Jastrzębski, D. Influence of the breathing pattern on the pulmonary function of endurance-trained athletes. *Sci. Rep.* **2024**, *14*, 1113. [CrossRef] [PubMed]
81. Migliaccio, G.M.; Russo, L.; Maric, M.; Padulo, J. Sports Performance and Breathing Rate: What Is the Connection? A Narrative Review on Breathing Strategies. *Sports* **2023**, *11*, 103. [CrossRef] [PubMed]

children

MDPI

Article

The Role of Capoeira in Improving Motor and Social Skills in Children with Autism

Roei Lev-Ari [1,*], Meir Lotan [2] and Liat Korn [1]

[1] Department of Health Systems Management, Faculty of Health Sciences, Ariel University, Ariel 40700, Israel; liatk@ariel.ac.il

[2] Department of Physiotherapy, Faculty of Health Sciences, Ariel University, Ariel 40700, Israel; meirlo@ariel.ac.il

* Correspondence: sababa.cdo@gmail.com

Highlights:

What are the main findings?

- Capoeira training improved motor skills such as coordination, balance, and body awareness in children with autism.
- Participation fostered social communication and peer interaction, enhancing children's confidence and engagement.

What is the implication of the main finding?

- Capoeira can serve as a culturally rich and inclusive physical activity program supporting both motor and social development.
- The findings suggest practical pathways for integrating children with autism into mixed-group physical education and community programs.

Abstract: Background: Children with Autism often face motor, sensory and communicational challenges that can hinder their participation in meaningful physical and social activities. This study explores the potential of Capoeira to support their development across these domains. Methods: This qualitative pilot study used semi-structured interviews with parents of children aged 7–15 with Autism Spectrum Disorder (ASD) who participated in group Capoeira programs. Data were analyzed through content categorization, leading to the development of thematic constructs. Results: Three central domains emerged regarding the perceived impact of Capoeira training on children with Autism: 1. Improvements in areas commonly affected in Autism, including sensory and auditory regulation, motor coordination, bodily awareness, compliance, and social communication. 2. Increased motivation, independence, sense of belonging and integration into mixed peer groups of typically developing (TD) children and children with ASD. 3. Broader developmental gains were also reported, such as increased self-confidence, initiative, awareness of others, and transfer of skills beyond the training context. Conclusions: The findings suggest that Capoeira may serve as an effective integrated intervention model, supporting physical and social development in children with ASD. Capoeira was reported to be associated with improved coordination, balance, body awareness, and gains in nonverbal interaction and social engagement, all within a collaborative, non-competitive framework. Future studies should explore the short and long-term impact of such interventions through quantitative outcome measures, as well as clarify the mechanisms that promote successful integration.

Keywords: autism; capoeira; inclusion; motor skills; social skills development; sensory regulation; adapted physical activity

1. Introduction

Autism Spectrum Disorder (ASD) is a neurodevelopmental condition. It is characterized by challenges in social communication, the presence of repetitive behaviors, and restricted interests [1]. Official definitions emphasize impairments in social-emotional reciprocity, nonverbal communicative behaviors, such as body language and eye contact, and difficulties in interpreting social cues [2,3]. Additional characteristics of ASD may include a pronounced insistence on routines, repetitive rituals, and atypical sensory sensitivities, which can involve unusual responses to sounds, tastes, or textures [4–6]. Such symptoms can contribute to significant challenges in personal, social, and occupational functioning. A fundamental aspect of ASD is the difficulty in establishing and maintaining friendships. These emotionally significant relationships necessitate intimacy, stability, and reciprocity, all of which depend on well-developed social-cognitive abilities [7,8]. Children diagnosed with ASD frequently encounter obstacles in expressing positive emotions, sharing experiences, maintaining eye contact, and engaging in cooperative interactions [9]. Consequently, their friendships are often fewer in number and inferior in quality compared to those of typically developing peers, which may adversely impact their present and future social and emotional well-being [4,5,10].

1.1. Motor Difficulties in Children with ASD

Approximately 87% of children with ASD struggle with age-appropriate motor tasks, particularly in areas such as ball skills, balance, and visuomotor coordination [11–14]. These challenges are clinically significant, affecting not only motor skills, but also social engagement, information processing, and executive functioning [15–17]. Moreover, the severity of the motor issues was found to correlate with the severity of core elements of ASD [18–20], while the presence of motor difficulties was found to negatively influence the advancement of children with ASD in regard to their core difficulties [20]. Research indicates that motor interventions, such as physical activity, swimming, therapeutic horseback riding, and hydrotherapy, can lead to improvements of 16% to 43% in skills like throwing, catching, manual dexterity, and balance [21–23]. Furthermore, enhancements in motor functioning have been linked to better executive functions, communication, and social behaviors, as well as increased serotonin uptake [24–29]. Despite the recognized importance of physical activity, children with ASD participate in such activities significantly less often than their peers. A study in the United States found that only 17% of boys with ASD engaged in daily physical activity, compared to 33% in the general population [30].

1.2. Gross Motor Skills and Social Competence in ASD

A meta-analysis incorporating 21 studies has established a significant relationship between gross motor impairments and deficiencies in social skills among individuals with ASD [17]. These motor impairments are posited to hinder participation in social activities, as evidenced by observations that children with poor gross motor skills exhibit lower social integration and diminished peer popularity [31]. Additionally, a systematic review and meta-analysis of 16 quantitative studies, comprising both randomized controlled trials (RCTs) and quasi-experimental designs, revealed that motor-based interventions, including adapted basketball, karate, therapeutic horseback riding, and swimming, resulted in notable improvements of up to 77% in social communication skills in children with ASD [32]. Evaluations of these improvements utilized standardized assessment instruments such as the Social Responsiveness Scale (SRS-2). Furthermore, notable advancements were observed in emotional regulation, self-awareness, and overall mood, alongside reductions in repetitive behaviors and rigidity, as assessed by tools like the Repetitive Behavior Scale-Revised (RBS-R). An RCT focusing on children with ASD indicated that participation in a 12-week running program markedly enhanced emotional regulation and led to a decrease in externalizing behaviors and overall behavioral issues, as measured by the Emotional Regulation Checklist (ERC) and the Child Behavior Checklist (CBCL). These findings may also imply indirect enhancements in social communication skills through the facilitation of improved emotional and behavioral functioning [33]. Moreover, gross motor skills have been linked to social-cognitive competencies, including executive functions (EF) and theory of mind (ToM), both of which are essential for effective social interactions [34]. These results emphasize the necessity for interventions that integrate motor, cognitive, and social-cognitive elements to foster optimal social functioning in children with ASD [35]. Previous literature has identified martial arts as efficacious interventions for bolstering executive functioning and social competencies in this population [36,37]. Within this paradigm, Capoeira, a motor-social activity that synthesizes physical, emotional, and cognitive dimensions emerges as a particularly promising intervention warranting further exploration.

1.3. Capoeira

Capoeira is a distinctive Afro-Brazilian martial art that emphasizes cooperation among participants. The Capoeira game is characterized by dynamic interaction, where practitioners move in sync, incorporating kicks, evasions, dance-like movements, and acrobatic elements. Unlike many other martial arts that focus on defeating an opponent, Capoeira aims to create a collaborative movement dialog [38]. As the central training strategy in Capoeira, the game requires coordinated physical interaction between two participants and serves as the foundational communicative framework of the practice, functioning as a form of "physical dialog" between players [39]. Dyadic practice plays a central role in the learning process, fostering motor synchronization from the earliest training stages. This synchronization is reinforced through rhythmic music and the paired practice of symmetrical movements, commonly seen in beginner-level instruction [40]. Due to its emphasis on acrobatic exercises, weight-bearing positions, and movements inspired by gymnastics, practitioners of Capoeira often develop high levels of strength and flexibility [41]. Beyond the physical aspects, research indicates that Capoeira improves posture, motor coordination, and significantly contributes to emotional, social, and psychological development [42–44]. A recent literature review has shown that Capoeira engages a wide range of brain regions, including areas linked to motor, cognitive, executive, and emotional functions, suggesting its potential to enhance integrated neurocognitive processing [45]. A qualitative study in Israel explored the therapeutic benefits of teaching Capoeira to children, adolescents, and young adults in marginalized settings. Interviews revealed that the combination of movement, music, and social interaction provides a nonviolent outlet for aggression, enhances self-efficacy, and fosters a sense of belonging within a supportive community. These factors indicate that Capoeira may be an effective approach for social and emotional rehabilitation, particularly for those facing exclusion or rejection [46]. A qualitative study conducted in Brazil examined the role of Capoeira in promoting inclusion, enhancing self-esteem, and improving social interactions among children with ASD [47]. Utilizing interviews and observations at two therapeutic centers for children with special needs, the research revealed that participation in Capoeira led to significant improvements in motor skills, social participation, and self-efficacy. The children demonstrated increased confidence, greater initiative in social interactions, and enhanced coping mechanisms. Furthermore, the integration of movement, music, rhythm, and play provided a rich sensory experience that facilitated emotional and social engagement. These findings underscore Capoeira's potential as an educational and rehabilitative space that supports the multidimensional development of children with ASD.

1.4. Capoeira and ASD in Israel

In Israel, it is estimated that approximately 10,000 school-aged children engage in Capoeira training across roughly 100 centers nationwide. Since the establishment of its activity over 35 years ago, the Israeli Capoeira community has developed comprehensive instructor training programs and routinely organizes professional conferences. During a national instructors' conference held in January 2023, attendees were queried regarding the inclusion of children diagnosed with ASD within their elementary-age groups. All respondents affirmed the integration of children with ASD in their programs, spanning a range of functional levels. Furthermore, some groups provided support for children requiring ongoing mediation through the assistance of aides during training sessions. It is estimated that around 200 children aged 7 to 12 with ASD consistently participate in community-based Capoeira classes, which are conducted in the afternoons, across the country. Despite the increasing scholarly interest in the prospective benefits of Capoeira for individuals with unique developmental profiles [46], and the rising acknowledgment of its contributions to psychological resilience, self-esteem, and social bonding [48,49], there remains a lack of systematic research investigating the specific advantages of inclusive Capoeira groups composed of both children with ASD and their typically developing peers.

The significance of the study lies in presenting Capoeira as a socio-rehabilitative model that integrates motor, sensory, and communicative interventions within a mixed group framework that includes both children with and without disabilities. Such a setting fosters an environment that combines social inclusion with the promotion of various developmental skills.

A preliminary review of the existing literature reveals a notable lack of studies addressing the connection between Capoeira and ASD. Most existing works focus on the historical evolution of Capoeira or on its contribution to motor development among typically developing populations.

Although physical activity interventions such as swimming, horseback riding, and martial arts have demonstrated benefits for children with ASD, Capoeira remains virtually unexplored. Its distinctive blend of rhythm, movement dialog, and non-competitive interaction suggests potential developmental value. This qualitative pilot study aimed to examine parents' perspectives on Capoeira's potential contributions to their children's motor, social, and sensory functioning, thereby providing preliminary insights to inform future research.

Beyond its theoretical contribution, this study also holds considerable practical potential. It may increase awareness among Capoeira instructors and trainers regarding the importance of including children with special needs in their programs, while also encouraging parents to consider enrolling their children in physically interactive activities that promote social engagement, emotional regulation, and a sense of belonging. In doing so, the study proposes an innovative framework for developing motor-social interventions grounded in rhythm, movement, play, and inclusion.

1.5. Research Aim

The current qualitative pilot study seeks to evaluate the suitability of existing measurement tools in preparation for a subsequent quantitative study that will examine the effectiveness of Capoeira training among children diagnosed with ASD. While established research-based instruments provide documented value, this study adopts a bottom-up, field-based approach aimed at exploring how participation in Capoeira is perceived to impact children's motor and social functioning, as reported by their parents. As a pilot study, the findings are exploratory and intended to inform future quantitative research.

The research questions address the daily challenges parents, and their children, face due to ASD, the success of integrating children into mixed-ability training groups, the meaning parents attribute to their child's participation, and the perceived motor and social changes resulting from the activity. Furthermore, the study investigates the instructional practices employed by Capoeira instructors, with the aim of identifying mechanisms and factors that contribute to successful group integration.

2. Materials and Methods

2.1. Procedure

This qualitative pilot study is based on semi-structured in-depth interviews with parents of children who had participated in Capoeira classes in Israel for at least one year. The study was approved by the university ethics committee (AU-HEA-LK-20240726). Following ethical approval, parents from across the country, whose children trained regularly with certified Capoeira instructors and who had voluntarily chosen to disclose their child's ASD diagnosis, were invited to participate.

Recruitment was carried out via an invitation message distributed by the Capoeira instructors to parents whose children met the study criteria. Upon scheduling the interview, participants voluntarily agreed to take part in the study and signed an informed consent form.

2.2. Participants

A convenience sample was composed of ten parents (seven mothers and three fathers) of children with ASD, aged 7 to 15 (Mean age 10.05 ± SD = 2.63), who regularly participate in Capoeira classes in Israel. All children had been diagnosed with ASD during early childhood, and the diagnosis had been openly disclosed to the group instructor by the parents as described in Table 1. Eligibility required that participants be parents of children with a confirmed ASD diagnosis, who had trained in Capoeira for at least one year and had participated in Capoeira during their elementary school years (ages 7–12). Families that did not meet these conditions, were unavailable for an interview, or declined to participate were excluded. In total, 16 families were invited through Capoeira instructors; 10 met the inclusion criteria and agreed to participate, while 6 did not meet the criteria or declined participation. Regarding educational placement, seven children were enrolled in special education classes, two attended mainstream classrooms with the support of an aide, and one was integrated into a mainstream classroom without ongoing support. After nine interviews, a noticeable decline in the emergence of new information was observed, indicating data saturation. Following this observation, the research team made a joint decision to discontinue data collection following the tenth interview. Potential data interpretation bias was addressed through peer debriefing and iterative discussions within the research team. This approach was considered suitable given the exploratory and pilot nature of the study.

Table 1. Socio-demographic and Capoeira participation details of children with ASD.

#	Child's Age (Years Months)	Sex	Age at Diagnosis	Autism Level	Age Started Capoeira	Capoeira Duration (Years)	Training Intensity (Recent)
1.	7.6	M	3	Mild-Moderate	4	3.5	1
2.	7	M	3	Mild-Moderate	6	1	1
3.	12	M	10	Mild	8	4	2
4.	9	M	3.5	Mild-Moderate	7	2	1
5.	10	F	9	Mild	5	4	2
6.	15	M	11.5	Mild	5	10	3
7.	10.7	M	2.5	Low Functioning	7	3.5	1
8.	13	M	3.9	Mild-Moderate	7	6	2
9.	9	M	8	Mild	4	5	2
10.	7.5	M	4	Mild	6	1.5	2
Mean ± (SD)	10.0 ± (2.6)		5.8 ± (3.4)		5.9 ± (1.3)	4.0 ± (2.6)	1.7 ± (0.6)

Note: Training intensity (recent) refers to the average weekly frequency of Capoeira sessions during the last year.

2.3. Research Instruments

Data was collected through in-depth interviews conducted by the first author (R.L.A). All interviews took place face-to-face and lasted between 20 and 50 min, with an average duration of approximately 35 min. The interviews were audio-recorded and transcribed with the participants' consent.

The interview protocol began with an overview of the study and its objectives, along with relevant ethical information required by the institutional review board. Following this, the interviewer collected essential demographic data about the participating child, including age, duration of Capoeira participation, and training frequency. Subsequent questions focused on the primary research areas while allowing flexibility for participants to elaborate. The interview guide included topics related to the child's background and diagnosis. Parents were initially asked to describe their child's autism diagnosis and developmental challenges, with prompts such as, "Please describe your child's autism; how does it manifest?" The conversation then shifted to the child's engagement with Capoeira, addressing behavioral and emotional responses before and after training. Sample questions included: "How does your child behave prior to training?" and "What do they say about the class at home?" Additionally, the guide prompted parents to reflect on perceived developmental, emotional, or behavioral changes linked to Capoeira participation. Key questions included, "Have you noticed any changes in your child due to Capoeira? Can you describe their emotional state before and after a session?" To further explore, parents were invited to share their understanding of how Capoeira instruction may contribute to these changes. Lastly, the interview addressed the parent-instructor relationship and how the Capoeira environment supported inclusion. Questions included, "What would you say to a parent with concerns about inclusion? How has your experience with the instructor been?" Each interview concluded with expressions of gratitude for the parent's participation and a brief note that a summary of the study's findings would be shared upon publication.

2.4. Interview Analysis

The recorded interviews were transcribed verbatim and analyzed using a thematic approach, following an inductive process to identify core themes emerging from the participants' narratives, including recurring language and patterns. Data analysis was conducted in accordance with established guidelines for thematic analysis [50].

Following an in-depth familiarization with the data, initial coding was performed manually by the first author, who repeatedly reviewed the transcripts and extracted illustrative quotations. The supervisory team (two senior researchers) subsequently reviewed the coding and transcripts, verified the appropriateness of quotations, and suggested refinements to the thematic structure. This was followed by the organization of participants' perceptions and experiences into key themes, which were grouped into conceptual categories. After reviewing the themes and checking for consistency, each identified theme was clearly defined and supported by direct quotations from the interviews, selected to faithfully reflect the essence of participants' views and the diversity of their perspectives. No qualitative data analysis software was used. The interviews were conducted in Hebrew only and there was no need for translation or re-translation during the data collection phase. In order to write the article in English, translation and scientific linguistic editing were performed accordingly.

2.5. Description of the Intervention—Participation in Capoeira Classes

The present study included parents of children diagnosed with ASD who regularly participate in Capoeira classes in cities across central Israel. The classes are led by certified Capoeira instructors licensed to teach, but do not have specialized training in working with children with special needs.

The autistic children are integrated into mixed-ability groups alongside typically developing peers of the same age. The majority of children represented in the sample (6 out of 10) train at least twice a week, with each session lasting a minimum of 45 min, and have been participating for over one year.

3. Results

This section is structured around three key themes that reflect the participants' perceptions of how Capoeira training has influenced their children's functioning. The main themes are the following:

(1) Common challenges associated with ASD;
(2) Experience of participating in Capoeira classes;
(3) Behavioral changes observed in the context of Capoeira.

Each overarching theme is further divided into sub themes that address specific topics highlighted by the interviewees, including: motor difficulties and sensory regulation; challenges in self-expression and social communication; preparation for and entry into training sessions; integration into mixed-ability groups; improvements in motor and sensory functioning; enhanced self-presentation; and increased understanding of others and social communication. All quotes included in this section are verbatim statements from the interviewees, enclosed in quotation marks and coded accordingly. Each code consists of a letter indicating the interview number and a numeral indicating the transcript page from which the quote was extracted, allowing for precise retrieval of the source material.

3.1. Common Challenges in ASD

This theme comprises two selected subthemes that address challenges commonly experienced by children with ASD, as reported by the interviewees. It focuses on difficulties in sensory regulation, motor functioning, alongside challenges in self-presentation and social communication.

3.1.1. Difficulties in Sensory Regulation and Motor Functioning

This sub-theme reflects interviewees' accounts of their children's sensory and motor challenges and the impact of these difficulties on daily functioning. Many of the participating children were described as having experienced, either currently or in the past, difficulties with sensory regulation, spatial orientation, and basic motor skills. These challenges, particularly heightened sensitivity to stimuli such as noise or touch, often led to avoidance of social and physical activities and required careful planning of daily routines and community participation.

Interviewees described challenges in interpreting bodily sensations, such as atypical responses to pain: "He didn't have a normal reaction to pain, he could get a bleeding open wound and just do nothing about it because he was busy with his own things" (A,2) and tactile sensitivities: "Hugs are impossible. He doesn't like hugging, he dislikes physical contact" (J,3) as well as sensitivity to noise and crowded environments: "If there's noise or lots of people, he wants to put on headphones and be alone" (B,4).

Such sensitivities often interfered with participation in social events and required families to carefully plan daily activities: "I really wanted to include him in the summer camp... but there were so many kids and such a range of ages, and it was very noisy... He just couldn't manage, and after an hour, I had to take him home. Maybe next year" (A,6).

Interviewees also described vestibular and proprioceptive regulation difficulties, as well as balance issues: "He constantly spins in place and bumps into things" (A,2); "He keeps falling" (B,5). Interviewees noted their child's motor challenges, especially when compared to peers of a similar age: "He had motor difficulties" (A,1); "At age three or four, he couldn't hold things properly. He couldn't grip a pencil the way he should" (I,5). Many of the children showed preference for sedentary activities and a general disinterest in physical activity: "He's not a sporty kid. If he had a choice, he'd sit on the couch playing with Lego, watching TV, or drawing" (I,6).

Interviewees emphasized that one of the reasons they chose Capoeira was that it does not involve uncomfortable physical touch: "One of the things that fascinated me about Capoeira is that there's no harsh or unpleasant touch" (A,6). Others emphasized previous difficulties with contact-based martial arts: "We tried judo, and he didn't like being touched. I remember thinking: in Capoeira they don't touch each other that much, maybe that'll work for him" (H,3).

3.1.2. Difficulties in Self-Presentation, Following Instructions, and Social Communication

This sub theme is directly related to the communication challenges often associated with ASD. Interviewees expressed concerns about these challenges and shared their desire to identify supportive strategies that could foster development in this area. Many interviewees indicated that recognizing these communication gaps prompted them to seek diagnostic evaluations and find activities that could promote social connection, openness to new situations, and motor development. Interviewees provided numerous examples of their children's difficulties in responding to verbal cues or instructions. For instance: "He did not really follow instructions. He did not fully understand them, even though his cognition is completely intact, he did not always hear or was able to concentrate" (A,1); "He barely spoke, did not talk to strangers, and did not always respond to his name" (A,2); "He tends to ignore; he is in his own world" (D,2); "In daycare she was quiet. Very quiet, anxious, nodding" (E,1). Interviewees described avoidant or withdrawn behaviors linked to anxiety or frustration: "He would hide under the table when something upset him, he would shut down, become stressed, and refuse to cooperate" (I,1). Interviewees also described patterns of avoiding communication with other children: "He always plays alone besides the other children, and if someone tries to join him, he gets upset. If an unfamiliar person tries to talk to him, he does not engage" (B,2); "He is very quiet, plays alone, and you can barely notice him" (D,1); "The gap between him and the other children in class keeps growing, in interests and in how they communicate" (C,1); "He did not engage with other children at all. Especially with younger ones, he just ignored them" (F,11). Some interviewees spoke about a sense of alienation resulting from their children's difficulties in developing effective social strategies: "Something is off about the way she communicates with her friends" (E,2); "He doesn't understand, and then there are a lot of misunderstandings and people get angry at him" (V,3); "He really wants friends and to fit in, but it seems like he doesn't know how", "He does things that trigger rejection and get him the opposite result" (C,2). In light of these prevalent challenges among children with ASD, interviewees expressed a strong desire to find meaningful out-of-home activities that could support both motor and social development while also helping to reduce anxiety.

3.2. The Experience of Participating in Capoeira Classes

This theme explores the experiences of interviewees regarding their children's participation in Capoeira classes and how these experiences contribute to their overall development and social integration. It includes two key subthemes: the process of preparing for and starting the activity, and the integration of children into mixed groups that include participants both with and without ASD.

An additional sub-theme not included here addresses the challenges of group integration and the supportive strategies implemented by instructors.

3.2.1. Preparation for and Entry into the Activity

Transitions and shifts between types of activity can present significant challenges for children with ASD and their families [51]. This sub-theme focuses on the process of preparing for Capoeira lessons from the moment the child arrives from school, through dressing in training clothes and their behavior prior to the session, to the moment of entering the training space. It also describes how parents and instructors support children when difficulties arise during entry into and integration within the activity.

Interviewees observed unusual functioning in their children's preparation for Capoeira, in contrast to the difficulties typically seen in other contexts. This was evident as early as school pickup: "When he knows it is for Capoeira, he is already waiting outside the classroom long before" (B,4); "When I pick him up from school, he shouts 'Capoeira! already at the school gate'" (G,3).

Interviewees described a strong willingness among the children to prepare independently: "He comes home, says, 'Dad, I have training today, I am going to get dressed, I am getting ready'" (J,7). They noted a clear contrast between the effort needed to prepare for other frameworks and the ease of preparation for Capoeira: "He comes home and asks me for the shirt and pants. It takes him one minute to get ready. So even though in the morning I have to dress him up, when it is for Capoeira, I do not need to do anything, not help at all," (B,4).

This independence was also reflected in readiness for class: "He already gets dressed on his own, gets ready on his own, takes a bottle on his own, maybe that is normal for other kids, but for us, it is not" (F,8).

Interviewees described strong anticipation for the training session and eagerness to participate: "He is happy, he is waiting, he knows when the class is" (A,1); "He truly looks forward for the training, really wants to go to Capoeira" (D,4). Interviewees also described a strong desire in their children to begin the activity: "He literally runs from the house to Capoeira" (B,4).

Few interviewees described challenges in getting the child out of the house when they were immersed in another activity: "It takes a push because when he is watching TV, it is hard to get him out, but (when it comes for Capoeira) it is not very hard. He likes the classes, he likes going" (I,5).

Interviewees emphasized the importance of a consistent and predictable structure, noting that disruptions to the training routine could lead to resistance: "If they move the day, he will suddenly start to struggle and will not want to go" (H,3).

Preparation strategies, such as pre-session reminders and priming, were described as essential tools for easing transitions: "When is it hard to leave? When I do not remind her in time" (E,5).

Additional challenges related to adjusting to the instructional staff were raised, particularly when there was an unexpected change of instructors. While adapted responses, such as assigning a personal mentor, supported successful engagement: "He has a mentor who helps him with the exercises" (G,2), the absence of such support could disrupt the entry into the session: "If the mentor were late or did not show up, there would be crying" (G,2).

Interviewees shared various strategies to manage staff transitions, such as receiving a photo of the substitute instructor in advance: "If there is a substitute teacher, we will only come after that teacher sends me a photo of himself" (G,3).

Another approach to easing transitions was arriving early to build familiarity: "We come fifteen minutes early, and the instructor comes outside and introduces himself to the child. He says, 'Do you want to be my assistant?' Then we go in fifteen minutes early to lay the groundwork" (G,3).

In general, interviewees described entry into the activity as a positive experience for their children: "I see that when he enters Capoeira, he suddenly feels calm" (G,2), and highlighted the independence their children demonstrated: "I arrive, he says hello, goes in, takes off his shoes, grabs his bottle, goodbye" (G,2); "He also wants to be independent, so when we arrive at the gym he tells me: 'I am going up by myself, do not come with me'" (D,4).

These findings suggest that participation in Capoeira elicits a unique sense of motivation in interviewees' children, reflected in exceptional cooperation during preparation, demonstrated independence when entering the session, and the ability to engage without ongoing support. Unlike other activities, Capoeira training was perceived as stimulating interest and commitment, serving as an opportunity to develop life skills and independence. However, alongside this enthusiasm and self-initiated participation, unexpected changes, lack of preparation, or disruptions to routine could hinder the child's ability to leave the house or participate effectively. Interviewees stressed the importance of proactive strategies such as verbal or visual priming, maintaining a consistent framework, and establishing familiarity with the instructional staff to support successful participation.

3.2.2. Integration into a Mixed Group

Programs designed for children with ASD typically focus on therapeutic or one-on-one settings, such as therapeutic horseback riding, hydrotherapy, speech therapy, or physiotherapy. While dedicated group settings allow for peer interaction among children with similar characteristics, research has shown that integrated groups, including children with typical development alongside those with ASD can significantly support the acquisition of life skills and communication through peer-mediated learning [7,52]. This subtheme presents the perspectives of interviewees regarding the challenges their children and instructors face when integrating children with ASD into mixed groups, as well as their impressions of the social environment in Capoeira classes. It also explores their views on their children's social experiences and how the core principles of Capoeira aid in successful inclusion. Interviewees emphasized the inclusive and nonjudgmental atmosphere of the group, where their children receive equal treatment, experience social successes, and develop a sense of belonging and self-expression. Capoeira's unique qualities, especially its focus on cooperation rather than competition, help create a social environment that enables children with ASD to actively participate, achieve success, and form friendships with their peers. These findings highlight the significant role of integrated settings in fostering belonging and helping children develop social skills within an inclusive environment.

Interviewees expressed a desire for their children to participate in a group-based, inclusive environment. One parent noted, "Group sports create social connections and a social circle, and that is what my child has been missing all his life" (F,12). However, they also shared concerns about integration in such settings. One interviewee remarked, "I see the children he is with, these are not children on the spectrum" (G,2), while another expressed worries about potential conflicts: "I was worried. I told the instructor: 'What if he starts fighting with the other kids? What if something does not work and he loses control? It will be hard for him'" (J,1). Some interviewees recognized the emotional challenge of placing their child in a group that differed from them: "To bring a child on the spectrum into a group of children who are not on the spectrum is already a challenge for the child" (J,8). From the interviews, it emerges that Capoeira classes are seen as socially inclusive environments. As one parent described, "He might start doing hand movements or dancing, things that typical kids do not usually do. Yes, they are very understanding, these kids" (J,8). Another parent shared, "It is his safe space, a place where they understand him, where being different is accepted. He does not feel different when he is there; that is one of his happiest things. The other kids say hello to him, he feels like one of the group" (G,4). Another noted, "They form a circle, and he steps in proudly and receives encouragement" (H,5). Interviewees also highlighted that this environment allows their children to learn appropriate behaviors from peers. One parent explained, "He tells me he can ask that kid or some of the others, if he is in a situation he does not understand. They will stop him and say, 'That is not appropriate', and he accepts it well" (F,3).

Capoeira is not a competitive sport; training for elementary-aged children emphasizes cooperation within the game. Interviewees viewed this aspect as a significant reason why Capoeira meets their children's needs, distinguishing it from other activities that are competitive: "There is no element of competition. You do your best relative to yourself." (E,8). Another said, "First of all, because it is not competitive, it is more of a social sport" (H,5). One parent remarked, "What I think works great for my child specifically is that it is not competitive. The goal is for everyone to succeed" (F,2). Another added, "I do not want him doing any competitive sport. Nothing. That would just make his anxiety worse. He had meltdowns when he lost at chess, he would be upset for days" (H,10). In Capoeira, however, the atmosphere is positive and supportive: "Here it is the opposite. If someone pulls off a move, 'Wow! That was awesome! How did he do that?' There is so much positive feedback, and it has always been that way" (F,12). Interviewees frequently described the sense of acceptance their children experience in Capoeira: "At some point, the girl from home also became the Capoeira girl. That means she feels very comfortable" (E,7). A parent shared, "My son is a bit reserved about his Autism, but there, it is like he came out of the closet. He does not hide it. The day he got the diagnosis, he walked into the studio and said, 'Hey, I am Asperger's. I am autistic...'" (F,4). Another parent noted, "I think it is the place where he feels free to express himself, to release energy and enjoy himself" (G,5). One interviewee reflected on how the social atmosphere of the group carried over beyond the class itself: "When it is our turn to drive them home, they laugh, there is this social vibe, something that usually does not happen at school. It really gives him a place to feel comfortable being himself, because he does not feel that way in most places in the world" (F,15). Interviewees indicated that Capoeira has become a meaningful social framework for their children: "Capoeira is her world, she is a part of it" (E,5). Another parent expressed, "Of course he loves it. It is like he found his place" (C,3). The parents emphasized the importance of having frameworks where their children can integrate without feeling excluded: "It means a lot because he is not supposed to feel different there. He already feels different in other areas, such as going to the park, playing with kids, or joining other activities, he needs to feel like everyone else" (G,9). These findings suggest that for the interviewees' children, Capoeira is not viewed merely as a physical activity but as a meaningful social space that allows for natural inclusion in a mixed group. As one parent put it, "In Capoeira he knows how to be with those who are better than him and those who are less good than him, without making a big deal of it, like he usually would in other situations" (C,6).

3.3. Changes Related to Being Involved in Capoeira

This theme presents interviewees' accounts of changes they observed in their children following participation in Capoeira classes, with a focus on sensory-motor functioning and social skills. It includes two selected sub-themes: improvement in sensory regulation, motor functioning, and enhancement of self-presentation and social communication.

3.3.1. Improvement in Sensory Regulation and Motor Functioning

This sub-theme presents the interviewees' observations of changes in their children following participation in Capoeira classes, specifically regarding their ability to cope with external stimuli, regulate sensory input, perceive their bodies in space, and improve motor development. According to the interviewees, Capoeira had a positive impact on their children's sensory regulation, evident in their improved responses to external stimuli, increased bodily awareness, and heightened calmness after training sessions. The music in Capoeira classes was viewed as a significant factor in enhancing auditory regulation and fostering a sense of social belonging.

Interviewees considered Capoeira a major contributor to their children's motor development, noting reduced clumsiness and notable improvements in coordination, balance, and overall movement abilities. In addition to physical progress, they emphasized that Capoeira expanded their children's movement repertoire and enhanced their sense of competence.

Most interviewees highlighted the importance of movement in responding to their children's need for physical stimulation, with one stating: "Of course, it gives him a lot in terms of sensory input. It is really important, he is a child who needs much physical stimulation, and the fitness and physical activity affect him very positively in every aspect, including his nervous system" (C,5). They described improvements in handling sensory challenges, such as wearing clothing: "In the last two times, he made an extra effort to come in long pants, which is totally uncharacteristic for him" (C,4).

Further improvement was observed in the children's ability to perceive their body's position in space and to act accordingly: "They feel their bodies better" (B,7) and "He really improved at that. For example, when he wants to do a cartwheel, in the past, if he tried, he would hit someone. Now he looks around, moves people out of the way, makes sure it is clear, and only then does it" (D,6)

Interviewees spoke about the unique role of music in supporting their children's auditory regulation. While loud environments are generally perceived as stressful or overwhelming, the music in Capoeira sessions was experienced differently: "There are

Capoeira songs he really likes" (G,2). One parent noted, "Usually, when there is noise, lots of things, people, he wants to wear headphones and be alone. Moreover, he usually stands at the side. That is what happened when we got there at first. But as soon as the music started, he took off the headphones and went in" (B,4). Another shared, "I can go with him to a family event, and he cannot stand the noise. But here, he is okay with the noise" (H, 6). It seems that the simple musical patterns played by participants themselves created a unique sense of belonging: "When they all stand and play music together, he really feels part of something, something he feels equal in. He feels like he is in rhythm with everyone. He does not experience that in other places" (C,4). Interviewees emphasized the significant motor improvements their children experienced through Capoeira, particularly given the motor challenges typically associated with ASD: "For my child, who is clumsy and not very physically active, it is great. It is exactly what he needs" (I,8); "His motor skills and physical abilities improved" (D,6) and "We saw his coordination improve. We noticed his body becoming smarter, with fewer injuries and bumping into things less, even when spinning" (A,3).

These improvements were evident in everyday functional tasks as well: "Now when he runs, he does not fall. I can see him doing things in a much more organized way" (B,5). Beyond physical improvement, interviewees reported that Capoeira greatly enhanced their children's confidence and sense of capability: "He enjoys it, he gets really excited if he suddenly manages to do a cartwheel" (A,4); "It gives him confidence and something to be proud of" (D,6). Additionally, Capoeira enabled children to engage in other movement-based activities: "It suddenly opened us up to a whole new world of body control that just did not exist before" (A,3); "This year, I signed him up for hip hop, and I am sure he would not have been able to do that if he had not gone through a year of Capoeira" (B,5). Interviewees also noted a sense of calmness in their children after Capoeira sessions: "When he comes out of there, it is like he took a breath" (B,5); "She comes back much more relaxed" (E,8).

3.3.2. Improvement in Self-Presentation, Understanding Others, and Social Communication

This sub-theme discusses the interviewees' reflections on the changes they observed in their children's self-presentation and communication skills after participating in Capoeira. The findings suggest that interviewees view Capoeira as an impactful tool that has significantly enhanced their children's social communication abilities, allowing them to present themselves positively and confidently to others. Through their membership in an inclusive community, showcasing personal skills, and engaging in teaching roles, children developed greater self-confidence and improved their ability to initiate social interactions. The movement-based interactions at the core of Capoeira were described as fostering awareness of others and enhancing adaptive communication skills. Interviewees highlighted Capoeira's contribution to developing cognitive flexibility and adaptability in dynamic social situations, noting that the skills learned in Capoeira present a carry-over and extend beyond the class applying to broader social contexts.

Interviewees expressed that Capoeira became a significant aspect of their children's identities: "Whenever someone asks him what he does in the afternoon, he says, 'I do Capoeira'" (H,3). They described how Capoeira's visual symbols, like the training uniform, act as tools for connection: "If he sees someone wearing a Capoeira shirt outside, he'll go straight over to talk to him, saying, 'I do Capoeira too; I play it too'" (C,4). Interviewees reported that their children use Capoeira skills to connect with others: "When we are in an open place with other people, he almost always demonstrates Capoeira moves, it gives him something positive to engage with and to present himself through" (C,5). They also noted increased social openness and a greater ability to engage with others in everyday situations: "I see he is more open, if someone talks to him, he does not shut down" (B,6). This improvement was linked to a rise in the children's self-confidence: "His confidence has significantly improved, he used to be very shy. Now he approaches other kids without any problem at all" (D,6).

Activities typical to Capoeira were experienced as supportive in understanding others' feelings: "There was a strong emphasis on whether your partner is ready, making eye contact. He knows how to look and wait to see if the other person is ready. That he can ask, 'Are you ready?'" (A,3); "In Capoeira, he has the opportunity to invite another person to practice or play, to understand boundaries, knowing when it is appropriate. You are doing something that reflects onto the other person, and you have to anticipate their movements while allowing them to anticipate yours. You are across from them, but not against them. It strengthens reciprocity, which he, as a child with ASD, really struggles with" (C,7).

The mutuality embedded in Capoeira was described as a catalyst for developing essential skills for communicative interaction: "There is a kind of dialog in Capoeira with the person you are with" (D,5); "It is like a type of interaction, only more movement-based" (I,9); "The whole structure of Capoeira, I feel like it gives him more cognitive flexibility. He understands that he has to go with the flow of the other person, for example, he has to duck so the kick passes over him. I actually see it as a metaphor for real-world relationships and interpersonal dynamics" (F,8).

Interviewees also shared how their children used Capoeira experiences to support others: "His brother was terrified, and he used Capoeira to show him how you train, try, try again, until you succeed, until you overcome the fear" (C,5). They expressed their impression of improvements in their children's behavior toward others: "I see how he acts toward others and how he eats, he has become more patient with other kids" (F,15). Interviewees spoke of their children's growing desire to share and teach what they have learned: "Sometimes he even offers to teach a little to younger kids" (C,5); "She likes to talk, demonstrate, and explain things to kids, she enjoys teaching" (E,6).

Opportunities to take on instructional roles were described as empowering moments: "The instructor uses her sometimes to demonstrate, and she feels responsible and committed, it boosts her confidence" (E,6). They emphasized the importance of the skills developed through instructional experience: "He was given the responsibility of being an assistant instructor, and that took him one step forward. Until then, he did not even know how to interact with little kids" (F,10).

3.4. Summary of the Findings

Through interviews with parents, four primary domains of functioning were identified in which their children exhibited notable changes following participation in Capoeira: motor functioning, sensory regulation, social communication, and sense of belonging. Parents reported advancements in their children's ability to manage external stimuli, enhanced bodily awareness concerning spatial orientation, decreased motor clumsiness, and improvements in coordination, balance, and overall movement capabilities. The incorporation of music within Capoeira was recognized as a significant factor in facilitating auditory regulation and strengthening the children's sense of social belonging.

In the area of social communication, parents observed improvements in their children's ability to initiate interactions, elevated self-confidence, and heightened awareness of others' emotional and social cues. Parents described Capoeira as a practice that cultivates cognitive flexibility and adaptability to dynamic social contexts, with the social skills acquired during training having a carryover effect, being applied outside of the class environment. Additionally, participation in Capoeira was noted to inspire a distinctive sense of motivation in the children. This was evident in their cooperation during preparation, their demonstration of independence upon entering class, and their ability to engage in the activity without requiring continuous support.

Another significant factor identified was the supportive social environment within the Capoeira group, which naturally facilitated the children's integration into a mixed setting. The inclusive atmosphere and equitable treatment contributed to positive social experiences, reinforced a sense of belonging, and encouraged the development of peer relationships, emphasizing cooperation over competition.

4. Discussion

The current study set out to explore the effect of Capoeira training on children with ASD. This qualitative pilot study is based on ten in-depth interviews with parents of children with ASD who participate in Capoeira classes. The aim was to explore the contributions of Capoeira across various domains, including motor and physical benefits, social skills development, experiences in mixed training groups, influences on executive functions, due to the activity. The significance of this study lies in its contribution to the limited understanding of Capoeira as a movement-based and social intervention for children with ASD, a topic that remains underexplored in the research literature. The findings suggest that Capoeira may positively impact all examined domains, with the most significant improvements observed in motor and social skills. Emerging evidence indicates that interventions focused on motor functioning may have broader positive effects on core symptoms of ASD, including social interaction, information processing, and executive functions [14,15]. According to parents' reports, the findings of this study support this assertion by presenting evidence of enhancements in movement abilities, sensory regulation, cognitive flexibility, functional independence, motivation, social communication, and social initiative. These results highlight Capoeira's potential as an integrated model that combines physical activity and social intervention.

From a motor perspective, interviewees reported that their children showed improvements in coordination, spatial body awareness, balance, and a reduction in falls. Additionally, they observed increased physical strength and a broader range of movement. These findings are consistent with a previous study [53], which highlighted the significant contribution of martial arts to the development of motor skills among children with ASD. The results suggest that participation in Capoeira enhanced the children's awareness of their body position in space, contributing to improved movement control, collision avoidance, sensory regulation, and the ability to perform movements in greater synchrony with the surrounding environment. Interviewees noted a significant reduction in motor clumsiness, including fewer collisions with objects and fewer falls and injuries. They also described greater bodily awareness, such as being mindful of their surroundings before attempting a cartwheel.

One of the distinctive aspects of Capoeira is its emphasis on reciprocal movement-based interactions, such as movement imitation and partner-based activity. These interactions require spatial awareness and promote motor synchronization. In Capoeira, children who struggle with spatial perception or motor coordination had the opportunity to explore adapted execution strategies while being encouraged to cooperate with their peers.

Additionally, Capoeira was found to expand the children's movement repertoire, thereby not only supporting motor functioning but also contributing to developing body awareness and a sense of competence. Interviewees described improvements in self-esteem, feelings of pride, and self-confidence, emphasizing the unique nature of Capoeira in offering a non-competitive opportunity for success based on personal progress.

In the domain of sensory regulation, the study points to the contribution of Capoeira participation in improving children's sensory self-regulation. This was reflected in better responses to external stimuli, increased body sensory awareness, and better management of internal tension. Movement during Capoeira training served as a regulatory tool, particularly for children with heightened needs for physical stimulation. Interviewees reported a heightened sense of calm following Capoeira sessions and described the training as a means for their children to release tension and regulate the elevated levels of physiological arousal often characteristic of some children with ASD. Similar sensory improvements following physical activity interventions have also been documented in other studies [54,55], especially when the intervention involved vestibular-related movements similar to those practiced in Capoeira [56].

Furthermore, the findings indicate that the music used during Capoeira sessions contributed to the children's sensory regulation, particularly among those with heightened sensitivity to noise. This outcome aligns with previous findings demonstrating that music can support sensory regulation and reduce auditory overload in children with ASD [57,58]. Moreover, music played a central role in strengthening the children's sense of social belonging. This effect is further supported by studies showing that participation in musical activities helps foster social bonding and a sense of inclusion within a group [59,60].

A common characteristic observed in children with ASD is difficulty transitioning between activities [2] and challenges in preparing for these activities [61]. The findings of the current study revealed a notable contrast between the difficulties these children faced when preparing for various activities and their high motivation and exceptional independence when preparing for Capoeira training. They also exhibited positive anticipation regarding their attendance and participation, which seems to be uniquely associated with Capoeira. Entry into the activity was found to be a significant phase in the integration process, during which the children showed initiative and autonomy, with little to no need for ongoing support. It appears that the structured and consistent framework of the training sessions provided a sense of security, reducing resistance to change. Specifically, priming, schedule consistency, and familiarity with instructors played vital roles in easing their transition into the activity.

In the social domain, the study highlights the unique contribution of Capoeira to developing social skills and a sense of belonging. Unlike most existing interventions, typically in one-on-one settings where the child mainly interacts with a therapist, Capoeira provides a natural group framework for social skills practice within a structured and supportive environment. Integration into a mixed group enabled the children to practice communicative skills while forming organic social connections with peers within the Capoeira sessions, as well as extending their social skills to social situations unrelated to the Capoeira training (in family gatherings and with small children). These findings reinforce previous research demonstrating that participation in integrated group settings contributes to acquiring life skills and improving social functioning of children with ASD [10,62].

An inclusive, accepting social climate was identified as a key factor in successful integration. Interviewees emphasized that the Capoeira environment was characterized by social acceptance and encouragement, which allowed the children to feel part of the group without being seen as different. This setting provided an opportunity to practice and improve social skills in real time while learning appropriate behaviors and understanding social norms. Compared to special education settings, where group sizes tend to be smaller and more structured, participation in larger and more diverse groups contributed to the children's ability to adapt to dynamic social environments outside the Capoeira setting and within daily situations.

The practice of Capoeira, commonly known as "the game," focuses on reciprocal movement interactions and has been shown to enhance nonverbal communication skills. Activities such as movement imitation, maintaining a shared rhythm, and coordinating with a partner enhanced the ability of children with ASD to interpret and respond to social cues while fostering awareness of others' emotional and physical states. Additionally, the absence of competition emerged as a significant advantage. While many sports activities focus on achievement and winning, Capoeira encourages cooperation, mutual empowerment, and personal success. The children learned to celebrate the achievements of others and to enjoy the process itself without experiencing the pressure or frustration often associated with losing. Interviewees noted that this characteristic reduced social anxiety and improved the children's ability to integrate into the group without fear of failure.

In addition to enhancing their ability to form social connections, Capoeira empowered the children to initiate interactions within the Capoeira setting but also beyond their Capoeira group and into daily situations. The children identified themselves as "Capoeira practitioners," using the skills they had acquired to present themselves to others and establish points of connection with their environment. Actions such as demonstrating movements for peers, assisting younger children, and taking on instructional roles within the Capoeira setting strengthened their self-confidence and ability to engage in social situations.

The findings indicate that Capoeira served as a supportive framework, allowing children to develop social skills in an inclusive and nonjudgmental environment. The combination of cooperative movement activities, group support, and the absence of competition created a safe space for forming relationships, practicing communication, and strengthening the sense of social belonging.

5. Conclusions and Recommendations

The findings of the present study underscore the potential and perceived contribution of Capoeira as an integrated model of physical, behavioral, sensory and social intervention for children with ASD. Parents reported that Capoeira was perceived to enhance motor skills, sensory regulation, social skills, ease of transitions, self-confidence, and a sense of belonging. It offers a unique framework that is non-competitive and instead based on cooperation and mutual empowerment.

Capoeira was described as providing motor benefits through perceived improvements in coordination, balance, and proprioceptive awareness, and a reduction in motor clumsiness. In the social domain, Capoeira was reported to provide an inclusive group environment that enabled the practice of nonverbal communication, social initiative, and adaptability to changing situations, while reinforcing the children's sense of belonging and self-worth.

These findings align with emerging evidence in the research literature, pointing to a possible link between improvements in motor functioning and gains in cognitive and social domains among children with ASD. They reinforce the understanding that motor intervention should not be viewed as an isolated goal but may contribute to broader functional outcomes. Given this understanding, it is advisable to explore the integration of Capoeira into educational and therapeutic interventions for children with ASD, especially within inclusive group settings that promote full participation with peers and in the broader community.

To enhance the success of inclusion in Capoeira specifically and in leisure activities more broadly, it is recommended that comprehensive professional training for Capoeira instructors in the field of Autism be provided, support systems tailored to the individual needs of each participant developed, and parents involved as active partners in the process. In addition, future research should examine the long-term effects of the intervention and identify the specific mechanisms that contribute to its success.

The findings of the current research suggest that in future studies regarding Capoeira and children with ASD, valid and objective outcome measures regarding individual goals (such as the goal attainment scale—GAS), sensory elements (such as the Short Sensory Profile—SSP), motor elements (such as the Movement Assessment Battery for Children—Movement ABC) and Autism severity (such as the Childhood Autism Rating Scale—CARS) should be used.

6. Limitations

The findings of this pilot study are based on interviews with parents of children with ASD, reflecting their perceptions through self-reporting. The goal of this study was to explore the full potential of content that may be beneficial for individuals with autism. However, as a qualitative pilot study, it does not permit causal inferences and given the small sample size and absence of a control group, its external validity remains limited. Therefore, it cannot be determined with certainty that the reported changes resulted directly from participation in Capoeira, as they may also be influenced by other factors, such as the child's age, their position on the Autism spectrum, or natural developmental progression.

Additionally, since no objective measures were used, and no comparison was made with a control group, this study cannot determine whether functional progress occurred specifically due to Capoeira. Recruitment via Capoeira instructors may also have introduced selection bias, as families with more positive attitudes toward Capoeira or stronger connections to the instructors may have been more likely to participate. As an exploratory pilot study, the conclusions should be understood as exploratory, pointing to possible directions for further investigation. Future quantitative research, including a control group and precise measurement tools, is essential to assess the actual contribution of Capoeira to improvements across various domains. Due to these limitations, further quantitative research is warranted to allow for the control of intervening variables such as those identified here. The study intends to pursue these directions in future investigations, after the benefits of capoeira for autism are detailed in this qualitative study.

Author Contributions: Conceptualization, R.L.-A., M.L. and L.K.; methodology, L.K.; investigation, R.L.-A.; data curation, R.L.-A.; formal analysis, R.L.-A. with guidance from L.K.; writing, original draft preparation, R.L.-A.; writing, review and editing, M.L. and L.K.; supervision, M.L. and L.K.; project administration, L.K. All authors have read and agreed to the published version of the manuscript.

Funding: This research received no external funding.

Institutional Review Board Statement: The study was conducted in accordance with the Declaration of Helsinki and approved by the Institutional Review Board of Ariel University (protocol code AU-HEA-LK 20240726, approved on 26 July 2024).

Informed Consent Statement: All participants signed a written informed consent form after the interviewer read aloud a standardized introduction. Participants were assured that their participation was voluntary, that all information shared would remain confidential and anonymous, and that they could skip questions or withdraw at any time.

Data Availability Statement: Due to the sensitive nature of the qualitative interviews and the need to preserve participant confidentiality, the data (full transcripts) are not publicly available. Summarized findings are presented in the article.

Acknowledgments: The author would like to thank the participating Capoeira instructors and centers for their assistance in facilitating access to the participating families.

Conflicts of Interest: The authors declare no conflicts of interest.

Abbreviations

The following abbreviations are used in this manuscript:

ASD	Autism Spectrum Disorder
TD	Typically Developing
SD	Standard Deviation
GAS	Goal attainment scale
SSP	Short Sensory Profile
Movement ABC	Movement Assessment Battery for Children
CARS	Childhood Autism Rating Scale

References

1. Lord, C.; Brugha, T.S.; Charman, T.; Cusack, J.; Dumas, G.; Frazier, T.; Jones, E.; Jones, R.; Pickles, A.; State, M.; et al. Autism spectrum disorder. *Nat. Rev. Dis. Primers.* **2020**, *6*, 5. [CrossRef]
2. American Psychiatric Association. *Diagnostic and Statistical Manual of Mental Disorders*, 5th ed.; American Psychiatric Publishing: Arlington, VA, USA, 2013.
3. World Health Organization. Autism Spectrum Disorders. 2023. Available online: https://www.who.int/news-room/fact-sheets/detail/Autism-spectrum-disorders (accessed on 28 June 2025).
4. World Health Organization. *International Classification of Diseases for Mortality and Morbidity Statistics*, 11th ed.; World Health Organization: Geneva, Switzerland, 2018.
5. Waizbard-Bartov, E.; Fein, D.; Lord, C.; Amaral, D.G. Autism severity and its relationship to disability. *Autism Res.* **2023**, *16*, 685–696. [CrossRef]
6. Gigliotti, F.; Giovannone, F.; Belli, A.; Sogos, C. Atypical Sensory Processing in Neurodevelopmental Disorders: Clinical Phenotypes in Preschool-Aged Children. *Children* **2024**, *11*, 875. [CrossRef]
7. Bauminger, N.; Solomon, M.; Aviezer, A.; Heung, K.; Gazit, L.; Brown, J.; Rogers, S.J. Children with Autism and Their Friends: A Multidimensional Study of Friendship in High-Functioning Autism Spectrum Disorder. *J. Abnorm. Child Psychol.* **2008**, *36*, 135–150. [CrossRef] [PubMed]
8. Bauminger, N.; Solomon, M.; Aviezer, A.; Heung, K.; Brown, J.; Rogers, S.J. Friendship in High-functioning Children with Autism Spectrum Disorder: Mixed and Non-mixed Dyads. *J. Autism Dev. Disord.* **2008**, *38*, 1211–1229. [CrossRef]
9. Bauminger-Zviely, N. *Social and Academic Abilities in Children with High-Functioning Autism Spectrum Disorders*; Guilford Press: New York, NY, USA, 2013; p. 338.
10. Mendelson, J.L.; Gates, J.A.; Lerner, M.D. Friendship in school-age boys with Autism spectrum disorders: A meta-analytic summary and developmental, process-based model. *Psychol. Bulletin.* **2016**, *142*, 601–622. [CrossRef]
11. Liu, T.; Breslin, C.M. Fine and gross motor performance of the MABC-2 by children with Autism spectrum disorder and typically developing children. *Res. Autism Spectr. Disorders.* **2013**, *7*, 1244–1249. [CrossRef]
12. Ament, K.; Mejia, A.; Buhlman, R.; Erklin, S.; Caffo, B.; Mostofsky, S.; Wodka, E. Evidence for Specificity of Motor Impairments in Catching and Balance in Children with Autism. *J. Autism Dev. Disord.* **2015**, *45*, 742–751. [CrossRef]
13. Bhat, A.N. Motor Impairment Increases in Children with Autism Spectrum Disorder as a Function of Social Communication, Cognitive and Functional Impairment, Repetitive Behavior Severity, and Comorbid Diagnoses: A SPARK Study Report. *Autism Res.* **2021**, *14*, 202–219. [CrossRef] [PubMed]
14. Ruggeri, A.; Dancel, A.; Johnson, R.; Sargent, B. The effect of motor and physical activity intervention on motor outcomes of children with Autism spectrum disorder: A systematic review. *Autism* **2020**, *24*, 544–568. [CrossRef] [PubMed]
15. Ludyga, S.; Pühse, U.; Gerber, M.; Mücke, M. Muscle strength and executive function in children and adolescents with Autism spectrum disorder. *Autism Res.* **2021**, *14*, 2555–2563. [CrossRef] [PubMed]
16. Zampella, C.J.; Wang, L.A.L.; Haley, M.; Hutchinson, A.G.; de Marchena, A. Motor Skill Differences in Autism Spectrum Disorder: A Clinically Focused Review. *Curr. Psychiatry Rep.* **2021**, *23*, 64. [CrossRef]
17. Wang, L.A.L.; Petrulla, V.; Zampella, C.J.; Waller, R.; Schultz, R.T. Gross motor impairment and its relation to social skills in Autism spectrum disorder: A systematic review and two meta-analyses. *Psychol. Bull.* **2022**, *148*, 273–300. [CrossRef]
18. Müller, A.; Bába, É.B.; Židek, P.; Lengyel, A.; Lakó, J.H.; Laoues-Czimbalmos, N.; Molnár, A.; Boda, E. The Experiences of Motor Skill Development in Children with Autism Spectrum Disorder (ASD) Reflected through Parental Responses. *Children* **2024**, *11*, 1238. [CrossRef]
19. MacDonald, M.; Lord, C.; Ulrich, D.A. The Relationship of Motor Skills and Social Communicative Skills in School-Aged Children with Autism Spectrum Disorder. *Adapt. Phys. Act. Q.* **2013**, *30*, 271–282. [CrossRef]

20. MacDonald, M.; Lord, C.; Ulrich, D.A. Motor Skills and Calibrated Autism Severity in Young Children with Autism Spectrum Disorder. *Adapt. Phys. Act. Q.* **2014**, *31*, 95–105. [CrossRef]
21. Omair, M.L. The Impact of Physical Exercise on the Overall Functioning of Children with Autism Spectrum Disorder (ASD) when Included with Non-Autistic Children Versus Segregated. Ph.D. Thesis, University of Leeds, Leeds, UK, 2020. Available online: https://etheses.whiterose.ac.uk/26985/ (accessed on 25 February 2024).
22. Rafiei Milajerdi, H.; Sheikh, M.; Najafabadi, M.G.; Saghaei, B.; Naghdi, N.; Dewey, D. The Effects of Physical Activity and Exergaming on Motor Skills and Executive Functions in Children with Autism Spectrum Disorder. *Games Health J.* **2021**, *10*, 33–42. [CrossRef] [PubMed]
23. Strofylla, G.; Charitou, S.; Asonitou, K.; Koutsouki, D. Efficacy of 6-Month Adapted Aerobic Program on Motor Proficiency, BMI and Cognitive Abilities of Students with Autism Spectrum Disorder: Three Case Reports. *Open J. Soc. Sci.* **2021**, *9*, 153–166. [CrossRef]
24. Aleksandrovic, M.; Jorgic, B.; Block, M.; Jovanovic, L. The Effects of Aquatic Activities on Physical Fitness and Aquatic Skills in Children with Autism Spectrum Disorders: A Systematic Review. *Facta Univ. Ser. Phys. Educ. Sport* **2016**, *13*, 351–362.
25. Azimigarosi, S.; Arjmandnia, A.; Mohseni Ezhei, A.; Asgari, M. Effectiveness of Hydrotherapy on Communication Skills of Children with Autism Spectrum Disorder: A Single Case Study. *Q. J. Child Ment. Health* **2020**, *6*, 35–50. [CrossRef]
26. Battaglia, G.; Agrò, G.; Cataldo, P.; Palma, A.; Alesi, M. Influence of a Specific Aquatic Program on Social and Gross Motor Skills in Adolescents with Autism Spectrum Disorders: Three Case Reports. *J. Funct. Morphol. Kinesiol.* **2019**, *4*, 27. [CrossRef] [PubMed]
27. Farahani, H.; Elmieh, A.; Samadi, S.A.; Shabani, R. The Effect of Hydrotherapy on Serum Serotonin in Autistic Children. *Sport Physiol. Manag. Investig.* **2020**, *12*, 49–59.
28. Lopes, J.; de Oliveira Camilo, A.; Nascimento, D.K.; de Mattos, G.P.; Stockler, G.A.; Mazur, T.B.; de Andrade, G.F. Efetividade da equoterapia na abordagem do transtorno do espectro autista: Revisão sistemática de ensaios clínicos/Effectiveness of hippotherapy in Autism spectrum disorder approach: A systematic review of clinical trials. *Braz. J. Health Rev.* **2021**, *4*, 27627–27641. [CrossRef]
29. Maresca, G.; Portaro, S.; Naro, A.; Crisafulli, R.; Raffa, A.; Scarcella, I.; Aliberti, B.; Gemelli, G.; Calabrò, R.S. Hippotherapy in neurodevelopmental disorders: A narrative review focusing on cognitive and behavioral outcomes. *Appl. Neuropsychol. Child* **2022**, *11*, 553–560. [CrossRef]
30. Gehricke, J.-G.; Chan, J.; Farmer, J.G.; Fenning, R.M.; Steinberg-Epstein, R.; Misra, M.; Parker, R.A.; Neumeyer, A.M. Physical activity rates in children and adolescents with Autism spectrum disorder compared to the general population. *Res. Autism Spectr. Disord.* **2020**, *70*, 101490. [CrossRef] [PubMed]
31. Herrmann, C.; Bretz, K.; Kühnis, J.; Seelig, H.; Keller, R.; Ferrari, I. Connection between Social Relationships and Basic Motor Competencies in Early Childhood. *Children* **2021**, *8*, 53. [CrossRef]
32. Wang, S.; Chen, D.; Yang, Y.; Zhu, L.; Xiong, X.; Chen, A. Effectiveness of physical activity interventions for core symptoms of Autism spectrum disorder: A systematic review and meta-analysis. *Autism Res.* **2023**, *16*, 1811–1824. [CrossRef]
33. Tse, A. Brief Report: Impact of a Physical Exercise Intervention on Emotion Regulation and Behavioral Functioning in Children with Autism Spectrum Disorder. *J. Autism Dev. Disord.* **2020**, *50*, 4191–4198. [CrossRef]
34. Estrugo, Y.; Bar Yehuda, S.; Bauminger-Zviely, N. Pathways to peer interaction in ASD and TD through individual and dyadic joint-action motor abilities. *Front. Psychol.* **2023**, *14*, 1234376. [CrossRef]
35. Estrugo, Y.; Bar Yehuda, S.; Bauminger-Zviely, N. Motor, cognitive, and socio-cognitive mechanisms explaining social skills in Autism and typical development. *Autism Res.* **2024**, *17*, 2319–2332. [CrossRef] [PubMed]
36. Bremer, E.; Crozier, M.; Lloyd, M. A systematic review of the behavioural outcomes following exercise interventions for children and youth with Autism spectrum disorder. *Autism* **2016**, *20*, 899–915. [CrossRef]
37. Phung, J.N.; Goldberg, W.A. Mixed martial arts training improves social skills and lessens problem behaviors in boys with Autism Spectrum Disorder. *Res. Autism Spectr. Disord.* **2021**, *83*, 101758. [CrossRef]
38. MacLennan, J. "To Build a Beautiful Dialogue": Capoeira as Contradiction. *J. Int. Intercult. Commun.* **2011**, *4*, 146–162. [CrossRef]
39. de Miranda, M.B. Jogo de capoeira: When actors play a 'physical dialogue'. *Theatre Danc. Perform. Train.* **2012**, *3*, 178–191. [CrossRef]
40. Barros, N.; Branco, M.; Catela, D. The basic foundations of capoeira' learning: Preliminary evaluation of a formative program. *Rev. Artes Marciales Asiát* **2019**, *14*, 9–20. [CrossRef]
41. Moreira, S.R.; Carvalho, F.O.; de Moraes, J.F.; da Silva Carvalho, R.G.; de Araújo, R.C.; Teixeira-Araújo, A.A.; Okano, A.H. Eight weeks of Capoeira progressive training program increases flexibility of beginners. *Sport. Sci. Health* **2016**, *12*, 329–337. [CrossRef]
42. Moreira, S.R.; Teixeira-Araujo, A.A.; Dos Santos, A.O.; Simões, H.G. Ten weeks of capoeira progressive training improved cardiovascular parameters in male practitioners. *J. Sports Med. Phys. Fit.* **2017**, *57*, 289–298. [CrossRef]
43. Teixeira, B.V.; da Mota, C.G. A prática da capoeira por pessoas com síndrome de Down: Uma revisão da literatura. *Acta Fisiátrica* **2018**, *25*, 40–45. [CrossRef]

44. Fernandes, V.R.; Ribeiro, M.L.S.; Araújo, N.B.; Mota, N.B.; Ribeiro, S.; Diamond, A.; Deslandes, A.C. Effects of Capoeira on children's executive functions: A randomized controlled trial. *Ment. Health Phys. Act.* **2022**, *22*, 100451. [CrossRef]
45. Monteiro-Junior, R.S.; da Rocha Fernandes, V.; Pereira Oliva, H.N.; Prudente, T.P.; Ribeiro, S. Capoeira and brain function: Hypotheses and perspectives from a systematic review. *Ment. Health Phys. Act.* **2025**, *28*, 100678. [CrossRef]
46. Amitay, G. Capoeira clubs as inclusive and therapeutic communities for youth and young adults experiencing social exclusion. *Int. J. Qual. Stud. Educ.* **2022**, *37*, 213–229. [CrossRef]
47. da Silva, R.F.; em Tea, E. Capoeira como espaço de inclusão e melhoria da autoestima e interação de estudantes com TEA: Capoeira as a space for inclusion and im-provement of the self-esteem and interaction of students with TEA. *Eur. J. Multidiscip. Res.* **2020**, *1*, 14–30.
48. Hacicaferoğlu, S.; Hacicaferoğlu, B.; Kayhan, R.F.; Doğanay, G. Examining the effect of Capoeira on socialization in terms of some variables. *Int. J. Sport Exerc. Train. Sci.—IJSETS* **2017**, *3*, 206–213. [CrossRef]
49. Momartin, S.; Miranda Eda, S.; Aroche, J.; Coello, M. Resilience building through alternative intervention: 'STARTTS "Project Bantu Capoeira Angola"'; On the road to recovery. *Intervention* **2018**, *16*, 154. [CrossRef]
50. Kiger, M.E.; Varpio, L. Thematic analysis of qualitative data: AMEE Guide No. 131. *Med. Teach.* **2020**, *42*, 846–854. [CrossRef] [PubMed]
51. Yerys, B.E.; Wallace, G.L.; Harrison, B.; Celano, M.J.; Giedd, J.N.; Kenworthy, L.E. Set-shifting in children with Autism spectrum disorders. *Autism* **2009**, *13*, 523–538. [CrossRef] [PubMed]
52. Tarr, B.; Launay, J.; Dunbar, R.I. Music and social bonding: "self-other" merging and neurohormonal mechanisms. *Front. Psychol.* **2014**, *5*, 1096. [CrossRef]
53. Amonkar, N.; Su, W.C.; Bhat, A.N.; Srinivasan, S.M. Effects of creative movement therapies on social communication, behavioral-affective, sensorimotor, cognitive, and functional participation skills of individuals with Autism spectrum disorder: A systematic review. *Front. Psychiatry* **2021**, *12*, 722874. [CrossRef] [PubMed]
54. Schaaf, R.C.; Benevides, T.; Mailloux, Z.; Faller, P.; Hunt, J.; Van Hooydonk, E.; Freeman, R.; Leiby, B.; Sendecki, J.; Kelly, D. An Intervention for Sensory Difficulties in Children with Autism: A Randomized Trial. *J. Autism Dev. Disord.* **2014**, *44*, 1493–1506. [CrossRef]
55. Yuan, H.-L.; Lai, C.Y.Y.; Wong, M.N.K.; Kwong, T.C.; Choy, Y.S.; Mung, S.W.Y.; Chan, C.C.H. Interventions for Sensory Over-Responsivity in Individuals with Autism Spectrum Disorder: A Narrative Review. *Children* **2022**, *9*, 1584. [CrossRef]
56. Wen, L.; Wu, Z. The impact of sensory integration based sports training on motor and social skill development in children with Autism spectrum disorder. *Sci. Rep.* **2025**, *15*, 19974. [CrossRef] [PubMed]
57. Applewhite, B.; Cankaya, Z.; Heiderscheit, A.; Himmerich, H. A Systematic Review of Scientific Studies on the Effects of Music in People with or at Risk for Autism Spectrum Disorder. *Int. J. Environ. Res. Public Health* **2022**, *19*, 5150. [CrossRef] [PubMed]
58. Ke, X.; Song, W.; Yang, M.; Li, J.; Liu, W. Effectiveness of music therapy in children with Autism spectrum disorder: A systematic review and meta-analysis. *Front. Psychiatry* **2022**, *13*, 905113. [CrossRef]
59. Lagasse, B.; Manning, R.; Crasta, J.; Gavin, W.; Davies, P. Assessing the Impact of Music Therapy on Sensory Gating and Attention in Children with Autism: A Pilot and Feasibility Study. *J. Music. Ther.* **2019**, *56*, 287–314. [CrossRef] [PubMed]
60. Savage, P.E.; Loui, P.; Tarr, B.; Schachner, A.; Glowacki, L.; Mithen, S.; Fitch, W.T. Music as a coevolved system for social bonding. *Behav. Brain Sci.* **2021**, *44*, e59. [CrossRef]
61. Schaaf, R.C.; Toth-Cohen, S.; Johnson, S.L.; Outten, G.; Benevides, T.W. The everyday routines of families of children with Autism: Examining the impact of sensory processing difficulties on the family. *Autism* **2011**, *15*, 373–389. [CrossRef]
62. Kasari, C.; Dean, M.; Kretzmann, M.; Shih, W.; Orlich, F.; Whitney, R.; Landa, R.; Lord, C.; King, B. Children with Autism spectrum disorder and social skills groups at school: A randomized trial comparing intervention approach and peer composition. *Child Psychol. Psychiatry* **2016**, *57*, 171–179. [CrossRef]

children

Article

Balance and Coordination Improvements in Children and Adolescents with Autism Spectrum Disorder (ASD), Resulting from a Hydrotherapy Intervention

Meir Lotan [1,*] and Marc Weiss [1,2]

1 Physical Therapy Department, Faculty of Health Sciences, Ariel University, Ariel 40700, Israel; marc.weiss@msmail.ariel.ac.il
2 Buot Hydrotherapy Center, Ashdod 7724004, Israel
* Correspondence: meirlo@ariel.ac.il

Highlights

What are the main findings?

- Hydrotherapy intervention improves motor challenges in children and adolescents with ASD.
- Hydrotherapy intervention improves communication, independence, as well as other core issues in children and adolescents with ASD.

What are the implications of the main findings?

- Hydrotherapy should be considered as a common therapeutic possibility for children and adolescents with ASD.

Abstract

Background/objective: Despite the fact that almost 87% of children with Autism Spectrum Disorder (ASD) have physical coordination issues, motor skills are not the primary concern when ASD is diagnosed. An aquatic environment can provide multisensory stimuli that might assist these children; however, studies related to hydrotherapy with children with ASD have not yet examined whether this environment has an effect on balance and coordination. Methods: A control vs. research group examined the effect of a weekly, three-month hydrotherapy program on the balance and coordination abilities of male children and adolescents diagnosed with high-functioning ASD. Children (N = 22) between the ages of 6 and 17 years (mean: 8.4 ± 2.4), participated in this study. Each participant's coordination and balance abilities were evaluated using the Movement Assessment Battery for Children-Second Edition (M-ABC-II). The initial evaluation (test one) was repeated (test two) after two months to establish improvement prior to intervention. The final evaluation (test three) was conducted at intervention termination. Individual functional goals were set for each patient using the Goal Attainment Scale (GAS). Results: No improvement was noted within the pre-intervention period (between tests one and two), yet there was a statistically significant improvement in the M-ABC-II Total Test score ($p = 0.0133$), in Manual Dexterity ($p = 0.0181$), and balance ($p = 0.0053$) post-intervention, between tests two and three. The mean GAS score for this study was 52.1, suggesting the achievement of prespecified functional goals. Conclusions: This study demonstrated a positive impact of a 12-week hydrotherapy program on balance and coordination and manual dexterity among children with ASD. A positive impact was also noted in patients' individual functional abilities.

 https://doi.org/10.3390/children13010094

Keywords: autism spectrum disorder (ASD); autism; Hydrotherapy; balance; coordination; movement assessment battery for children -second edition (M-ABC-II); goal attainment scale (GAS)

1. Introduction

Autism Spectrum Disorder (ASD) is a complex developmental condition that poses motor challenges, as well as the better-known social/emotional, speech and nonverbal communication challenges [1]. The incidence of ASD is constantly rising, with incidence reported recently by the Centers for Disease Control (CDC) at 1:31 children [2]. Since the main focus of therapeutic interventions in ASD is on behavioral, emotional, and communicational issues, scarce research has been conducted to date on the influence of aquatic treatments on challenges in the motor realm. Furthermore, studies related to hydrotherapy that have been performed in children diagnosed with ASD have not examined the effect of hydrotherapy on balance and/or coordination [3–9].

Most children with ASD (86.9%) have physical coordination issues [10]. Despite such high prevalence, motor skills are not the primary concern when ASD is diagnosed, and only 31.6% of children with ASD receive physical therapy services [11]. Children and adults with ASD (aged from 7 to 32 years) have shown poor upper-limb coordination during visuomotor and manual dexterity tasks, and poor lower-limb coordination during tasks requiring balance, agility, and speed [12]. Difficulties in motor skills include poor upper-limb and lower-limb coordination, including bilateral coordination and visuomotor coordination [12]. Moreover, the literature suggests that there are correlations between the severity of motor difficulties presented by children with ASD, and the severity of ASD; therefore, children with poorer motor skills have greater deficits in social communicative skills [13]. The impact of motor difficulties in childhood may also contribute to reduced participation with peers during play and sports, and, as a result, may further hamper social interaction and social development [11,14]. Bhat et al. propose that early motor delays within the first two years of life may contribute to the social impairments of children with ASD [12]. These primary and secondary difficulties highlight the need for early, intensive, appropriate therapeutic intervention for this group of children. Therefore, motor impairments should be addressed early, with the use of timely assessments and appropriate and effective interventions [12]. One of the suggested therapeutic approaches for this group of patients is hydrotherapy.

Hydrotherapy is the use of water in any of its forms (water, ice, steam) for health promotion or treatment of various diseases. It is one of the naturopathic treatment modalities used widely in ancient cultures, including India, Egypt, China, as well as others [3]. Hydrotherapy incorporates exercises (active and passive) performed in water and takes advantage of the effects of water on the body (e.g., temperature, density, buoyancy, hydrostatic pressure).

According to the American Physical Therapy Association [3], hydrotherapy provides stability to the patient's body, enhanced ease of movement, enhanced proprioceptive awareness, and enhanced sensory feedback. Hydrotherapy's positive effects on the human body in populations other than ASD were found to include relaxation [15,16], improved ability to participate in training exercises, high-intensity exercise and greater comfort [17,18], motor control, and functional mobility and swimming skills [19,20].

An aquatic environment provides stability and uniform sensorial support, allowing ease of movement and improved body awareness [5,11], which in turn allows an individual to practice important movement skills with fewer body constraints. Therefore, children

https://doi.org/10.3390/children13010094

with movement difficulties may experience more success in attaining movement skills in an aquatic environment [11].

Studies on children with ASD show increasing evidence that hydrotherapy may be effective in improving core elements of ASD, such as social interactions, communication skills, sensory processing, behavior [5,7], as well as aquatic skills [5,8,9], physical fitness [11], object control, and locomotor skills [6]. Yet, only few of those studies focused on motor elements such as balance [21], yet most of the recent meta-analysis performed in relation to motor achievements related to hydrotherapy intervention with children with ASD report methodological issues and heterogeneity between different studies, enabling but little scientific rigor regarding out-of-water motor achievements [22,23].

The most reliable assessments [24] and commonly used assessment tools for motor assessment in children with neurotypical development [25], which also include the most psychometrically suitable motor assessment tools for children with ASD [26] are: Movement Assessment Battery for Children—(MABC-2) [24,26], Test of Gross Motor Development, Second Edition—(TGMD-2) [24,27], Peabody Developmental Motor Scales, Second Edition—(PDMS-2) [28] and Bruininks–Oseretsky Test of Motor Proficiency, Second edition—(BOT-2) [29]. All of these scales have been found with good psychometric values for neurotypical children as well as for children with disabilities [26,29] and have been previously used in scientific papers assessing motor abilities of children with ASD.

PDMS-2 (aged 0–7 Y) and TGMD-2 (3–10 Y) could not be used as they do not cover the full age range of possible participants within the current study (6–16 Y). The BOT-2 covers the age range of participants within the current study but requires 45-60 min to be fully administered [29], while MABC-2 takes only minutes to be administered [29]. Therefore, the MABC-2 was selected to be the preferred motor scale in the current study as it covers the full age range of the participants (6–16 Y) and is the most frequently used by examiners to test the gross motor performance in children [24].

While current research suggests that hydrotherapy can improve gross motor skills among children diagnosed with ASD [3–5,7–9], these studies focused mainly on aquatic skills while mostly ignoring issues related to transfer of aquatic intervention into land skills, such as balance and coordination. Therefore, we found this topic appropriate for the current research project.

2. Methods

Ethical approval statements: The study was conducted in accordance with the Declaration of Helsinki. The research was conducted after receiving ethical permission from the Ariel University IRB (AU-HEA-ML-20231011) on 11 October 2023and authorization from the Buot hydrotherapy center's management; all parents and some of the participants (Diagnosed with high-functioning ASD) signed an informed consent form.

Research goal: Examine the effect of a once weekly three-month hydrotherapy program on the balance and coordination abilities of children and adolescents with ASD.

Research hypothesis: A three-month hydrotherapy program will significantly improve the motor skills of balance and coordination among children and adolescents diagnosed with ASD.

Methods: This study comprised a control group (children not receiving hydrotherapy intervention) and the same children served as their own comparison group (study group), which was identical (same children) to the study group, thereby eliminating clinical heterogeneity typical of those with ASD as they both were the same individuals, once measured without the therapeutic intervention (control), and once after receiving the therapeutic intervention (study group). The pre–post method, which uses the participants as their own control group (with and without treatment), is consistent with previous stud-

 https://doi.org/10.3390/children13010094

ies conducted on this population and accounts for considerable inter-variability between ASD patients [4,5,7,8,13].

Participants: The study included 22 male participants between the ages of 6 and 17 years (mean, 8.4 ± 2.4), who were diagnosed with high-functioning ASD, according to the DSM-5 (level 1) or ADOS-II (mild ASD), and ability to understand simple instructions and comply with these instructions during a hydrotherapy session. (see Table 1 for demographic details and scores.)

Table 1. General data—all participants.

Participant #	Age in Months	SRS Score	GAS Goals	Initial M-ABC-II Total Score	Post-Intervention M-ABC-II Total Score
1	187	122		1	1
2	99	104	45.4	1	5
3	140	77	59.1	0.5	0.5
4	88	67	50	0.5	1
5	98		63.7	5	37
6	76	53	50	1	2
7	128	113	59.1	0.1	1
8	78	104	31.9	0.1	0.1
9	73	70	64.5	0.5	16
10	118	59	39.1	0.1	0.1
11	72	47	50	0.1	1
12	117	96	68.1	5	9
13	75	70	50	0.5	9
14	73	133	60.9	2	37
15	92	70	42.8	0.1	0.1
16	107	71	50	1	1
17	84	114	54.6	0.1	0.1
18	69	88	45.4	1	16
19	124	113	59.1	2	9
20	150	72	42.8	0.5	0.1
21	86	89	68.1	0.5	0.5
22	89	96	40.9	2	9
Mean	101.05	85.76	52.17	1.12	7.07
Min–Max (±SD)	189–69 (±59)	133–47 (±43)	68.1–31.9 (±18.1)	5–0.1 (±2.5)	37–0.1 (±18.5)
Index	SRS—Social Responsiveness Scale II		GAS—Goal attainment scaling		
	M-ABC-II—Movement Assessment Battery for Children—Second Edition				

Inclusion and Exclusion Criteria

Inclusion Criteria: Male children (aged 6–17 years) diagnosed with ASD according to ADOS or ADI-R, demonstrating full cooperation and presenting an average M-ABC-II score below the 15th percentile (see extended explanation below), and able to understand and follow instructions.

Exclusion Criteria: Children who suffer from an additional severe chronic medical disorder in addition to ASD (e.g., neurological, psychiatric, metabolic, genetic, or orthopedic disorder), children with hearing impairments as a result of acquired trauma, children who take anti-anxiety medications, children in the middle of physical therapy or any type of intervention meant to improve balance and coordination (including hippotherapy and hydrotherapy), children who have difficulty cooperating and could not fully cooperate with the researcher's instructions, and children presenting fear of water (based on the Humphries Assessment of Aquatic Readiness [HAAR] measure).

3. Procedure

Recruitment and Baseline Assessments: (presented visually in Figure 1): Only children officially diagnosed with ASD were recruited to participate in the study. This was performed by advertising on social media platforms, through the social services departments

https://doi.org/10.3390/children13010094

in the municipalities of the cities Ashdod and Ashkelon, with the help of colleagues, and directly through Buot Hydrotherapy Center.

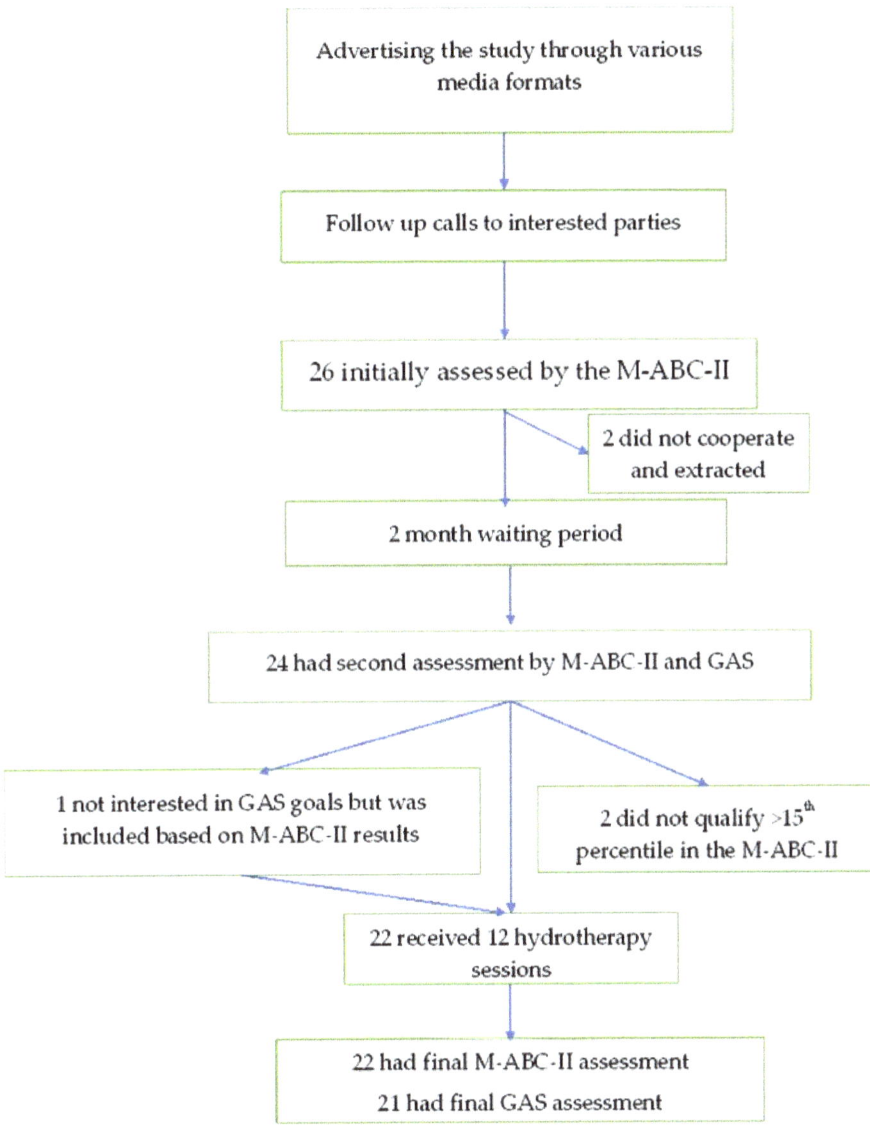

Figure 1. Flowchart of recruitment and intervention.

After initial contact was made, interested families signed informed consent forms, and an initial evaluation using the M-ABC-II was chosen to determine a baseline score. All evaluations were conducted by the researcher (the first author, M.W.) in the offices at Buot Center. After the initial evaluation, a date was immediately set for the second evaluation two months later. The time frame of a two-month waiting period, where no intervention was conducted, was chosen based on the clinical experience of the authors conducting the study in order to establish a comparison between the control (no treatment) and the study (with treatment). On completion of the second evaluation, the scores were averaged

 https://doi.org/10.3390/children13010094

to establish a steady baseline score, percentile rank, and level of function. Participants were included in the research study if their average score was below the 15th percentile on M-ABC-II. Personal goals were established, while consulting the participants and their families, using the Goal Attainment Scale (GAS) after the baseline assessments and before the commencement of treatment sessions in the water. All evaluations were recorded for review by an independent and objective professional (an occupational therapist who has many years of experience implementing the M-ABC-II).

Each participant received a three-month hydrotherapy weekly intervention, as was performed in previous intervention protocols with children with ASD (4,8,9), with each therapeutic session lasting 30 min and divided into two equal parts, focusing on the two specific aspects of the study goals (balance and motor coordination). Minor adaptations were made to accommodate the individual needs and interests of each participant. In each therapeutic section, each exercise moved from a lower to a higher difficulty level after the participant had achieved control over the previous level (see Supplemental Materials—Therapeutic protocol of the hydrotherapy program).

The treatment was conducted by the Primary Investigator (PI. MW), an experienced pediatric physical therapist working as a licensed hydro-therapist. Each participant was exposed to an intervention program designed and constructed by the researchers, based on physical therapy principles used in the treatment of children in a clinical setting, combined with the principles of treatment in hydrotherapy to address the goals of the program. The plan and structure of the hydrotherapy intervention were based on protocols previously used in hydrotherapy for children with ASD, as well as the experience of the PI, who specialized in the field of early intervention and pediatric neuromuscular disorders for 27 years and who has been working as a hydro-therapist for the past 10 years, with various populations, including children with ASD. Hydrotherapy sessions were provided once weekly for 30 min, including exercises that focused on balance and coordination that progressed to higher levels of difficulty, depending on how each participant responded. At the end of the 12 session series, a final evaluation was conducted using the M-ABC-II. The individual goals achieved were evaluated through the use of the GAS. The final evaluations were also recorded for review by an independent and objective professional.

4. Outcome Measures

4.1. *Movement Assessment Battery for Children*

Movement Assessment Battery for Children—Second Edition (M-ABC-II): The M-ABC-II is a valid and reliable assessment of fine and gross motor skills [30–32] that has been used in children diagnosed with ASD [14,22]. The M-ABC-II includes eight tasks within three domains—manual dexterity, ball skills (aiming and catching), and static and dynamic balance. The strengths of the M-ABC-II include its ability to assess children using a different combination of fine and gross motor skill items appropriate for three different age groups within the age range from 3 to 16 years (age bands [AB]): AB1, three–six years; AB2, 7–10 years; and AB3, 11–16 years [31]. Within studies that use the M-ABC-II, children vary in age, but they are mainly within AB1 and AB2 [32–36]. The duration of a full assessment is in the range of 20–40 min, depending on the age of the child, the level of the child's functioning, the cooperation of the child, and the skill of the examiner. One study showed high intra- and inter-rater reliability in the M-ABC-II performed in children in AB 2 [36]. In a study conducted on Thai children, inter-rater reliability was moderate to good (intra-class correlation coefficient of inter-rater reliability ranged from 0.71 to 1.00) [35]. Each item within the M-ABC-II is assigned a raw score; within each domain, the raw scores of the items are summed to reach a raw domain score, which is converted into a standard score and corresponding percentile. The scores for each of the

https://doi.org/10.3390/children13010094

three domains are summed into a standardized total score and percentiles. The percentiles are further classified: ≤5th percentile is the red zone, indicating significant movement difficulty; a score between the 5th and 15th percentile is classified as the amber zone, indicating being at risk of movement difficulty; and a score > 15th percentile is classified as the green zone, indicating no movement difficulty detected. The M-ABC-II presents high psychometric values, with test reliability found to be moderate to high [31]. One study demonstrated low sensitivity (41%) and acceptable specificity (88%) [32], while another study showed that the M-ABC-II at age 4 years had high sensitivity (79%) and specificity (93%) for predicting motor impairment at age 8 years [25]. The M-ABC-II has been tested in numerous populations with various functional disabilities, including ASD [22]. In this study, which included 30 children with ASD (age 3–16 years; 25 males, 5 females), the authors concluded that children with ASD would be delayed in fine and gross motor skill development, compared to their age-matched typically developing peers [31].

In the current study, the PI administered all of the tasks according to the M-ABC-II manual, including detailed verbal descriptions and demonstrations prior to the participants' motor skill performances. To reduce the possibility of bias from the PI during M-ABC-II administration, each exam was recorded and reevaluated by an experienced professional (an OT working with children with ASD for over 15 years, trained in the use of the M-ABC) blinded to the time and place of the test within the research timeframe. The mean score of the PI and professional was used for statistical analysis. The primary focus of the treatment sessions was to improve balance and coordination; therefore, the score in the category of Balance was the main focal point, and therefore, the treatment program was designed for that purpose as well. Secondary analysis included the other domains of the M-ABC-II as well as the Total Test score.

4.2. Goal Attainment Scaling

Goal attainment scaling (GAS) is a method of scoring the extent to which one achieves individual goals throughout the intervention [37]. Each patient has their own outcome measure that is scored in a standardized way to allow for statistical analysis. Traditional standardized measures include a standard set of tasks/items, each rated on a standard level. In GAS, goals are individually established to suit the patient (and are therefore highly appropriate for children with ASD presenting vast clinical heterogeneity), and therefore, the levels are individually set around their current (pre-intervention) and expected (post-intervention) levels of performance. An important feature of GAS is the "a priori" establishment of criteria for a "successful" outcome in each individual, which is agreed upon by the patient and family before the intervention starts. Each goal is rated on a 5-point scale, with the degree of attainment captured for each goal area:

If the patient achieves the expected level, this is scored at 0. If they achieve a worse-than-expected outcome, this is scored at −1 (somewhat worse) or −2 (much worse/no change from baseline). If they achieve a better-than-expected outcome, this is scored as +1 (somewhat better) or +2 (much better).

Goals may be weighted (weight = importance × difficulty) to account for the relative importance of the goal to the participating individual and/or the anticipated difficulty of achieving the goal. A final score of approximately 50 represents a high-quality GAS outcome and indicates that functional goals were achieved. A final score below 50 implies that the set goals may have been too difficult to achieve, while a score over 50 implies that the goals were too easy to achieve [37].

The set goals followed the SMART principles (i.e., Specific, Measurable, Attainable, Realistic, and Timely).

https://doi.org/10.3390/children13010094

4.3. Social Responsiveness Scale II—(SRS-2)

The SRS-second edition [38] is a 65-item questionnaire, measuring the severity of autism spectrum symptoms as they occur in natural social settings. The scale is completed by parents, and it is appropriate for use with children aged 4–18 years, with higher scores indicating more autistic symptoms. The SRS forms can also be used when complete information regarding ASD diagnosis (ADOS; ADI-R) is missing. There are five sub-scales: social awareness (ability to recognize social cues), social cognition, social/reciprocal communication, social motivation interests, and stereotypy. The sum of all items is calculated to provide a total score (max of 195). T-scores are interpreted as follows: ≤59 T, within normal limits; 60–65 T, mild; 66–75 T, moderate; and ≥76 T, severe range. Cronbach's alpha was 0.97. Global scores are calculated by averaging responses across items, with higher scores indicating more severe symptoms (max of 6) [39]. SRS-2 has been shown to be sensitive to changes in social functioning among children with ASD [40]. The scale was translated to Hebrew and is officially recommended for use with autistic children by the Ministry of Health [41]. The SRS-II was used at the initial assessment of the participants in the current research, enabling future research protocols a possibility to compare their participants' level of autism with the participants of the current study.

4.4. Eligibility for Aquatic Intervention

This study included a hydrotherapy intervention, which requires a certain level of comfort in an aquatic environment. Participants and their parents were asked about their comfort in the water. In the eventuality that participants were not fully acclimated to an aquatic environment, the Humphries Assessment of Aquatic Readiness (HAAR) was used to assess eligibility for the hydrotherapeutic intervention. The HAAR, based on the principles of the Halliwick method, as well as components of popular aquatic assessments, is an evaluation used to measure one's capabilities and functional performance in the water [42]. It takes into consideration the hydrotherapeutic needs and ability levels of people with various disabilities and is appropriate for use in ASD [9].

5. Statistical Analysis

All analyses were conducted with a significance threshold of $\alpha = 0.05$. Normality of the dependent variables was first assessed using the Shapiro–Wilk test. Because the outcome variables (M-ABC-II domain scores and Total Test score) did not follow a normal distribution and instead exhibited a distributional pattern Poisson-like distribution (skewed, variance linked to mean), a repeated measures ANOVA was considered but rejected.

The primary inferential method was therefore Poisson regression with repeated measures, chosen to accommodate the non-normal distributional characteristics of the data and the repeated design across three time points (baseline, pre-intervention, post-intervention). Results are reported as Incidence Rate Ratios (IRR = exp(β)) with 95% confidence intervals, which quantify the relative change in performance following intervention.

Inter-rater reliability of the M-ABC-II scoring was evaluated using a Type C Intra-Class Correlation (ICC), based on a two-way mixed-effects model for consistency (ICC (3,1)). ICC values were computed from ANOVA mean squares (MSR, MSC, MSE) and are reported with point estimates and confidence intervals. This analysis served as a methodological quality check rather than an inferential test of treatment efficacy.

Finally, goal attainment scaling (GAS) scores were calculated according to the accepted statistical formula (Formula (1)) [37]. A mean GAS score of approximately 50 with a standard deviation of 10 is considered an indicator of appropriate goal setting and successful attainment and was used here as a complementary measure of functional improvement.

https://doi.org/10.3390/children13010094

6. Results

6.1. M-ABC-II

The calculation regarding the M-ABC-II results refers to Standard Scores as these provide a measure of how far a participant's raw score is from the average (mean) score of a normative population, we also used present results by percentiles, as these indicate the percentage of a participant in a normative sample and provide an easy-to-understand measure of a child's relative standing compared to their peers.

Inter-rater reliability was tested by using ICC when comparing the results of the percentile ranks of the three domains separately, as well as the total percentile score, between the scoring of the PI (MW) and the independent observer. The average ICC (3,1) was 0.968 with a 95% confidence from 0.932 to 1.0 ($p < 0.001$), suggesting very high inter-rater reliability for all tests. This value is consistent with previous studies that were conducted using the M-ABC-II [26,27].

Table 2 presents Poisson regression coefficients for the three evaluated domains (Manual Dexterity, Aiming and Catching, and Balance), each assessed using two scoring formats (Standard Score and Percentile).

Table 2. Comparison of all MABC-II domains within the study and control groups.

Dependent Variable	Score Type	Parameter	β	95% Wald Confidence Interval	Hypothesis Test	Exp(B) = OR	95% Wald Confidence Interval for Exp(B)		
				Lower	Upper	Wald X^2 Sig.		Lower	Upper
Manual Dexterity Evaluation	Standard	Intercept	1.363	1.152	1.575	0.000	3.909	3.164	4.829
		Study Group	0.325	0.047	0.602	0.022	1.384	1.049	1.826
		Control Group	0.067	−0.227	0.361	0.653	1.070	0.797	1.435
	Percentile	Intercept	1.533	1.324	1.742	0.000	4.632	3.758	5.708
		Study Group	1.269	1.032	1.505	0.000	3.557	2.808	4.506
		Control Group	0.277	−0.003	0.558	0.053	1.319	0.997	1.746
Aiming and Catching Evaluation	Standard	Intercept	1.705	1.527	1.883	0.000	5.500	4.602	6.573
		Study Group	−0.008	−0.261	0.244	0.949	0.992	0.770	1.277
		Control Group	0.087	-0.160	0.334	0.489	1.091	0.852	1.396
	Percentile	Intercept	2.561	2.439	2.683	0.000	12.950	11.465	14.627
		Study Group	0.189	0.018	0.360	0.030	1.208	1.018	1.434
		Control Group	0.091	−0.075	0.258	0.282	1.096	0.928	1.294
Balance Evaluation	Standard	Intercept	0.841	0.566	1.115	0.000	2.318	1.762	3.050
		Study Group	0.741	0.408	1.075	0.000	2.098	1.503	2.929
		Control Group	0.243	−0.124	0.609	0.195	1.275	0.883	1.839
	Percentile	Intercept	1.476	1.145	1.807	0.000	4.375	3.141	6.093
		Study Group	1.418	1.066	1.770	0.000	4.130	2.904	5.872
		Control Group	−0.036	−0.495	0.424	0.879	0.965	0.610	1.528
Total Test Score Evaluation	Standard	Intercept	0.916	0.652	1.181	0.000	2.500	1.919	3.256
		Study Group	0.481	0.145	0.817	0.005	1.618	1.156	2.265
		Control Group	0.136	−0.226	0.497	0.462	1.145	0.798	1.645
	Percentile	Intercept	0.742	0.314	1.170	0.001	2.100	1.369	3.221
		Study Group	1.587	1.131	2.043	0.000	4.889	3.099	7.713
		Control Group	−0.049	−0.615	0.517	0.866	0.952	0.541	1.677

In all models, the Baseline category serves as the Reference group and is therefore not displayed in the table: its regression coefficient is always 0 and its odds ratio (OR = Exp(β)) is always 1. Accordingly, only the values for the intercept, study group, and control group are shown.

This means that each β and OR reported in the table represents a direct comparison against the baseline. Positive β values and ORs greater than 1 indicate a higher likelihood

https://doi.org/10.3390/children13010094

of success relative to the baseline, while negative β values and ORs below 1 indicate a lower likelihood of success relative to the baseline.

Consistently, the study group demonstrates statistically significant advantages across all domains, whereas the control group shows significantly reduced odds of success. These findings highlight the overall effectiveness of the intervention in improving motor performance outcomes

Figure 2 presents a visual representation of the table above.

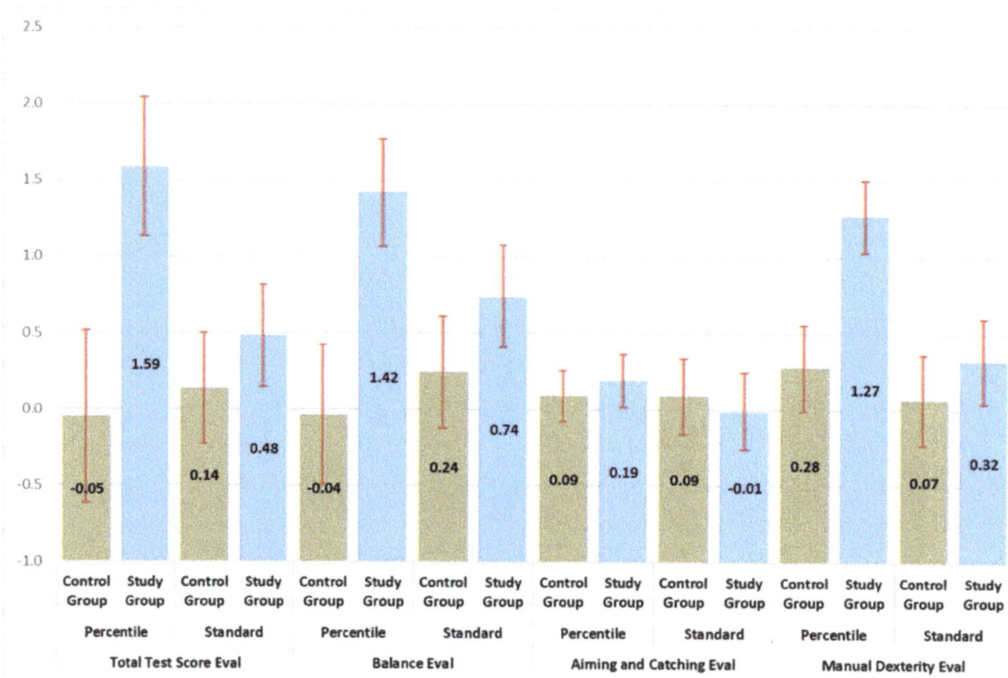

Figure 2. M-ABC-II, all fassonian coefficients in comparison to the baseline (no treatment).

Table 3 divides the participants between the three age groups according to the M-ABC-II and indicates which subjects improved by moving up a category according to the M-ABC-II between their baseline average percentile score (pre-intervention) and percentile score of the third evaluation (post-intervention). These results were not statistically significant and inconclusive, due to the small subgroups.

Figure 3 shows that a 5/7 children (71%) of the younger age group moved up a category according to the M-ABC-II, while 7/12 (58%) of the middle age group and only 1/3 (33%) of the older age group children showed the same phenomenon (for better visual effect, age groups are written in black, improvement rates are in red color).

https://doi.org/10.3390/children13010094

Table 3. Age division of all participants.

AB	Participant #	Balance Baseline Average	Balance 3ed Evaluation Percentile	Change in Percentile Ranking
AB1 (3–6 yrs.)	11	0.1	0.5	No
	6	0.5	5	Yes
	18	0.75	37	Yes
	9	3.5	37	Yes
	13	4.55	5	Yes
	14	7	63	Yes
	8	0.1	0.1	No
AB2 (7–10 yrs.)	10	0.1	0.1	No
	12	0.1	5	Yes
	15	0.1	0.1	No
	17	0.1	0.5	No
	16	0.3	2	No
	4	0.5	2	No
	21	0.55	1	No
	7	2.5	25	Yes
	5	3	37	Yes
	22	3	25	Yes
	19	4.75	9	Yes
	2	5	9	No
AB3 (11–16 yrs.)	3	0.1	0.1	No
	20	0.1	0.1	No
	1	2.55	9	Yes

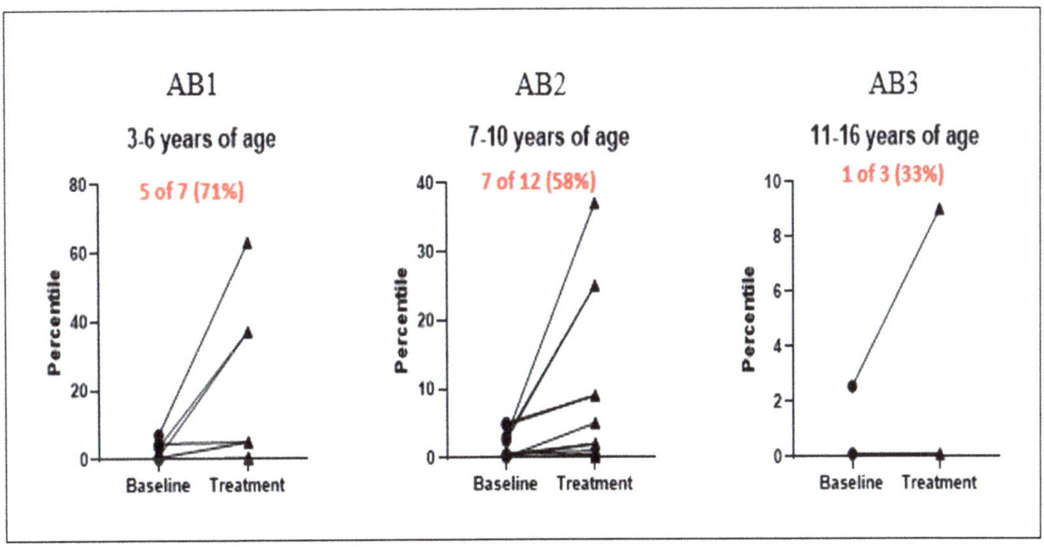

Figure 3. Number (%) of participants jumping a percentile, by age group.

6.2. GAS

The GAS score had a normal distribution, with a mean of 52.1 for this study, which implies improved function with the achievement of pre-established goals (see Figure 4 each dot in the Figure represents one participating child). Since 1 participant was not interested in participating in this part of the study, the average total GAS

https://doi.org/10.3390/children13010094

was based on 21 participants. Each point in Figure 4 represents the post-treatment score for each participant.

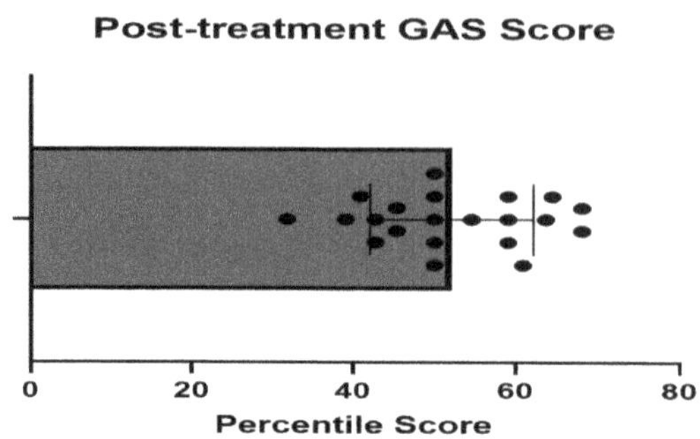

Figure 4. Post-intervention GAS scores.

7. Discussion

This study focused on improving functional and motor abilities in children and adolescents with ASD and evaluated the impact of 12 weekly hydrotherapy sessions on the functional, balance, and coordination abilities of children diagnosed with ASD.

The results were based on a group of participants that were measured as their own comparison group to avoid the clinical diversity presented by all children with ASD. After a 12-session hydrotherapy intervention, the Total Score of the M-ABC-II improved by 5.8%, while the Balance and Coordination domain of the M-ABC-II increased significantly by 10.6% from the baseline measurements. Therefore, the main results suggest participants' improvement during the intervention period, but not during the pre-intervention period. Upon examining secondary goals and sub-scales of the M-ABC-II, a significant improvement from baseline was also seen in the Manual Dexterity domain, while the Aiming and Catching domain (which was not a goal of the current intervention) showed no significant change. The mean GAS score for this study was 52.1, suggesting achievement of planned individual goals.

7.1. M-ABC-II Scores

The percentile and standard values of the Total Test score demonstrated statistically significant improvement from baseline, suggesting that a 12-session hydrotherapy intervention program, when performed by a licensed hydro-therapist, can yield functional improvements for children and adolescents with ASD.

The primary component of interest for this study, the Balance domain of the M-ABC-II, showed significant improvement from baseline. The importance of such a change is due to the fact that proper balance and postural control allow a person to participate in sports, kick a ball, and negotiate stairs [43]. In contrast, poor balance as a result of poor postural control, leads to a greater risk of falling, which affects the development of advanced motor skills and reduced participation. Moreover, adequate postural control enables a child to better manage educational activities and activities of daily living (ADL) [44]. Therefore, the authors adhere to the assumption that enhancing postural control (indicated by improved balance) might yield improved results for other functions [45]. A previous single case report [46] showed that balance and agility improved after a 10-week intervention of swimming training and water exercise, which is in line with our results. Recent meta-analysis and RCT evaluating motor improvements (among other areas) due to hydrotherapy intervention in children with ASD. Most of the improvements presented refer to in-water improvements (such as factors related to rotation, balance and control, and independent

https://doi.org/10.3390/children13010094

movement in water) [22,23], while the current intervention presented carryover from the hydrotherapy sessions to land improvements in balance and manual dexterity, which is a novel discovery, supporting previous reports [22,23] and extending the call of previous data related to the potential of hydrotherapy in improving motor skills of the ASD population.

Battaglia, in a study involving three participants diagnosed with low-functioning ASD, demonstrated that a 12-week aquatic program yielded improvement in running, hopping, and horizontal jumps [4]. As our study included 22 high-functioning participants, the combined results (which require further empirical support) suggest that this type of intervention might be promising for individuals with ASD at all functional levels.

Among the secondary domains that we scored, the Manual Dexterity domain also showed significant improvement from baseline. Manual dexterity, as defined by the Encyclopedia of Clinical Neuropsychology [47], is the ability to make coordinated hand and finger movements to grasp and manipulate objects. Functionally, it allows a person to perform precise movements (executive functions) such as writing, buttoning, and picking up small items. This skill develops primarily during childhood and can be affected by neurological disorders. Grip strength, which is considered an objective measure of upper extremity function, is essential for independence in early childhood functional tasks [48]. The findings suggest that improved manual dexterity can result from a motor-type intervention, such as hydrotherapy extending beyond the scope of the water to on-land improvements. Manual dexterity is also a function of core muscle stability, with coincides with the improvement in balance also achieved by the participants in the current study. These findings are in accordance with previous research [49].

No change was seen in the Aiming and Catching domain of the M-ABC-II. The current intervention was not aimed toward this goal, and we did not anticipate any change in this domain. This specific result strengthens our current findings, suggesting that using hydrotherapy to focus on specific treatment goals can yield positive results within the planned intervention goals. Previous research has suggested that water exercise programs can improve both social and aquatic skills in children with ASD [3–5,7–9]. A few of these studies addressed gross motor skills, but none explicitly measured manual dexterity or catching/throwing skills. One exception was a study by Battaglia that did not use hydrotherapy but included an aquatic intervention and demonstrated effectiveness for enhancing object control and locomotor skills, including tasks such as catching a ball with a tennis racket, stationary bounce, catching, kicking, and overhand throw [4].

7.2. GAS Scores

Scientific, valid, and reliable evaluation tools such as the M-ABC-II assess functions in specific areas and, therefore, reflect a child's ability and achievements on a specific set of skills. However, they do not necessarily acknowledge the individuality of children with ASD, nor do they reflect the functional ability of the child within daily activities, thereby limiting assessment to the domains covered by the scale chosen by the researcher. Due to the individual clinical variability of children with ASD, a more individualized evaluation and approach that focuses on specific, individually tailored functional skills is warranted. The point of view of prioritizing personal variability among research participants has been promoted by the World Health Organization (WHO) with the presentation of the International Classification of Functioning (ICF) [50]. To address this issue, we used the GAS as a standardized test to establish individual functional goals for each participant, which were selected as important to each participant and/or their family [37]. Since the focus of this study was balance and coordination, the individual and functional goals were related. The functional goals established in cooperation with the children and their families revolved around playing sports, which included running, jumping, kicking, and/or

 https://doi.org/10.3390/children13010094

hopping with the goal of improving the ability to play football, as well as running faster without falling. The average final GAS score was 52.1, and all but one child achieved their goals. The GAS has been used in prior studies related to hydrotherapy and other land-based exercise programs, specifically with children with Intellectual and Developmental Disability [51,52] and was suggested by others to be used as a measurement tool when assessing research outcomes with participants with ASD [53] in numerous situations; therefore, the current findings support the use of GAS within the ASD population and support its use in future intervention projects and within active therapeutic interventions in hydrotherapy and physical therapy [54,55].

7.3. Association Between Improvement and Patient Age

M-ABC-II scores can be quantified by the number of participants who moved up in percentile ranking categories, as well as the ages at which they did so. In the category of Balance, 11 children (50%) had improvements in the percentile ranking category. Five of seven children (71%) in the youngest age group AB1 (aged 3–6 y), five of twelve children (42%) in at age group AB2 (aged 7–10 y), while only one of three (33%) children in category AB3 (aged 11–16 y) moved up a category. These findings indicate that the youngest participants (<6) gained more from the intervention program than older participants. Despite these findings, our results were statistically inconclusive, probably as a result of a small group of participants within the AB3 group. Despite these inconclusive findings, previous evidence suggests that acquiring gross motor skills at the appropriate young age creates a solid foundation for further growth and can result in the development of more advanced milestones [56]. The current findings, in accordance with many previously reported intervention programs with children with ASD, suggest that early intervention is crucial for children with ASD, as it improves their overall prognosis [12,31,57]. Review articles published after the termination of the current study are also in alliance with the findings presented by the current study [58,59]

7.4. Additional Improvements as a Result of Hydrotherapy Intervention

Of note, while the hydrotherapy intervention was designed to improve Balance and Coordination, there was a significant improvement in the Manual Dexterity domain, but not in Aiming and Catching. A potential explanation for this could be that improved postural control reduces the need for participants to manage postural stability, thereby enabling them to direct their focus toward manual dexterity tasks [39,40,60], with a stable body acting as a proper base for limb-accurate activity. Alternatively, it is possible that with a longer hydrotherapy intervention, the Aiming and Catching domain would also have improved.

7.5. Qualitative Observation

The use of hydrotherapy as an intervention tool may result in improvements in other areas of function. Anecdotally, in recorded individual summation conversations, parents reported seeing improvement in other areas not directly connected with the direct goals of the current research. These improvements included general behavior, success at school, improved ability of participants to communicatively express themselves, improved ability to fall asleep at night, and an increased sense of independence, which was demonstrated by using public transportation independently for the first time. Numerous families reported improved self-confidence in social situations, including but not limited to initiating conversation and by the participants expressing their desires more coherently. Progress was also noted in school, specifically in terms of increased participation in class and better communication with the teacher. The oldest participant in the study acknowledged his difficulties with changes to his daily schedule and commented that now he feels he can

https://doi.org/10.3390/children13010094

"contain the fire", while his mother said he is more flexible in his thinking and his ability to adapt to change. In addition, while he had difficulty getting out of bed in the morning, he is now able to get up immediately after he wakes up.

These anecdotal findings are supported by results from Mills et al. [61] as well as by recent meta-analysis and RCT's [22,23], who demonstrated that children with ASD may benefit from a hydrotherapy program to improve their anxiousness and challenging behaviors, as well as reduce ill thoughts and overcome attentional difficulties. Other studies also acknowledged improvements in core ASD issues, such as social interactions and behaviors [7,9] as well as significantly decreased autistic behaviour in children with ASD [23] due to motor-type interventions including hydrotherapy [23,24].

7.6. Clinical Implications

The use of the M-ABC-II as a measuring tool was useful and is feasible as a measurement scale appropriate for measuring progress during a hydrotherapy intervention. This assumption coincides with previous suggestions by researchers exploring the field of ASD and motor-type interventions [31]. Due to the clinical versatility of individuals with ASD, we advise the use of the GAS when performing future hydrotherapy interventions for children and adolescents with ASD. The use of GAS allows assessment of the attainment of specific and personalized functional goals. The results of this study suggest that younger children (<6 years) experience greater improvements than older children. Despite their non-conclusiveness, these findings support the advancement of early motor-based intervention for children with ASD, in accordance with previous studies [12,31,56,57]. While the intervention itself was tailored to each individual participant, the hydrotherapeutic pool was occupied by other therapeutic sessions occurring concurrently. In some situations, there were up to 16 people (therapists and clients) working in parallel to the sessions of the study. This type of setting was found to disturb some of the participants and prevented them from fully cooperating, thereby preventing them from achieving their full potential. This suggests that children with ASD would gain more from an intervention in a more secluded therapeutic setting, as has been previously suggested [56]. The current results suggest that high-functioning children with ASD are inclined to achieve good results when introduced to a hydrotherapy program. Our clinical experience during the course of the current project suggests the need to construct favorable conditions for clients with ASD when involved in a therapeutic setting. For example, using a more secluded therapeutic environment (fewer surrounding interferences), an intensive intervention program (more therapeutic sessions per week), and a longer intervention period (more than 12 sessions). An important element that allowed this study to be successful was the relationship with the PI and the rapport built with the child and his family. Cooperation and trust between therapist and client are the cornerstones that encourage progress, especially with this population of children with ASD [62].

7.7. Limitations

Due to the clinical heterogeneity of children with autism, the authors found it inappropriate to select a different group of children (presenting a completely different picture of ASD despite having the same diagnosis) to serve as a control. Therefore, the same children were used as a control group (pre-intervention) and as a study group (with intervention).

While this study included a relatively larger number of participants than previous studies of hydrotherapy in ASD, a larger sample would allow us to draw better conclusions and more easily generalize them to the ASD population.

A more homogenous age group might yield more consistent results from which we can draw better conclusions, yet with less ability to generalize to the whole ASD spectrum.

https://doi.org/10.3390/children13010094

While all participants were at the same diagnosed level of ASD, their individual conduct and ability to focus were important factors that affected their experience of the intervention. Cooperation could enhance or impede any treatment program, including hydrotherapy sessions.

Due to the specific nature of the hydrotherapy center (which serves ultra-orthodox clients, as well as the general population, the hours in the center are divided between the two genders, both therapists and clients). As the therapist was male, all the clients recruited for the current research had to be males as well. Therefore, the results of the current research's findings can only be generalized to children and adolescents males with the diagnosis of ASD.

The exclusion of non-cooperating children narrowed the research population to include only high-functioning participants. Future research should also examine the results of a similar intervention program regarding less cooperating, low functioning, children with ASD.

8. Conclusions

The results of the current study demonstrated a positive impact of a 12-week hydrotherapy program; therefore, this type of intervention is suitable and recommended for this group of clients (high-functioning male children and adolescents with ASD). We recommend further studies on this topic should compare the interventions of hydrotherapy to other physical-motor type interventions, while also implementing hydrotherapy interventions with longer intervention period, with a larger sample population, including low-functioning children with ASD as well as females with the same diagnosis. As the incidence of ASD is constantly increasing worldwide, the necessity for continued research and intervention involving this group of clients is ever more important.

Supplementary Materials: The following supporting information can be downloaded at: https://www.mdpi.com/article/10.3390/children13010094/s1, Therapeutic protocol of the hydrotherapy program.

Author Contributions: The first author (M.L.) is the supervisor of the reported work, assisting in planning, conducting, writing, and other functions. The second author (M.W.) is the PI who performed the actual research including data collection and intervention. All authors have read and agreed to the published version of the manuscript.

Funding: This research received no external funding.

Institutional Review Board Statement: The study was conducted in accordance with the Declaration of Helsinki and approved by the Institutional Review Board of Ariel University (protocol code (AU-HEA-ML-20230415 on 15 April 2023).

Informed Consent Statement: Informed consent for participation was obtained from the subjects' guardians involved in the study, see complete detail under "ethics" section.

Data Availability Statement: Data is unavailable due to privacy restrictions.

Acknowledgments: The authors would like to thank the children and their families for their cooperation and the Buot hydrotherapy center for enabling the conduct of the current research.

Conflicts of Interest: The authors declare no conflict of interest. The authors declares no potential conflicts of interest with respect to the research, authorship, and/or publication of this article.

References

1. American Psychiatric Association. What is Autism Spectrum Disorder? Updated August 2018. Available online: https://www.psychiatry.org/patients-families/autism/what-is-autism-spectrum-disorder (accessed on 2 July 2021).

https://doi.org/10.3390/children13010094

2. Centers for Disease Control and Prevention. What is Autism Spectrum Disorder?. Updated March 2020. Available online: https://www.cdc.gov/autism/index.html (accessed on 4 July 2021).
3. APTA. Academy of Aquatic Physical Therapy. The Benefits of Aquatic Physical Therapy for Children. Updated 2021. Available online: https://aquaticpt.org/Files/Aquatic-Peds-Fact-Sheet.pdf (accessed on 15 July 2021).
4. Battaglia, G.; Agro, G.; Cataldo, P.; Palma, A.; Alesi, M. Influence of a specific aquatic program on social and gross motor skills in adolescents with autism spectrum disorders: Three case reports. *J. Funct. Morphol. Kinesiol.* **2019**, *4*, 27. [CrossRef]
5. Chu, C.H.; Pan, C.Y. The effect of peer- and sibling-assisted aquatic program on interaction behaviors and aquatic skills of children with autism spectrum disorders and their peers/siblings. *Res. Autism Spectr. Disord.* **2012**, *6*, 1211–1223. [CrossRef]
6. Ennis, E. The effects of a physical therapy-directed aquatic program on children with autism spectrum disorders. *J. Aqua. Phy. Ther.* **2011**, *19*, 4–10.
7. Mortimer, R.; Privopoulos, M.; Kumar, S. The effectiveness of hydrotherapy in the treatment of social and behavioral aspects of children with autism spectrum disorders: A systematic review. *J. Multidiscip. Health* **2014**, *3*, 93–104. [CrossRef]
8. Pan, C.Y. Effects of water exercise swimming program on aquatic skills and social behaviors in children with autism spectrum disorders. *Autism* **2010**, *14*, 9–28. [CrossRef]
9. Pan, C.Y. The efficacy of an aquatic program on physical fitness and aquatic skills in children with and without autism spectrum disorders. *Res. Autism Spectr. Disord.* **2011**, *5*, 657–665. [CrossRef]
10. Bhat, A.N. Is motor impairment in autism spectrum disorder distinct from developmental coordination disorder? A report from the SPARK Study. *Phys. Ther.* **2020**, *100*, 633–644. [CrossRef]
11. Caçola, P.; Miller, H.L.; Williamson, P.O. Behavioral comparisons in autism spectrum disorder and developmental coordination disorder: A systematic literature review. *Res. Autism Spectr. Disord.* **2017**, *38*, 6–18. [CrossRef] [PubMed]
12. Bhat, A.N.; Landa, R.J.; Galloway, J.C. Current perspectives on motor functioning in infants, children, and adults with autism spectrum disorders. *Phys. Ther.* **2011**, *91*, 1116–1129. [CrossRef] [PubMed]
13. MacDonald, M.; Lord, C.; Ulrich, D.A. The relationship of motor skills and social communicative skills in school-aged children with autism spectrum disorder. *Adapt. Phys. Act. Q.* **2013**, *30*, 271–282. [CrossRef]
14. Stins, J.F.; Emck, C. Balance performance in autism: A brief overview. *Front. Psychol.* **2018**, *5*, 901. [CrossRef]
15. Castro-Sánchez, A.M.; Matarán-Peñarrocha, G.A.; Lara-Palomo, I.; Saavedra-Hernández, M.; Arroyo-Morales, M.; Moreno-Lorenzo, C. Hydrotherapy for the treatment of pain in people with multiple sclerosis: A randomized controlled trial. *Evid.-Based Complement. Altern. Med.* **2012**, *2012*, e473963. [CrossRef]
16. Calandre, E.P.; Rodriguez-Claro, M.L.; Rico-Villademoros, F.; Vilchez, J.S.; Hidalgo, J.; Delgado-Rodriguez, A. Effects of pool-based exercise in fibromyalgia symptomatology and sleep quality: A prospective randomized comparison between stretching and Ai Chi. *Clin. Exp. Rheumatol.* **2009**, *27*, S21–S28. [PubMed]
17. King, M.R. Principles and application of hydrotherapy for equine athletes. *Vet. Clin. Equine Pract.* **2016**, *32*, 115–126. [CrossRef]
18. Torres-Ronda, L.; Del Alcázar, X.S. The properties of water and their applications for training. *J. Hum. Kinet.* **2014**, *44*, 237–248. [CrossRef] [PubMed]
19. Geytenbeek, J. Evidence for effective hydrotherapy. *Physiotherapy* **2002**, *88*, 514–529. [CrossRef]
20. Pinto, C.; Salazar, A.P.; Marchese, R.R.; Stein, C.; Pagnussat, A.S. The effects of hydrotherapy on balance, functional mobility, motor status, and quality of life in patients with parkinson disease: A systematic review and meta-analysis. *J. Inj. Funct. Rehabil.* **2019**, *11*, 278–291. [CrossRef]
21. Ansari, S.; Hosseinkhanzadeh, A.A.; AdibSaber, F.; Shojaei, M.; Daneshfar, A. The effects of aquatic versus kata techniques training on static and dynamic balance in children with autism spectrum disorder. *J. Autism Dev. Disord.* **2021**, *51*, 3180–3186.
22. Shariat, A.; Najafabadi, M.G.; Dos Santos, I.K.; Anastasio, A.T.; Milajerdi, H.R.; Hassanzadeh, G.; Nouri, E. The Effectiveness of Aquatic Therapy on Motor and Social Skill as Well as Executive Function in Children with Neurodevelopmental Disorder: A Systematic Review and Meta-analysis. *Arch. Phys. Med. Rehabil.* **2024**, *105*, 1000–1007. [CrossRef] [PubMed]
23. Van t Hooft, P.; Moeijes, J.; Hartman, C.; Van Busschbach, J.; Hartman, E. Aquatic Interventions to Improve Motor and Social Functioning in Children with ASD: A Systematic Review. *Rev. J. Autism Dev. Disord.* **2024**, 1–21. [CrossRef]
24. Griffiths, A.; Toovey, R. Psychometric properties of gross motor assessment tools for children: A systematic review. *BMJ Open* **2018**, *8*, e021734. [CrossRef] [PubMed]
25. Palisano, R.; Orlin, M.; Schreiber, J. *Campbell's Physical Therapy for Children Expert Consult*, 5th ed.; Saunders: Amsterdam, The Netherlands; Elsevier: Amsterdam, The Netherlands, 2016; ISBN 9780323390187.
26. Downs, S.J.; Boddy, L.M. Motor competence assessments for children with intellectual disabilities and/or autism: A systematic review. *BMJ Open Sport Exerc. Med.* **2020**, *6*, e000902. [CrossRef]
27. Cancer, A.; Minoliti, R. Identifying Developmental Motor Difficulties: A Review of Tests to Assess Motor Coordination in Children. *J. Funct. Morphol. Kinesiol.* **2020**, *5*, 16. [CrossRef] [PubMed]
28. Rebelo, M.; Serrano, J. Evaluation of the Psychometric Properties of the Portuguese Peabody Developmental Motor Scales-2 Edition: A Study with Children Aged 12 to 48 Months. *Children* **2021**, *8*, 1049. [CrossRef]

 https://doi.org/10.3390/children13010094

29. Baharudin, N.S.; Harun, D. An Assessment of the Movement and Function of Children with Specific Learning Disabilities: A Review of Five Standardised Assessment Tools. *Malays. J. Med. Sci.* **2020**, *27*, 21–36.
30. Ellinoudis, T.; Evaggelinou, C.; Kourtessis, T.; Konstantinidou, Z.; Venetsanou, F.; Kambas, A. Reliability and validity of age band 1 of the movement assessment battery for children–second edition. *Res. Dev. Disabil.* **2011**, *32*, 1046–1051.
31. Liu, T.; Breslin, C.M. Fine and gross motor performance of the MABC-2 by children with autism spectrum disorder and typically developing children. *Res. Autism Spectr. Disord.* **2013**, *7*, 1244–1249. [CrossRef]
32. Schoemaker, M.M.; Niemeijer, A.S.; Flapper, B.C.; Smits-Engelsman, B.C.M. Validity and reliability of the movement assessment battery for children-2 checklist for children with and without motor impairments. *Dev. Med. Child Neurol.* **2012**, *54*, 368–375. [CrossRef] [PubMed]
33. Engel-Yeger, B.; Rosenblum, S.; Josman, N. Movement assessment battery for children (M-ABC): Establishing construct validity for Israeli children. *Res. Dev. Disabil.* **2010**, *31*, 87–96. [CrossRef]
34. Griffiths, A.; Morgan, P.; Anderson, P.J.; Doyle, L.W.; Lee, K.J.; Spittle, A.J. Predictive value of the movement assessment battery for children-second edition at 4 years, for motor impairment at 8 years in children born preterm. *Dev. Med. Child Neurol.* **2017**, *59*, 490–496. [CrossRef]
35. Jaikaew, R.; Satiansukpong, N. Movement assessment battery for children-second edition (MABC2): Cross-cultural validity, content validity, and interrater reliability in thai children. *Occup. Ther. Int.* **2019**, *2019*, e4086594. [CrossRef]
36. Holm, I.; Tveter, A.T.; Aulie, V.S.; Stuge, B. High intra- and inter-rater chance variation of the movement assessment battery for children 2, age band 2. *Res. Dev. Disabil.* **2013**, *34*, 795–800. [CrossRef] [PubMed]
37. Turner-Stokes, L. Goal attainment scaling (GAS) in rehabilitation: A practical guide. *Clin. Rehabil.* **2009**, *23*, 362–370. [CrossRef] [PubMed]
38. Constantino, J.N.; Gruber, C.P. *Social Responsiveness Scale–Second Edition (SRS-2)*; Western Psychological Services: Torrance, CA, USA, 2012.
39. Lang, K.; Larsson, E.; Mavromara, L.; Simic, M.; Treasure, J.; Tchanturia, K. Diminished facial emotion expression and associated clinical characteristics in anorexia nervosa. *Psych. Res.* **2016**, *236*, 165–172. [CrossRef]
40. Wood, J.J.; Drahota, A.; Sze, K.; Van Dyke, M.; Decker, K.; Fujii, C.; Bahng, C.; Renno, P.; Hwang, W.-C.; Spiker, M. Brief Report: Effects of Cognitive Behavioral Therapy on Parent-Reported Autism Symptoms in School-Age Children with High-Functioning Autism. *J. Autism Dev. Disord.* **2009**, *39*, 1608–1612. [CrossRef] [PubMed]
41. Department of Child Development and Rehabilitation, Ministry of Health. An On-Line Guide For Child Development Units. 2023. Available online: https://www.gov.il/en/departments/units/child_development_and_rehabilitation_unit/govil-landing-page (accessed on 16 February 2024). (In Hebrew)
42. Humphries, K.M. Humphries' Assessment of Aquatic Readiness. Master's Thesis, Texas Women's University, Denton, TX, USA, 2008.
43. Fong, S.S.M.; Chung, L.M.Y.; Bae, Y.H.; Vackova, D.; Ma, A.W.W.; Liu, K.P.Y. Neuromuscular processes in the control of posture in children with developmental coordination disorder: Current evidence and future research directions. *Curr. Dev. Disord. Rep.* **2018**, *5*, 43–48. [CrossRef]
44. Fong, S.S.M.; Tsang, W.W.N.; Ng, G.Y.F. Altered postural control strategies and sensory organization in children with developmental coordination disorder. *Hum. Mov. Sci.* **2012**, *31*, 1317–1327. [CrossRef] [PubMed]
45. Westcott, S.L.; Burtner, P. Postural control in children: Implications for pediatric practice. *Phys. Occup. Ther. Pediatr.* **2010**, *24*, 5–55. [CrossRef] [PubMed]
46. Yilmaz, I.; Yanardag, M.; Birkan, B.; Bumin, G. Effects of swimming training on physical fitness and water orientation in autism. *Pediatr. Int.* **2004**, *46*, 624–626. [CrossRef]
47. Makofskee, B. Manual dexterity. In *Encyclopedia of Clinical Neuropsychology*, 2nd ed.; Kreutzer, J.S., DeLuca, J., Caplan, B., Eds.; Springer: Cham, Switzerland, 2018; pp. 2080–2081. [CrossRef]
48. Abu-Dahab, S.M.N.; Skidmore, E.R.; Holm, M.B.; Rogers, J.C.; Minshew, N.J. Motor and tactile-perceptual skill differences between individuals with high-functioning autism and typically developing individuals ages 5–21. *J. Autism Dev. Disord.* **2012**, *43*, 2241–2248. [CrossRef]
49. Hassani, F.; Shahrbanian, S.; Shahidi, S.H.; Sheikh, M. Playing games can improve physical performance in children with autism. *Int. J. Dev. Disabil.* **2022**, *68*, 219–226. [CrossRef]
50. McDougall, J.; Wright, V. The icf-cy and goal attainment scaling: Benefits of their combined use for pediatric practice. *Disabil. Rehabil.* **2009**, *31*, 1362–1372. [CrossRef] [PubMed]
51. Jones, M.C.; Walley, R.M.; Leech, A.; Paterson, M.; Common, S.; Metcalf, C. Using goal attainment scaling to evaluate a needs-led exercise program for people with severe and profound intellectual disabilities. *J. Intellect. Disabil.* **2006**, *10*, 317–335. [CrossRef] [PubMed]
52. Materne, M.; Frank, A.; Arvidsson, P. The utility of goal attainment scaling in evaluating a structured water dance intervention for adults with profound intellectual and multiple disabilities. *Heliyon* **2021**, *7*, e07902. [CrossRef] [PubMed]

https://doi.org/10.3390/children13010094

53. Staunton, H.; McIver, T.; Tillmann, J.; Clinch, S.; Hanrahan, V.; Ewens, B.; Averius, C.; Barsdorf, A.I.; Baranger, A.; Berry Kravis, E.; et al. Development of a Goal Attainment Scale (GAS) outcome measure for clinical interventional studies in paediatric autism. *Autism* **2025**, *29*, 2975–2990. [CrossRef] [PubMed] [PubMed Central]
54. Lee, C.E.; Shogren, K.A.; Segal, J.; Pezzimenti, F.; Aleman-Tovar, J.; Taylor, J.L. Goal attainment scaling—Community-based: A method to incorporate personalized outcomes into intervention research with youth and adults on the autism spectrum. *Autism* **2021**, *26*, 178–187. [CrossRef]
55. Ruble, L.; McGrew, J.; Dale, B.; Yee, M. Goal attainment scaling: An idiographic measure sensitive to parent and teacher report of IEP goal outcome assessment for students with ASD. *J. Autism Dev. Disord.* **2022**, *52*, 3344–3352. [CrossRef]
56. MacDonald, M.; McIntyre, L.L. The relationship of age early motor skills and observable child behaviors in young children with developmental delays. *Res. Dev. Disabil.* **2019**, *93*, 103445. [CrossRef]
57. National Institute of Child Health and Human Development. Early Intervention for Autism. Updated 19 April 2021. Available online: https://www.nichd.nih.gov/health/topics/autism/conditioninfo/treatments/early-intervention (accessed on 16 October 2023).
58. Vodakova, E.; Chatziioannou, D.; Jesina, O.; Kudlacek, M. The Effect of Halliwick Method on Aquatic Skills of Children with Autism Spectrum Disorder. *Int. J. Environ. Res. Public Health* **2022**, *19*, 16250. [CrossRef] [PubMed] [PubMed Central]
59. Movahedi, A.; Bahrami, F.; Marandi, S.M.; Abedi, A. Improvement in social dysfunction of children with autism spectrum disorder following long term kata techniques training. *Res. Autism Spectr. Disord.* **2013**, *7*, 1054–1061. [CrossRef]
60. Mills, W.; Kondakis, N.; Orr, R.; Warburton, M.; Milne, N. Does Hydrotherapy Impact Behaviours Related to Mental Health and Well-Being for Children with Autism Spectrum Disorder? A Randomised Crossover-Controlled Pilot Trial. *Int. J. Environ. Res. Public Health* **2020**, *17*, 558. [CrossRef] [PubMed] [PubMed Central]
61. Brewe, A.M.; Mazefsky, C.A.; White, S.W. Therapeutic alliance formation for adolescents and young adults with autism: Relation to treatment outcomes and client characteristics. *J. Autism Dev. Disord.* **2021**, *51*, 1446–1457. [CrossRef] [PubMed]
62. Cools, W.; Martelaer, K.D. Movement skill assessment of typically developing preschool children: A review of seven movement skill assessment tools. *J. Sports Sci. Med.* **2009**, *8*, 154–168. [PubMed]

https://doi.org/10.3390/children13010094

children

MDPI

Article

Exploring Self-Reported Physical Activity Levels and Physical Fitness in Italian Children: A Mediation and Moderation Analysis

Domenico Monacis [1,*], Italo Sannicandro [2] and Dario Colella [3]

[1] Department of Education and Sport Sciences, Pegaso Telematic University, 80143 Naples, Italy
[2] Department of Clinical and Experimental Medicine, University of Foggia, 71122 Foggia, Italy; italo.sannicandro@unifg.it
[3] Department of Biological and Environmental Sciences and Technologies, University of Salento, 73100 Lecce, Italy; dario.colella@unisalento.it
* Correspondence: domenico.monacis@unipegaso.it

Abstract: Background/Objectives: Skill-related physical fitness is a crucial factor influencing health status during childhood. Starting from the lack of knowledge in the field of skill-related physical fitness and levels of physical activity in Southern Italy, this cross-sectional study aims to explore the mediating and moderating influence of PAL on the association between BMI and skill-related physical fitness. Methods: The sample (N = 387 students; male = 196, age = 12.2 ± 0.87 yrs; female = 191, age = 12.3 ± 0.93) was recruited from schools in the Apulia Region. The assessment included standing long jump (SLJ), 2 kg medicine ball throw (MBT) and 10 × 5 shuttle run (10 × 5) as indicators of physical fitness, and a self-report for measuring daily physical activity (PAL). A 2 (gender) × 3 (BMI cutoff)-factorial ANOVA was performed to highlight differences between groups for physical fitness components and PAL. Then, mediation and moderation models were created, establishing BMI as the independent variable, physical fitness tests as dependent variables, and PAL as the mediator and moderator variable. Results: The findings showed higher physical fitness and PAL in male and female normal-weight groups than in those who were overweight and obese. Mediation analysis revealed that higher PAL improved performance in SLJ (b = 0.091, $p < 0.01$, $R^2 = 17.16\%$), led to a modest understanding of the variation in MBT ($\Delta R^2 = 0.026$), and significantly reduced the time spent to perform 10 × 5 ($p < 0.0$, $R^2 = 10.72\%$). Conclusions: Despite the obtained results, future research is needed to further understand the association between physical fitness and the sociocultural determinants of physical activity to guide institutional policies and interventions to prevent poor health habits.

Keywords: regional observatory of motor assessment; physical fitness; obesity; sedentary behavior; daily physical activity

1. Introduction

The advantages of physical activity and healthy lifestyles during the lifespan have been widely documented in international public health research [1,2]. The enhanced functioning of the cardiovascular, respiratory, and immune systems [3] and improved brain development and synaptogenesis [4,5], muscle and bone health, body weight management, and metabolism [6,7] are among the main benefits. Additionally, active lifestyles and healthy behaviors throughout life best contribute to a significant decrease in the risk of cardiovascular and metabolic diseases, and type-2 diabetes [8]. Moreover, they also lower the risk of several types of cancer (e.g., colon, stomach, lung, bladder, etc.) [9], as well as the onset of anxiety, stress, and depression [10].

However, despite the WHO guidelines [11] recommending that children and adolescents should be engaged in at least 60 min of moderate to vigorous daily physical activity (MVPA), recent studies indicate that boys and girls between 11 and 17 years old do not engage in sufficient physical activity daily [12,13]. The increasing adoption of sedentary lifestyles and sitting activities is among the main reasons for what has been termed as one of the major public health issues of the 21st century [12–15].

Epidemiological data are even more worrying when considered in view of the effects of the recent COVID-19 pandemic. The restrictions implemented during quarantine have resulted in an even greater reduction in opportunities for physical activity [16–18] and the rise in psychological diseases (e.g., anxiety, depression, and eating disorders, etc.) among young people [19,20]. These negative trends, besides being significant for the rise in the percentage of overweight and obesity in children and adolescents, are among the main determinants of the decline in levels of physical activity as well as motor skill development and coordination [21].

This negative trend results in restricted opportunities for the development of physical fitness, defined as a positive state of well-being influenced by regular physical activity, genetic makeup, and nutritional adequacy, which includes aerobic endurance, muscular strength, muscular endurance, joint flexibility, and body composition [22,23]. Additionally, physical fitness is categorized into two main components: health-related physical fitness, which encompasses muscular strength and endurance, cardiovascular endurance, flexibility, and body composition, and skill-related physical fitness, which includes agility, coordination, power, speed, and balance [22–25].

During the last few decades, the association between physical fitness and health effects has emerged in international scientific debate, alongside attitudes and changes toward physical activity, becoming a significant indicator of health status from childhood to adolescence [26,27]. Thus, the global decline in physical fitness and rising pandemic of overweight and obesity can be interpreted in the light of unhealthy habits and poor lifestyles defined as activities with an energy expenditure of 1.5 METs (metabolic equivalent tasks) or lower (e.g., increased screen time, addiction to smartphones and social media, unbalanced diet, increased automobile travel, sitting time, etc.) [11], which are significant predictors of sedentary behavior and poor health in adulthood [28,29]. Despite the fact that higher fitness and levels of physical activity (PALs) lead to the minimization of negative consequences associated with high body mass index and contribute to positive effects on health [30], recent international monitoring and surveillance of physical activity reported that approximately 32% to 8–9-year-old Italian children achieved the sufficient physical activity levels recommended by the WHO [11]. These epidemiological data highlight the concerning and alarming reduction in the percentage of children who are physically active: in the eleven-year-old age group, only 11.9% engaged in sufficient daily physical activity, while among thirteen- and fifteen-year-olds, the percentages are approximately 9.3% and 6.8%, respectively [31]. Cross-sectional research studies carried out on Italian children suggest that reduced daily physical activity and higher BMI have a negative impact on children's physical fitness and overall health status [32,33].

Moreover, recent findings showed an international and widespread inverse dose–response association between the improvement of cardiorespiratory fitness and all causes of mortality, including cardiovascular disease and cancer, independent of gender, age, and race [34,35]. A study conducted on 378 Portuguese children aged 9–11 years highlighted the important role of muscle strength in attenuating the effects of physical inactivity on metabolic risk: children classified as inactive but stronger had lower metabolic risk than inactive and "low-strength" peers [36]. In fact, lower levels of physical activity and physical fitness are associated with overweight and obesity, as an expression of reduced levels of motor skill development. Moreover, findings revealed that this unhealthy association is stronger in boys than in girls [37–39].

Despite this well-known association between health-related physical fitness and PAL, there is a lack of knowledge in the field of skill-related physical fitness and PAL in children in Southern Italy.

The literature analysis posed the following research questions:

(R1) Do skill-related physical fitness and PAL differ according to gender and BMI cutoffs in Italian children?

(R2) Does PAL mediate and moderate the relationship between BMI and skill-related physical fitness components? Which components of physical fitness can be best influenced by PAL?

To test the hypothesis that BMI may contribute to explaining variance in physical fitness, and that this association could be indirect via PAL, mediation models were created. Furthermore, moderation models were developed to determine whether the association between BMI and physical fitness was dependent on PAL.

2. Materials and Methods

2.1. Participants

This study was supported by the University of Salento (Lecce, Apulia). The study population was composed of Italian secondary schoolchildren, with no disabilities or mental/physical impairments or disorders. Participants were recruited from schools that joined the ROMA Project (Regional Observatory of Motor Assessment) in the Apulia Region of Southern Italy. The sampling strategy was based on the choice of the authors to control for specific variables that could add significant confounding factors to the study, as highlighted in international literature on the topic [40,41]

Before starting this study, a priori power calculations were conducted with G*Power [42,43] to identify the minimum number of participants required to achieve sufficient power ($\alpha = 0.05$; expected power = 0.95). This study utilized a cross-sectional design. A multistage sampling procedure was applied to recruit participants (N = 400 students; male = 200, female = 200) from six Apulian provinces (Foggia, BAT, Bari, Lecce, Brindisi, and Taranto) to enhance the representativeness in the Apulia target population. However, the total sample consisted of 387 children aged 11–14 years (male = 196; female = 191), as 13 children did not attend all assessment procedures. The Committee established by the University of Salento regarding data collection on humans concerns psychological-medical research. All other types of research do not include an Ethics Committee. Informed consent was obtained from all children involved in the project before data collection.

2.2. Assessment Procedure

After recording weight and height, participants were classified as normal weight, overweight, or obese according to Cole's Scale [44]. For the physical fitness assessment, lower- and upper-limb muscular strength were evaluated with standing long jump (SLJ) and 2 Kg medicine ball throw (MBT) tests, respectively [45,46], while speed and agility were assessed through the 10×5 m shuttle run test [47]. These physical fitness tests are reliable and field-based assessments for evaluating lower- and upper-limb explosive strength, and speed–agility [48], for skill-related fitness assessment as in previous studies in the Apulia Region [49]. Furthermore, data on these components of physical fitness are indirectly linked with middle-to-low motor development during adolescence [45].

Additionally, children were asked to complete the Italian version of the Physical Activity Questionnaire for Older Children [50–54] to evaluate self-reported daily physical activity practice over the last week. Physical education teachers in the Apulia Region and graduates in Sports Sciences were initially recruited in the ROMA Project and trained on the assessment procedure. Subsequently, they conducted the evaluations from October to December 2023. Assessments were carried out only in the schools that participated in the ROMA Project during curricular physical education lessons.

2.3. Statistical Analysis

After testing normality with the Kolmogorov–Smirnov test (sample size > 50), descriptive statistics for all anthropometric data, physical fitness tests, and levels of physical activity were conducted out in terms of mean, standard deviation, minimum, and maximum. Furthermore, a 2 (gender) × 3 (BMI cutoff)-factorial ANOVA was performed to highlight differences between groups for physical fitness components and levels of physical activity. Levene's test was used to assess the equality of variance assumption. Both the main effect and interaction effect of gender (male/female) and BMI cutoff (normal weight/overweight/obese) on physical fitness tests and levels of physical activity were carried out. Since group sizes were unequal, Gabriel's procedure was applied to conduct post hoc analysis. Moreover, partial eta squared (ηp2) and Cohen's d were calculated as measures of effect size as follows: ηp2 = 0.01 (small effect); ηp2 = 0.06 (small effect), and ηp2 = 0.14 (large effect); Cohen's d = 0.2 for small effect, Cohen's d = 0.5 for medium effect, and Cohen's d = 0.8 for large effect [55]

Then, Pearson's r coefficient was used to highlight significant relationships between variables; the results were interpreted as follows: small correlation < 0.30; 0.30 < medium correlation < 0.50; and large correlation > 0.50.

After verifying the relationship between variables, the mediation analysis was applied to assess if physical activity levels (mediation variable) mediate the relationship between BMI, as the independent variable, and physical fitness tests as the dependent variable. The analysis was conducted according to the Preacher and Hayes methods [56]. Results were interpreted as follows: mediation was defined as partial if the indirect effect was significant, while it was defined as total if the indirect effect was non-significant. Significance was verified with the Bootstrapping method of Preacher and Hayes [55,56].

Moreover, according to Hayes (2018), the moderation analysis was carried out to study the interaction effect between BMI and PAL to explain the direction or magnitude of the relationship between BMI and physical fitness components, after adding the moderation variable [57]. All significant indices were set at p-value < 0.05. SPSS software vers. 26.0 for Windows and the PROCESS macro for SPSS were used for data analysis.

3. Results

The results of descriptive statistics have been reported in Table 1 according to gender and BMI cutoff. Due to missing values (male = 4, female = 9) in anthropometric characteristics and the physical fitness assessment, the final sample consists of 387 children. The main results of the descriptive analysis reveal better physical fitness indicators and PAL for both male and female normal-weight groups compared to overweight and obese ones.

Table 1. Sample's anthropometric profile.

Male n **= 196**						
	Nw = 114		**Ow = 58**		**Ob = 24**	
	M ± SD	**Min–Max**	**M ± SD**	**Min–Max**	**M ± SD**	**Min–Max**
Age	12.27 ± 0.87	11–14	12.05 ± 0.85	11–14	12.04 ± 0.95	11–14
Height (m)	1.53 ± 0.09	1.29–1.79	1.57 ± 0.08	1.40–1.77	1.57 ± 0.96	1.38–1.78
Weight (Kg)	43.58 ± 8.93	24.00–71.80	57.38 ± 7.48	44.00–71.00	71.00 ± 9.42	54.00–92.00
BMI (kg/m^2)	18.17 ± 2.01	13.47–21.86	22.98 ± 1.39	20.50–26.10	28.40 ± 2.35	25.22–35.41
SLJ (m)	1.56 ± 0.25	0.70–2.17	1.38 ± 0.22	1.00–2.20	1.30 ± 0.28	0.87–1.90
MBT Kg2 (m)	4.93 ± 1.16	2.50–8.24	5.14 ± 1.18	3.35–8.13	5.16 ± 1.24	2.90–8.10
10 × 5 (s)	18.52 ± 3.57	11.32–26.68	20.16 ± 3.83	13.83–32.73	21.29 ± 3.80	13.73–26.39
PAL	2.91 ± 0.75	1.16–4.37	2.62 ± 0.78	1.39–4.58	2.05 ± 0.41	1.57–2.85
Female n **= 191**						
	Nw = 126		**Ow = 53**		**Ob = 12**	
	M ± SD	**Min–Max**	**M ± SD**	**Min–Max**	**M ± SD**	**Min–Max**
Age	12.37 ± 0.96	11–14	12.23 ± 0.82	11–14	12.17 ± 1.19	11–14
Height (m)	1.53 ± 0.08	1.28–1.77	1.55 ± 0.08	1.31–1.73	1.59 ± 0.04	1.52–1.67
Weight (Kg)	44.20 ± 8.37	25.00–65.20	57.98 ± 8.60	40.00–76.90	73.67 ± 5.67	65.00–85.00
BMI (kg/m^2)	18.46 ± 2.21	13.14–22.70	23.87 ± 1.60	20.77–27.34	29.13 ± 2.40	25.65–35.84
SLJ (m)	1.32 ± 0.21	0.67–2.05	1.21 ± 0.17	0.80–1.51	1.11 ± 0.19	0.86–1.55
MBT Kg2 (m)	4.13 ± 0.91	2.30–7.20	4.47 ± 0.86	2.75–7.00	5.30 ± 1.45	3.20–8.40
10 × 5 (s)	20.48 ± 4.01	12.82–31.50	22.54 ± 4.17	14.78–32.84	26.22 ± 2.64	19.18–29.39
PAL	2.47 ± 0.74	1.00–4.57	2.26 ± 0.61	1.32–4.14	2.35 ± 0.64	1.43–3.24

Moreover, the F value for gender has a significant main effect on SLJ (F = 38.604, $p < 0.01$), MBT (F = 8.525, $p < 0.01$), and 10 × 5 (F = 32.736, $p < 0.01$), but not on PAL, while BMI cutoff significantly affects SLJ (F = 24.824, $p < 0,01$), MBT (F = 7.363, $p < 0.01$), 10 × 5 (F = 22.234, $p < 0.01$), and PAL (F = 8.229, $p < 0.01$), as can be seen in Table 2. No significant interaction effects between factors were found, except for PAL (F = 3.452, $p < 0.01$).

Table 2. Effect of gender and BMI cutoff on physical fitness and PAL.

	Gender				**CutOff**				**Gender × Cutoff**			
	df	**F**	p	η^2	**df**	**F**	p	η^2	**df**	**F**	p	η^2
SLJ	1	38.604	<0.01	0.082	2	24.824	<0.01	0.105	2	1.058	0.348	0.004
MBT	1	8.525	<0.01	0.021	2	7.363	<0.01	0.036	2	2.761	0.065	0.013
10 × 5	1	32.736	<0.01	0.071	2	22.234	<0.01	0.096	2	2.101	0.124	0.009
PAL	1	2.251	0.113	0.008	2	8.229	<0.01	0.050	2	3.452	<0.01	0.021

Since the main effects of gender and cutoff are almost all significant, post hoc analysis was performed to determine the simple effects of each variable (see Table 3).

Table 3. Post hoc analysis.

	Gender	**Groups**
SLJ	Female < male; $p < 0.01$; $d = 0.824$	Nw > Ow; $p < 0.01$; $d = 0.530$ Nw > Ob; $p < 0.01$; $d = 0.774$ Ow > Ob; $p = 0.130$; $d = 0.244$
MBT	Female < male; $p < 0.01$; $d = 0.622$	Nw < Ow; $p = 0.064$; $d = 0.277$ Nw < Ob; $p < 0.01$; $d = 0.620$ Ow < Ob; $p = 0.118$; $d = 0.343$
10 × 5	Female > male; $p < 0.01$; $d = 0.512$	Nw < Ow; $p < 0.01$; $d = 0.436$ Nw < Ob; $p < 0.01$; $d = 0.843$ Ow < Ob; $p < 0.01$; $d = 0.407$
PAL	Female < male; $p = 0.113$; $d = 0.428$	Nw > Ow; $p < 0.05$; $d = 0.302$

Table 3. *Cont.*

	Gender					Groups				
						Nw > Ob; $p < 0.01$; $d = 0.720$ Ow > Ob; $p = 0.238$; $d = 0.418$				
	Male					Female				
	F	p	ηp^2	Groups		F	p	ηp^2	Groups	
SLJ	16.771	<0.01	0.148	Nw > Ow Nw > Ob Ow > Ob	<0.01 <0.01 0.380	9.150	<0.01	0.089	Nw > Ow Nw > Ob Ow > Ob	<0.01 <0.01 0.299
MBT	0.786	0.457	0.008	Nw < Ow Nw < Ob Ow < Ob	0.520 0.665 0.997	9.827	<0.01	0.095	Nw < Ow Nw < Ob Ow < Ob	0.067 <0.01 0.017
10 × 5	7.682	<0.01	0.074	Nw < Ow Nw < Ob Ow < Ob	0.017 <0.01 0.417	14.231	<0.01	0.131	Nw < Ow Nw < Ob Ow < Ob	<0.01 <0.01 0.012
PAL	11.850	<0.01	0.129	Nw > Ow Nw > Ob Ow > Ob	0.069 <0.01 <0.01	1.456	0.236	0.019	Nw > Ow Nw > Ob Ow < Ob	0.214 0.837 0.917

The results highlighted that boys performed significantly better in all physical fitness tests and were more physically active than girls. Moreover, Nw showed overall significantly higher physical fitness and PAL compared to Ow and Ob in all tests, except for MBT.

In the male sample, ANOVA analysis revealed significant differences in SLJ ($F = 16.771$, $p < 0.01$; $\eta p^2 = 0.148$) and PAL ($F = 11.850$, $p < 0.01$; $\eta p^2 = 0.129$) with large effect sizes according to BMI cutoff. A significant effect was also reported for 10 × 5 ($F = 7.682$, $p < 0.01$) with a medium effect size ($\eta p^2 = 0.074$). In females, BMI cutoff significantly influenced SLJ ($F = 9.150$, $p < 0.01$; $\eta p^2 = 0.089$), MBT ($F = 9.827$, $p < 0.01$; $\eta p^2 = 0.095$), and 10 × 5 ($F = 14.231$, $p < 0.01$; $\eta p^2 = 0.131$). No significant differences were highlighted for MBT in males and PAL in females.

The correlation matrix between BMI and other variables is reported in Table 4. The results show an inverse significant association between BMI, SLJ ($r = -0.257$, $p < 0.01$), and PAL ($r = -0.228$, $p < 0.01$). At the same time, increasing BMI increases motor performance in MBT ($r = 0.289$, $p < 0.01$) and the time required to perform 10 × 5 ($r = 0.224$, $p < 0.01$). Subsequently, the mediation analysis was performed based on the correlation matrix.

Table 4. Correlation between variables.

	SLJ	MBT	10 × 5	PAL
BMI	−0.257 **	0.289 **	0.224 **	−0.228 **
SLJ	/	0.429 **	−0.356 **	0.334 **
MBT	/	/	−0.090	0.089
10 × 5	/	/	/	−0.233 **

** = $p < 0.01$.

Table 5 provides a synthetic description of the three mediation models created. All models assume BMI as the IV, PAL as the MV, and physical fitness tests (SLJ, MBT, and *10 × 5*) as DVs. Since all indirect effects were significant, PAL is a partial mediator between variables. In the first model (IV = SLJ), BMI is inversely associated with SLJ ($c = -0.019$, $p < 0.01$), explaining about 10% of the total variance of SLJ ($R^2 = 9.92\%$). Moreover, an increase in PAL (Figure 1) results in better performance in SLJ ($b = 0.091$, $p < 0.01$) with higher variance across lower-limb strength ($R^2 = 17.16\%$). The same applies to Model 2 (Figure 2), where MBT is the IV: higher BMI improves motor performance in MBT (c = 0.087, $p < 0.01$), and higher self-reported PA enhances results in MBT (b = 0.250, $p < 0.01$). However, the addition of the mediation variable allowed for a slight understanding of the variation in upper-limb strength ($\Delta R^2 = 0.0262$). The third mediation model (Figure 3) assumes 10 × 5 as the IV. BMI negatively affects the 10 × 5 shuttle run (c = 0.248, $p < 0.01$), while children who are more physically active demonstrate a significant reduction in time spent performing the test (b = −0.837, $p < 0.01$), explaining more than 10.72% of the total variance.

Table 5. Analysis of indirect effect of Models 1, 2, and 3.

	Direct Effect					Indirect Effect					
	R^2	Value	LLCI	Bootstrap ULCI	p	R^2_1	Value	LLCI	Bootstrap ULCI	p	ΔR^2
Model 1	0.099	−0.016	−0.026	−0.013	<0.01	0.171	−0.003	−0.006	−0.002	<0.01	0.0724
Model 2	0.091	0.098	0.057	0.117	<0.01	0.117	−0.011	−0.206	−0.004	<0.01	0.0262
Model 3	0.076	0.211	0.153	0.342	<0.01	0.107	0.037	0.013	0.068	<0.01	0.0303

LLCI = lower limit of confidence interval; ULCI = upper limit of confidence interval.

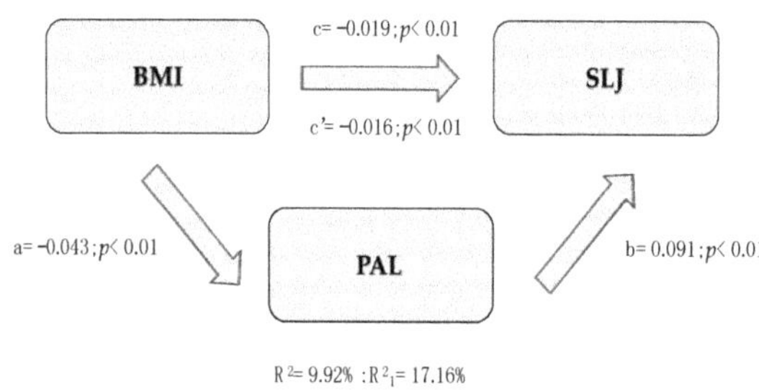

Figure 1. Representation of Mediation Model 1.

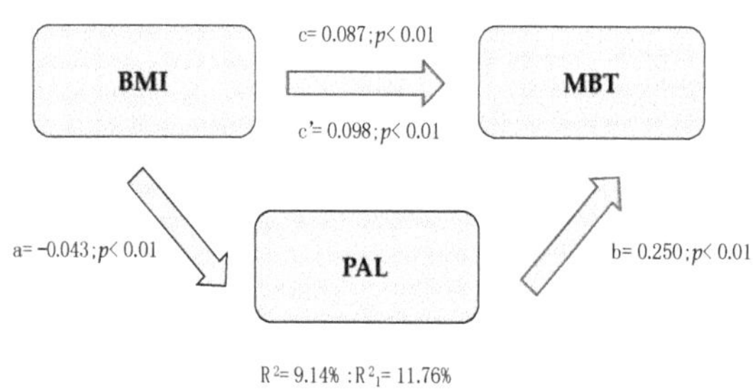

Figure 2. Representation of Mediation Model 2.

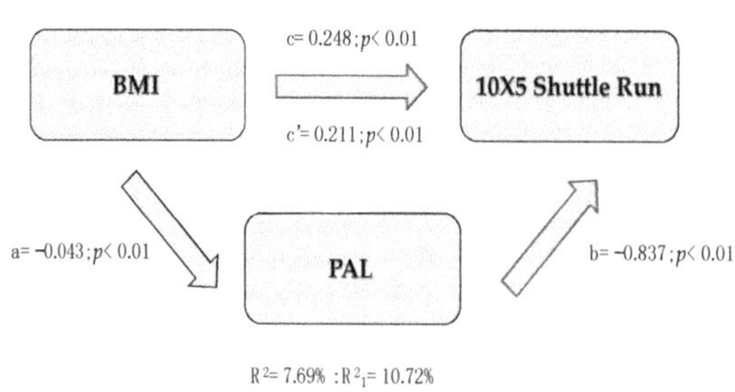

Figure 3. Representation of Mediation Model 3.

In Figures 1–3, c = total effect of independent variable on dependent variable; c′ = direct effect of independent variable on dependent variable adjusted per mediation variable; a = effect of independent variable on mediation variable; b = effect of mediation variable on dependent variable controlled per independent variable; a × b = indirect effects of independent variable on mediation variable, and mediation variable on dependent variable.

The moderation analysis according to Preacher and Hayes' method is reported in Table 6. Despite the interaction term between BMI and PAL accounting for a certain proportion of the children's physical fitness components (R2 Model 1 = 16.94%; R2 Model 2 = 12.84% and R2 Model 3 = 10.64%), these results are non-significant. Interaction plots (Figures 4 and 5 show an enhancing effect whereby, as PAL increased and BMI decreased, lower-limb strength and agility improved. In contrast, both the increase in BMI and PAL led to better performance in MBT (Figure 6). All results, even if non-significant, confirm that an increase in PAL contributes to enhancing each component of physical fitness.

Table 6. Moderation analysis and interaction effect between BMI and PAL (INT) in Models 1, 2, and 3.

Moderation Analysis						
				Bootstrap		
		Value	LLCI	ULCI	p	R^2
Model 1	BMI	−0.023	−0.048	0.0023	0.074	16.94
	PAL	0.032	−0.169	0.2347	0.752	
	INT	0.003	−0.007	0.0127	0.568	
Model 2	BMI	0.017	−0.100	0.1355	0.770	12.84
	PAL	−0.389	−1.339	0.561	0.421	
	INT	0.033	−0.013	0.079	0.161	
Model 3	BMI	0.146	−0.226	0.517	0.441	10.64
	PAL	−1.374	−4.364	1.617	0.367	
	INT	0.027	−0.119	0.0173	0.719	

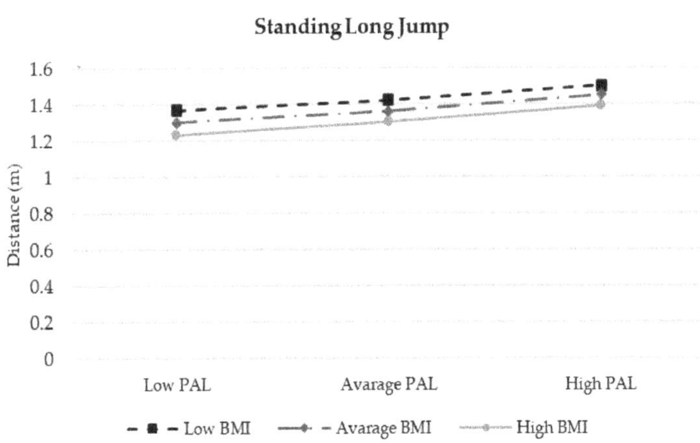

Figure 4. Moderation Model 1.

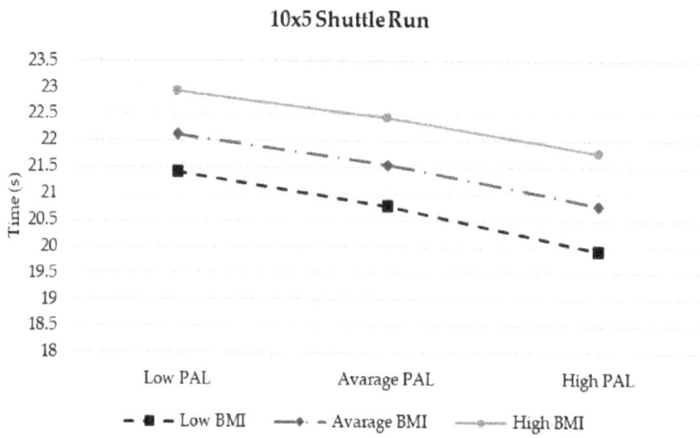

Figure 5. Moderation Model 3.

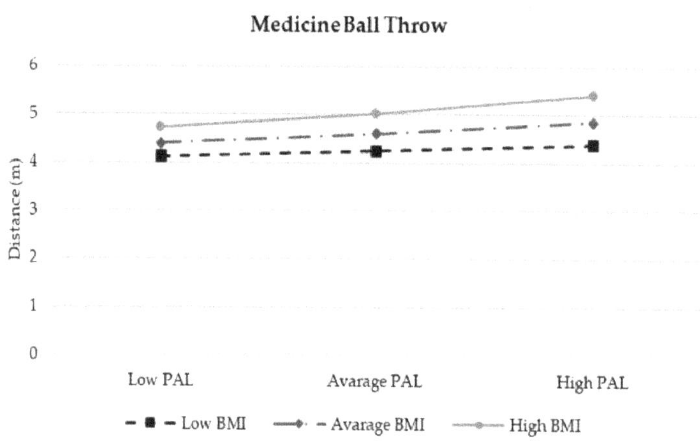

Figure 6. Moderation Model 2.

4. Discussion

The present study provides (R1) an analysis of physical fitness components and levels of physical activity in secondary schoolchildren according to gender and BMI cutoff. Results highlight that lower BMI is positively associated with higher lower-limb explosive strength, aerobic endurance, and levels of physical activity in both boys and girls, while upper-limb strength is directly associated with an increase in BMI. However, the findings reveal significant simple main effects for all variables according to BMI cutoff and gender (except for PAL), and a significant interaction effect for PAL.

The results of the present study are consistent with other studies conducted in Apulia as part of the ROMA Project, whose main findings revealed that increased BMI is negatively associated with motor performance [49,58].

Recent findings in the same field revealed that obese children showed better motor performance and explosive power compared to normal-weight children, while lower body weight was negatively associated with musculoskeletal strength [32]. As demonstrated in the present research, the study by Tsolakis et al. [26] highlighted that BMI was positively associated with upper-limb strength (assessed via the Hand Grip test), and negatively associated with cardiorespiratory fitness, lower-limb explosive strength, and trunk muscle endurance. Furthermore, sedentary lifestyles and reduced levels of physical activity led to an increase in overweight and obesity and a reduction in performance indicators of physical fitness components [59,60].

The second research question (R2) concerns the analysis of the mediating and moderating role of PAL between BMI and the development of physical fitness. In fact, although scientific evidence agrees that there is a negative association between BMI and physical fitness, the nature of this association remains to be clarified when considering the mediating and/or moderating effects of daily physical activity practice.

The results highlighted that PAL partially mediates the association between BMI and skill-related physical fitness. Data analyses revealed an inverse association between BMI, SLJ, and 10×5 and a positive correlation between BMI and MBT, but these models are mediated by daily practice of physical activity.

The findings in this paper are similar to those obtained in a previous study conducted in Apulia, but in just a single province: the results showed, in fact, a total mediating effect between BMI and the different components of physical fitness [49].

Findings in the literature confirm that higher levels of physical activity and physical fitness levels lead to a possible reduction in genetic predisposition to being overweight or obese during adulthood [61]. Moreover, studies reveal that structured physical activity interventions can improve body composition in children with overweight or obesity, regardless of age [62]. According to Wisnieski et al. [63], the development of aerobic capacity and the functionality of the cardiovascular system is a mediating factor between MVPA and body mass index (BMI). Furthermore, cross-sectional studies have already demonstrated that the incidence of overweight and obesity is strictly related to lower levels of physical activity [64,65]

A recent study [66] highlighted the importance of cardiorespiratory fitness as a full mediator between motor competence and daily physical activity in both boys and girls. Moreover, cardiorespiratory fitness serves as a complete mediator between obesity and PAL [67].

Findings from the present study align with other research in the same field, which indicates that the negative association between BMI, PAL, and physical fitness is closely related to the significant decline in MVPA in the 3-to-18-year age groups [68].

The obtained results gain significance when considering that higher speed–agility and muscle strength are also linked to other domains in children and adolescents, beyond the physical one. In fact, these physical fitness components play a mediating role in the negative association between excessive body weight and academic performance in children [69].

In addition, the moderation analysis showed no significant results. This may be due to inaccuracies in self-reporting physical activity levels by children, as reported by other studies [70,71]. These results also suggest a further reflection of the intensity of physical activity. According to Sardinha et al. [72], energy expenditure during vigorous physical activity was inversely associated with total and abdominal fat mass indices in obese children, independent of cardiorespiratory fitness levels. Moreover, recent findings highlighted the importance of balancing volume and intensity during PA to achieve different goals: increased volume is linked to improved bone-mineral content in children, and reduced fat mass in males, while intensity is associated with lean mass and fatness in both males and females [73].

In summary, although the results emphasize the negative association between increased BMI and motor performance, the scientific literature on the subject seems to attribute a significant role (e.g., direct or indirect effect) to physical activity practice.

4.1. Methodological and Didactic Implications for Physical Education Teachers

The results of the present study should be interesting and add to a better understanding of PE teachers' behavior in the school setting, where the teacher is primarily responsible for enabling mediation functions among the students, the motor tasks, and the environment in which the motor experiences occur [74,75]. Furthermore, these findings assign significant value to the choice and the teachers' reflection on the content and the organizational modalities to increase the levels of physical activity and the time of motor engagement during practice [76].

A thorough examination of teaching methodologies and organizational strategies in physical education is needed to enhance motor engagement during physical education classes and lessons. In fact, there is a positive association between time spent in moderate to vigorous physical activity and extended opportunities for motor skill learning [75].

Another study evaluated the effects of an experimental intervention protocol based on the learning of motor skills in a sample of overweight and obese children aged 6–7 years concerning the children's routines at home, self-perception, body mass index, motor development, and the time spent in physical activity during physical education lessons [77]. The findings showed a decrease in television viewing and total screen time, and enhanced perceived motor competence, participation in physical activity, and motor skills, as well as a decrease in BMI [77]. In addition, the study by Ługowska et al. (2023) showed that an increase in PA at school (10 h per week) effectively improved physical fitness levels assessed using standing long jump, shuttle run, and core strength in adolescents aged 11–12 years old [78].

Further opportunities to promote and enhance time for motor engagement in school might include family involvement [79,80], as well as the proposal of multi-component projects at school [81,82] and experimental interventions aimed at developing PE teachers' training courses regarding variables that may lead to an increase or decrease in PAL, such as self-perception, self-perceived competence, enjoyment, and motivation, as suggested in other studies [83–87].

4.2. Study Limitations and Future Research

This study highlights significant differences based on gender and BMI cutoff groups, as well as significant indirect effects of PAL in the association between BMI and physical fitness, suggesting a foundation for future scientific research. However, some limitations emerged and should be adequately considered. First, although the authors used cluster sampling to recruit the sample, the cutoff groups are quite unequal, making it difficult to generalize the results. Despite the authors applying Gabriel's procedure for conducting post hoc analysis, the presence of unequal group sizes may still lead to higher variability that could influence the robustness of the findings. Future studies should use a stratified sampling approach.

Additionally, in this study, the authors used Cole's classification [44] for normal weight, overweight, and obesity. Subsequent studies could, for example, classify children through percentile z-scores or the addition of other assessment tools (e.g., waist circumference, plicometry, etc.). Regarding the assessment methods, despite the authors proposing a validated questionnaire for assessing self-reported physical activity, the instrument may still introduce recall bias or inaccuracies, particularly in children, who may struggle to report their activity levels accurately.

A further limitation is the lack of additional covariates, in this specific case age. The authors' objective was, in fact, to create a possible explanatory model applicable to secondary schools in Italy. Future research will focus on defining specific age-dependent models of mediation and moderation, as well as the assessment of the mediating and/or moderating effects of different activities conducted during physical education classes on physical fitness. Moreover, to validate these preliminary findings, future research should employ longitudinal designs to examine differences among various age groups and genders, including children with disabilities and/or physical/cognitive impairments. Finally, it would be interesting to conduct and assess the effectiveness of experimental interventions in schools for enhancing physical fitness and promoting healthy behaviors in adolescents.

5. Conclusions

The present study suggests the important role of physical activity in mediating the association between BMI and physical fitness in Italian children. Despite the non-significant moderation effect, the findings indicate that higher levels of physical activity result in better motor performance in children with higher BMI compared to those with average and low BMI. The developed mediation models confirm the effect of BMI on physical fitness components via PAL, suggesting that BMI affects PAL, which in turn influences motor performance. Instead, the results of moderation models show no significant conditional effect, suggesting that the influence of BMI on physical fitness depends on the PAL (as a moderator). However, these data should be properly interpreted in light of the mentioned limitations of this study. Future research should also be performed using different research designs and a deeper analysis of sociocultural determinants of physical activity for the generalization of the results.

Author Contributions: Conceptualization, D.M.; methodology, D.M. and I.S.; data curation, D.M. and I.S.; formal analysis, D.M.; writing—original draft preparation, D.M. and I.S.; writing—review and editing, D.C.; supervision, D.C.; project administration, D.M. and D.C. All authors have read and agreed to the published version of the manuscript.

Funding: This research received no external funding.

Institutional Review Board Statement: The Committee envisaged by the University of Salento for data collection on humans concerns psychological–medical research. All other types of research do not include the Ethics Committee. The manuscript discusses an educational research study that was not related to clinical treatment. As stated in Article 9 of Regulation (EU) 679/2016, commonly referred to as the General Data Protection Regulation (GDPR), ethical approval is not required since no sensitive data are gathered in this kind of research. This study was conducted in accordance with the Declaration of Helsinki. Ethical review and approval were waived for this study because it was an educational research study that did not involve clinical treatment.

Informed Consent Statement: Informed consent was obtained from all subjects involved in the study.

Data Availability Statement: The data presented in this study are available on request from the corresponding author. Data are unavailable due to privacy or ethical restrictions.

Conflicts of Interest: The authors declare no conflicts of interest.

Abbreviations

The following abbreviations are used in this manuscript:

BMI	Body mass index
SLJ	Standing long jump
MBT	Medicine ball throw
10×5	Shuttle run 10×5
PAL	Level of physical activity
WHO	World Health Organization
MET	Metabolic equivalent task

References

1. Malm, C.; Jakobsson, J.; Isaksson, A. Physical Activity and Sports—Real Health Benefits: A Review with Insight into the Public Health of Sweden. *Sports* **2019**, *7*, 127. [CrossRef] [PubMed]
2. Singh, R.; Pattisapu, A.; Emery, M.S. US Physical Activity Guidelines: Current State, Impact and Future Directions. *Trends Cardiovasc. Med.* **2020**, *30*, 407–412. [CrossRef] [PubMed]
3. Barker, A.R.; Gracia-Marco, L.; Ruiz, J.R.; Castillo, M.J.; Aparicio-Ugarriza, R.; González-Gross, M.; Kafatos, A.; Androutsos, O.; Polito, A.; Molnar, D.; et al. Physical Activity, Sedentary Time, TV Viewing, Physical Fitness and Cardiovascular Disease Risk in Adolescents: The HELENA Study. *Int. J. Cardiol.* **2018**, *254*, 303–309. [CrossRef] [PubMed]
4. Di Liegro, C.M.; Schiera, G.; Proia, P.; Di Liegro, I. Physical Activity and Brain Health. *Genes* **2019**, *10*, 720. [CrossRef]
5. Hillman, C.H.; Logan, N.E.; Shigeta, T.T. A Review of Acute Physical Activity Effects on Brain and Cognition in Children. *Transl. J. Am. Coll. Sports Med.* **2019**, *4*, 132–136. [CrossRef]
6. Bourdier, P.; Simon, C.; Bessesen, D.H.; Blanc, S.; Bergouignan, A. The Role of Physical Activity in the Regulation of Body Weight: The Overlooked Contribution of Light Physical Activity and Sedentary Behaviors. *Obes. Rev.* **2023**, *24*, e13528. [CrossRef]
7. Julian, V.; Bergsten, P.; Forslund, A.; Ahlstrom, H.; Ciba, I.; Dahlbom, M.; Furthner, D.; Gomahr, J.; Kullberg, J.; Maruszczak, K.; et al. Sedentary Time Has a Stronger Impact on Metabolic Health than Moderate to Vigorous Physical Activity in Adolescents with Obesity: A Cross-Sectional Analysis of the Beta-JUDO Study. *Pediatr. Obes.* **2022**, *17*, e12897. [CrossRef]
8. US Preventive Services Task Force. Behavioral Counseling Interventions to Promote a Healthy Diet and Physical Activity for Cardiovascular Disease Prevention in Adults Without Cardiovascular Disease Risk Factors: US Preventive Services Task Force Recommendation Statement. *JAMA* **2022**, *328*, 367–374. [CrossRef]
9. Mao, J.J.; Pillai, G.G.; Andrade, C.J.; Ligibel, J.A.; Basu, P.; Cohen, L.; Khan, I.A.; Mustian, K.M.; Puthiyedath, R.; Dhiman, K.S.; et al. Integrative Oncology: Addressing the Global Challenges of Cancer Prevention and Treatment. *CA Cancer J. Clin.* **2022**, *72*, 144–164. [CrossRef]
10. Singh, B.; Olds, T.; Curtis, R.; Dumuid, D.; Virgara, R.; Watson, A.; Szeto, K.; O'Connor, E.; Ferguson, T.; Eglitis, E.; et al. Effectiveness of Physical Activity Interventions for Improving Depression, Anxiety and Distress: An Overview of Systematic Reviews. *Br. J. Sports Med.* **2023**, *57*, 1203–1209. [CrossRef]
11. Bull, F.C.; Al-Ansari, S.S.; Biddle, S.; Borodulin, K.; Buman, M.P.; Cardon, G.; Carty, C.; Chaput, J.-P.; Chastin, S.; Chou, R.; et al. World Health Organization 2020 Guidelines on Physical Activity and Sedentary Behaviour. *Br. J. Sports Med.* **2020**, *54*, 1451–1462. [CrossRef] [PubMed]
12. Guthold, R.; Stevens, G.A.; Riley, L.M.; Bull, F.C. Worldwide Trends in Insufficient Physical Activity from 2001 to 2016: A Pooled Analysis of 358 Population-Based Surveys with 1.9 Million Participants. *Lancet Glob. Health* **2018**, *6*, e1077–e1086. [CrossRef]
13. World Health Organization (WHO). Overweight and Obesity. Available online: https://www.who.int/news-room/fact-sheets/detail/obesity-and-overweight (accessed on 13 September 2024).
14. Katzmarzyk, P.T. Expanding Our Understanding of the Global Impact of Physical Inactivity. *Lancet Glob. Health* **2023**, *11*, e2–e3. [CrossRef] [PubMed]
15. Blair, S.N. Physical Inactivity: The Biggest Public Health Problem of the 21st Century. *Br. J. Sports Med.* **2009**, *43*, 1–2.
16. Caputo, E.L.; Reichert, F.F. Studies of Physical Activity and COVID-19 During the Pandemic: A Scoping Review. *J. Phys. Act. Health* **2020**, *17*, 1275–1284. [CrossRef] [PubMed]
17. Robinson, E.; Boyland, E.; Chisholm, A.; Harrold, J.; Maloney, N.G.; Marty, L.; Mead, B.R.; Noonan, R.; Hardman, C.A. Obesity, Eating Behavior and Physical Activity during COVID-19 Lockdown: A Study of UK Adults. *Appetite* **2021**, *156*, 104853. [CrossRef] [PubMed]
18. Zenic, N.; Taiar, R.; Gilic, B.; Blazevic, M.; Maric, D.; Pojskic, H.; Sekulic, D. Levels and Changes of Physical Activity in Adolescents during the COVID-19 Pandemic: Contextualizing Urban vs. Rural Living Environment. *Appl. Sci.* **2020**, *10*, 3997. [CrossRef]
19. Puccinelli, P.J.; da Costa, T.S.; Seffrin, A.; de Lira, C.A.B.; Vancini, R.L.; Nikolaidis, P.T.; Knechtle, B.; Rosemann, T.; Hill, L.; Andrade, M.S. Reduced Level of Physical Activity during COVID-19 Pandemic Is Associated with Depression and Anxiety Levels: An Internet-Based Survey. *BMC Public Health* **2021**, *21*, 425. [CrossRef]
20. Ingram, J.; Maciejewski, G.; Hand, C.J. Changes in Diet, Sleep, and Physical Activity Are Associated With Differences in Negative Mood During COVID-19 Lockdown. *Front. Psychol.* **2020**, *11*, 588604. [CrossRef]
21. Hills, A.P.; Andersen, L.B.; Byrne, N.M. Physical Activity and Obesity in Children. *Br. J. Sports Med.* **2011**, *45*, 866–870. [CrossRef]
22. Goodway, J.D.; Ozmun, J.C.; Gallahue, D.L. *Understanding Motor Development: Infants, Children, Adolescents, Adults*; Jones & Bartlett Learning: Burlington, MA, USA, 2019.
23. Human Kinetics. What Is Physical Fitness? Available online: https://us.humankinetics.com/blogs/excerpt/what-is-physical-fitness#:~:text=Physical%20fitness%20refers%20to%20the,with%20the%20least%20effort%20possible (accessed on 12 December 2024).
24. Britton, Ú.; Issartel, J.; Fahey, G.; Conyngham, G.; Belton, S. What Is Health-Related Fitness? Investigating the Underlying Factor Structure of Fitness in Youth. *Eur. Phys. Educ. Rev.* **2019**, *26*, 782–796. [CrossRef]

25. Lamb, K.L.; Brodie, D.A.; Roberts, K. Physical Fitness and Health-Related Fitness as Indicators of a Positive Health State. *Health Promot. Int.* **1988**, *3*, 171–182. [CrossRef]
26. Tsolakis, C.; Cherouveim, E.D.; Skouras, A.Z.; Antonakis-Karamintzas, D.; Czvekus, C.; Halvatsiotis, P.; Savvidou, O.; Koulouvaris, P. The Impact of Obesity on the Fitness Performance of School-Aged Children Living in Rural Areas-The West Attica Project. *Int. J. Environ. Res. Public Health* **2022**, *19*, 11476. [CrossRef] [PubMed]
27. García-Hermoso, A.; Izquierdo, M.; Ramírez-Vélez, R. Tracking of Physical Fitness Levels from Childhood and Adolescence to Adulthood: A Systematic Review and Meta-Analysis. *Transl. Pediatr.* **2022**, *11*, 474–486. [CrossRef]
28. Kallio, P.; Pahkala, K.; Heinonen, O.J.; Tammelin, T.H.; Pälve, K.; Hirvensalo, M.; Juonala, M.; Loo, B.-M.; Magnussen, C.G.; Rovio, S.; et al. Physical Inactivity from Youth to Adulthood and Adult Cardiometabolic Risk Profile. *Prev. Med.* **2021**, *145*, 106433. [CrossRef]
29. Dalton, E.D.; Hammen, C.L.; Brennan, P.A.; Najman, J.M. Pathways Maintaining Physical Health Problems from Childhood to Young Adulthood: The Role of Stress and Mood. *Psychol. Health* **2016**, *31*, 1255–1271. [CrossRef]
30. Ortega, F.B.; Ruiz, J.R.; Castillo, M.J. Physical activity, physical fitness, and overweight in children and adolescents: Evidence from epidemiologic studies. *Endocrinol. Nutr. Organo. Soc. Esp. Endocrinol. Nutr.* **2013**, *60*, 458–469. [CrossRef]
31. World Health Organization. *2021 Physical Activity Factsheets for the European Union Member States in the WHO European Region*; World Health Organization, Regional Office for Europe: Copenhagen, Denmark, 2021.
32. Vandoni, M.; Calcaterra, V.; Carnevale Pellino, V.; De Silvestri, A.; Marin, L.; Zuccotti, G.V.; Tranfaglia, V.; Giuriato, M.; Codella, R.; Lovecchio, N. "Fitness and Fatness" in Children and Adolescents: An Italian Cross-Sectional Study. *Children* **2021**, *8*, 762. [CrossRef]
33. Fiori, F.; Bravo, G.; Parpinel, M.; Messina, G.; Malavolta, R.; Lazzer, S. Relationship between Body Mass Index and Physical Fitness in Italian Prepubertal Schoolchildren. *PLoS ONE* **2020**, *15*, e0233362. [CrossRef] [PubMed]
34. Han, M.; Qie, R.; Shi, X.; Yang, Y.; Lu, J.; Hu, F.; Zhang, M.; Zhang, Z.; Hu, D.; Zhao, Y. Cardiorespiratory Fitness and Mortality from All Causes, Cardiovascular Disease and Cancer: Dose–Response Meta-Analysis of Cohort Studies. *Br. J. Sports Med.* **2022**, *56*, 733–739. [CrossRef] [PubMed]
35. Peter, K.; Charles, F.; Henry, S.I.B.; Andreas, P.; Michael, D.; Rayelynn, M.; Heimall, M.S.; Xuemei, S.; Jiajia, Z.; Jonathan, M. Cardiorespiratory Fitness and Mortality Risk Across the Spectra of Age, Race, and Sex. *J. Am. Coll. Cardiol.* **2022**, *80*, 598–609. [CrossRef]
36. Gomes, T.N.; dos Santos, F.K.; Katzmarzyk, P.T.; Maia, J. Active and Strong: Physical Activity, Muscular Strength, and Metabolic Risk in Children. *Am. J. Hum. Biol.* **2017**, *29*, e22904. [CrossRef] [PubMed]
37. Colley, R.C.; Clarke, J.; Doyon, C.Y.; Janssen, I.; Lang, J.J.; Timmons, B.W.; Tremblay, M.S. Trends in Physical Fitness among Canadian Children and Youth. *Health Rep.* **2019**, *30*, 3–13. [CrossRef]
38. Milanovic, I.; Radisavljevic-Janic, S.; Zivkovic, M.Z.; Mirkov, D.M. Health-Related Physical Fitness Levels and Prevalence of Obesity in Serbian Elementary Schoolchildren. *Nutr. Hosp.* **2019**, *36*, 253–260. [CrossRef] [PubMed]
39. Kretschmer, L.; Salali, G.D.; Andersen, L.B.; Hallal, P.C.; Northstone, K.; Sardinha, L.B.; Dyble, M.; Bann, D.; Andersen, L.B.; Anderssen, S.; et al. Gender Differences in the Distribution of Children's Physical Activity: Evidence from Nine Countries. *Int. J. Behav. Nutr. Phys. Act.* **2023**, *20*, 103. [CrossRef]
40. Ma, Y.; Liu, M.; Liu, Y.; Liu, D.; Hou, M. Exploring Physical Activity in Children and Adolescents with Disabilities: A Bibliometric Review of Current Status, Guidelines, Perceived Barriers, and Facilitators and Future Directions. *Healthcare* **2024**, *12*, 934. [CrossRef]
41. Martin Ginis, K.A.; van der Ploeg, H.P.; Foster, C.; Lai, B.; McBride, C.B.; Ng, K.; Pratt, M.; Shirazipour, C.H.; Smith, B.; Vásquez, P.M.; et al. Participation of People Living with Disabilities in Physical Activity: A Global Perspective. *Lancet* **2021**, *398*, 443–455. [CrossRef] [PubMed]
42. Faul, F.; Erdfelder, E.; Buchner, A.; Lang, A.-G. Statistical Power Analyses Using G* Power 3.1: Tests for Correlation and Regression Analyses. *Behav. Res. Methods* **2009**, *41*, 1149–1160. [CrossRef] [PubMed]
43. Faul, F.; Erdfelder, E.; Lang, A.-G.; Buchner, A. G* Power 3: A Flexible Statistical Power Analysis Program for the Social, Behavioral, and Biomedical Sciences. *Behav. Res. Methods* **2007**, *39*, 175–191. [CrossRef]
44. Cole, T.J.; Bellizzi, M.C.; Flegal, K.M.; Dietz, W.H. Establishing a Standard Definition for Child Overweight and Obesity Worldwide: International Survey. *BMJ* **2000**, *320*, 1240. [CrossRef]
45. Ruiz, J.R.; Castro-Piñero, J.; España-Romero, V.; Artero, E.G.; Ortega, F.B.; Cuenca, M.M.; Jimenez-Pavón, D.; Chillón, P.; Girela-Rejón, M.J.; Mora, J.; et al. Field-Based Fitness Assessment in Young People: The ALPHA Health-Related Fitness Test Battery for Children and Adolescents. *Br. J. Sports Med.* **2011**, *45*, 518–524. [CrossRef]
46. Morrow, J.J.R.; Mood, D.; Disch, J.; Kang, M. *Measurement and Evaluation in Human Performance, 5E*; Human Kinetics: Champaign, IL, USA, 2015.
47. Council of Europe. Committee for the Development of Sport. In *Eurofit: Handbook for the Eurofit Tests of Physical Fitness*, 2nd ed.; Council of Europe: Strasbourg, France, 1993.

48. Marques, A.; Henriques-Neto, D.; Peralta, M.; Martins, J.; Gomes, F.; Popovic, S.; Masanovic, B.; Demetriou, Y.; Schlund, A.; Ihle, A. Field-Based Health-Related Physical Fitness Tests in Children and Adolescents: A Systematic Review. *Front. Pediatr.* **2021**, *9*, 640028. [CrossRef]
49. Monacis, D.; Pascali, G.; Colella, D. Mediating Role of Physical Activity Levels on Physical Fitness in Overweight and Obese Children When Body Mass Index Is Not a Determining Factor. *Pedagog. Phys. Cult. Sports* **2024**, *28*, 192–200. [CrossRef]
50. Crocker, P.R.; Bailey, D.A.; Faulkner, R.A.; Kowalski, K.C.; McGrath, R. Measuring General Levels of Physical Activity: Preliminary Evidence for the Physical Activity Questionnaire for Older Children. *Med. Sci. Sports Exerc.* **1997**, *29*, 1344–1349. [CrossRef] [PubMed]
51. Crocker, P.R.; Eklund, R.C.; Kowalski, K.C. Children's Physical Activity and Physical Self-Perceptions. *J. Sports Sci.* **2000**, *18*, 383–394. [CrossRef]
52. Kowalski, K.C.; Crocker, P.R.E.; Donen, R.M. The Physical Activity Questionnaire for Older Children (PAQ-C) and Adolescents (PAQ-A) Manual. *Coll. Kinesiol. Univ. Sask.* **2004**, *87*, 1–38.
53. Gobbi, E.; Elliot, C.; Varnier, M.; Carraro, A. Psychometric Properties of the Physical Activity Questionnaire for Older Children in Italy: Testing the Validity among a General and Clinical Pediatric Population. *PLoS ONE* **2016**, *11*, e0156354. [CrossRef]
54. Monacis, D.; Annoscia, S.; Colella, D.; Limone, P. Measuring Validity and Reliability of the Italian Version of Physical Activity Questionnaire for Older Children in Overweight and Obese Children. *Front. Educ.* **2024**, *9*, 1414126. [CrossRef]
55. Cohen, J. *Statistical Power Analysis for the Behavioral Sciences, Revised*; Academic Press: New York, NY, USA, 2013.
56. Preacher, K.J.; Hayes, A.F. SPSS and SAS Procedures for Estimating Indirect Effects in Simple Mediation Models. *Behav. Res. Methods Instrum. Comput. J. Psychon. Soc. Inc.* **2004**, *36*, 717–731. [CrossRef] [PubMed]
57. Hayes, A.F. *Introduction to Mediation, Moderation, and Conditional Process Analysis: A Regression-Based Approach*, 2nd ed.; Guilford Publications: New York, NY, USA, 2018.
58. Monacis, D.; Colella, D.; Kolimechkov, S. Regional Observatory of Physical Fitness in Children and Adolescents in Southern Italy: A Thirty-Year Comparison Between 1990–2020. *Kinesiol. Slov.* **2023**, *29*, 122–137. [CrossRef]
59. Müller, A.; Nagy, Z.; Kovács, S.; Szőke, S.; Bendíková, E.; Ráthonyi, G.; Ráthonyi-Ódor, K.; Szabados, G.; Gabnai, Z.; Bába, É.B. Correlations between Physical Fitness and Body Composition among Boys Aged 14-18-Conclusions of a Case Study to Reverse the Worsening Secular Trend in Fitness among Urban Youth Due to Sedentary Lifestyles. *Int. J. Environ. Res. Public Health* **2022**, *19*, 8765. [CrossRef]
60. Evaristo, S.; Moreira, C.; Lopes, L.; Oliveira, A.; Abreu, S.; Agostinis-Sobrinho, C.; Oliveira-Santos, J.; Póvoas, S.; Santos, R.; Mota, J. Muscular Fitness and Cardiorespiratory Fitness Are Associated with Health-Related Quality of Life: Results from Labmed Physical Activity Study. *J. Exerc. Sci. Fit.* **2019**, *17*, 55–61. [CrossRef] [PubMed]
61. Todendi, P.F.; Brand, C.; de Castro Silveira, J.F.; Gaya, A.R.; Agostinis-Sobrinho, C.; Fiegenbaum, M.; Burns, R.D.; Valim, A.R.d.M.; Reuter, C.P. Physical Fitness Attenuates the Genetic Predisposition to Obesity in Children and Adolescents. *Scand. J. Med. Sci. Sports* **2021**, *31*, 894–902. [CrossRef]
62. Soares, R.; Brasil, I.; Monteiro, W.; Farinatti, P. Effects of Physical Activity on Body Mass and Composition of School-Age Children and Adolescents with Overweight or Obesity: Systematic Review Focusing on Intervention Characteristics. *J. Bodyw. Mov. Ther.* **2023**, *33*, 154–163. [CrossRef]
63. Wisnieski, L.; Dalimonte-Merckling, D.; Robbins, L.B. Cardiorespiratory Fitness as a Mediator of the Association between Physical Activity and Overweight and Obesity in Adolescent Girls. *Child. Obes.* **2019**, *15*, 338–345. [CrossRef] [PubMed]
64. Syam, Y.; Erika, K.A.; Fadilah, N.; Syahrul, S. Physical Activity among Obese School-Aged Children: A Cross-Sectional Study. *Enferm. Clin.* **2021**, *31*, S704–S708. [CrossRef]
65. Kumari Ekanayake, H.D.; Salibi, D.G.; Tzenios, N. Analysis of Association between Childhood Overweight/Obesity with Screen Time, Sedentary Life Style and Low Levels of Physical Activity. *Spec. J. Med. Acad. other Life Sci.* **2023**, *1*, 1–17. [CrossRef]
66. Kaioglou, V.; Dania, A.; Kambas, A.; Venetsanou, F. Associations of Motor Competence, Cardiorespiratory Fitness, and Physical Activity: The Mediating Role of Cardiorespiratory Fitness. *Res. Q. Exerc. Sport* **2023**, *94*, 361–367. [CrossRef] [PubMed]
67. González-Gálvez, N.; López-Martínez, A.B.; López-Vivancos, A. Clustered Cardiometabolic Risk and the "Fat but Fit Paradox" in Adolescents: Cross-Sectional Study. *Nutrients* **2024**, *16*, 606. [CrossRef]
68. Farooq, A.; Martin, A.; Janssen, X.; Wilson, M.G.; Gibson, A.-M.; Hughes, A.; Reilly, J.J. Longitudinal Changes in Moderate-to-Vigorous-Intensity Physical Activity in Children and Adolescents: A Systematic Review and Meta-Analysis. *Obes. Rev.* **2020**, *21*, e12953. [CrossRef] [PubMed]
69. Muntaner-Mas, A.; Palou, P.; Vidal-Conti, J.; Esteban-Cornejo, I. A Mediation Analysis on the Relationship of Physical Fitness Components, Obesity, and Academic Performance in Children. *J. Pediatr.* **2018**, *198*, 90–97.e4. [CrossRef] [PubMed]
70. Healey, E.L.; Allen, K.D.; Bennell, K.; Bowden, J.L.; Quicke, J.G.; Smith, R. Self-Report Measures of Physical Activity. *Arthritis Care Res.* **2020**, *72* (Suppl. 10), 717–730. [CrossRef]

71. Cerin, E.; Cain, K.L.; Oyeyemi, A.L.; Owen, N.; Conway, T.L.; Cochrane, T.; Van Dyck, D.; Schipperijn, J.; Mitáš, J.; Toftager, M.; et al. Correlates of Agreement between Accelerometry and Self-Reported Physical Activity. *Med. Sci. Sports Exerc.* **2016**, *48*, 1075–1084. [CrossRef] [PubMed]
72. Sardinha, L.B.; Magalhães, J.P.; Santos, D.A.; Hetherington-Rauth, M. Intensity Matters: Impact of Physical Activity Energy Expenditure at Moderate and Vigorous Intensity on Total and Abdominal Obesity in Children. *Eur. J. Clin. Nutr.* **2023**, *77*, 546–550. [CrossRef] [PubMed]
73. Skinner, A.M.; Vlachopoulos, D.; Barker, A.R.; Moore, S.A.; Rowlands, A.V.; Soininen, S.; Haapala, E.A.; Väistö, J.; Westgate, K.; Brage, S.; et al. Physical Activity Volume and Intensity Distribution in Relation to Bone, Lean and Fat Mass in Children. *Scand. J. Med. Sci. Sports* **2023**, *33*, 267–282. [CrossRef]
74. Arufe-Giráldez, V.; Sanmiguel-Rodríguez, A.; Ramos-Álvarez, O.; Navarro-Patón, R. News of the Pedagogical Models in Physical Education—A Quick Review. *Int. J. Environ. Res. Public Health* **2023**, *20*, 2586. [CrossRef]
75. Webster, E.K.; Martin, C.K.; Staiano, A.E. Fundamental Motor Skills, Screen-Time, and Physical Activity in Preschoolers. *J. Sport Health Sci.* **2019**, *8*, 114–121. [CrossRef] [PubMed]
76. Monacis, D.; Trecroci, A.; Invernizzi, P.L.; Colella, D. Can Enjoyment and Physical Self-Perception Mediate the Relationship between BMI and Levels of Physical Activity? Preliminary Results from the Regional Observatory of Motor Development in Italy. *Int. J. Environ. Res. Public Health* **2022**, *19*, 12567. [CrossRef] [PubMed]
77. Berleze, A.; Valentini, N.C. Intervention for Children with Obesity and Overweight and Motor Delays from Low-Income Families: Fostering Engagement, Motor Development, Self-Perceptions, and Playtime. *Int. J. Environ. Res. Public Health* **2022**, *19*, 2545. [CrossRef] [PubMed]
78. Ługowska, K.; Kolanowski, W.; Trafialek, J. Increasing Physical Activity at School Improves Physical Fitness of Early Adolescents. *Int. J. Environ. Res. Public Health* **2023**, *20*, 2348. [CrossRef]
79. Ha, A.S.; Ng, J.Y.Y.; Lonsdale, C.; Lubans, D.R.; Ng, F.F. Promoting Physical Activity in Children through Family-Based Intervention: Protocol of the "Active 1 + FUN" Randomized Controlled Trial. *BMC Public Health* **2019**, *19*, 218. [CrossRef] [PubMed]
80. Santos, F.; Sousa, H.; Gouveia, É.R.; Lopes, H.; Peralta, M.; Martins, J.; Murawska-Ciałowicz, E.; Żurek, G.; Marques, A. School-Based Family-Oriented Health Interventions to Promote Physical Activity in Children and Adolescents: A Systematic Review. *Am. J. Health Promot.* **2022**, *37*, 243–262. [CrossRef]
81. Mannocci, A.; D'Egidio, V.; Backhaus, I.; Federici, A.; Sinopoli, A.; Ramirez Varela, A.; Villari, P.; La Torre, G. Are There Effective Interventions to Increase Physical Activity in Children and Young People? An Umbrella Review. *Int. J. Environ. Res. Public Health* **2020**, *17*, 3528. [CrossRef]
82. Messing, S.; Rütten, A.; Abu-Omar, K.; Ungerer-Röhrich, U.; Goodwin, L.; Burlacu, I.; Gediga, G. How Can Physical Activity Be Promoted Among Children and Adolescents? A Systematic Review of Reviews Across Settings. *Front. Public Health* **2019**, *7*, 55. [CrossRef]
83. Colella, D.; Morano, M.; Robazza, C.; Bortoli, L. Body Image, Perceived Physical Ability, and Motor Performance in Nonoverweight and Overweight Italian Children. *Percept. Mot. Ski.* **2009**, *108*, 209–218. [CrossRef] [PubMed]
84. Morano, M.; Colella, D.; Capranica, L. Body Image, Perceived and Actual Physical Abilities in Normal-Weight and Overweight Boys Involved in Individual and Team Sports. *J. Sports Sci.* **2011**, *29*, 355–362. [CrossRef]
85. Morano, M.; Colella, D.; Rutigliano, I.; Fiore, P.; Pettoello-Mantovani, M.; Campanozzi, A. Changes in Actual and Perceived Physical Abilities in Clinically Obese Children: A 9-Month Multi-Component Intervention Study. *PLoS ONE* **2012**, *7*, e50782. [CrossRef]
86. Morano, M.; Colella, D.; Rutigliano, I.; Fiore, P.; Pettoello-Mantovani, M.; Campanozzi, A. A Multi-Modal Training Programme to Improve Physical Activity, Physical Fitness and Perceived Physical Ability in Obese Children. *J. Sports Sci.* **2014**, *32*, 345–353. [CrossRef]
87. Monacis, D.; Annoscia, S.; Limone, P.; Colella, D. Examining the Effects of Reproductive and Productive Teaching Styles Interventions on Primary Schoolchildren. What Implications for Physical Education Teachers? *Phys. Educ. Theory Methodol.* **2023**, *23*, 839–849. [CrossRef]

children

MDPI

Article

An Assessment of Motor Skills in Infants at Risk of Atypical Psychomotor Development Using the Vojta Method

Robert Podstawski [1,*], Katarzyna Balewska-Juras [1], Krzysztof Borysławski [2], Attila Szabo [3] and Jadwiga Snarska [4]

[1] Human Wellness Research Laboratory, Department of Physiotherapy, School of Public Health, University of Warmia and Mazury in Olsztyn, 10-957 Olsztyn, Poland; kbalewska.juras@wp.pl
[2] Institute of Health, Angelus Silesius University of Applied Sciences in Wałbrzych, 58-300 Wałbrzych, Poland; kboryslawski@ans.edu.pl
[3] Faculty of Health and Sport Sciences, Széchenyi István University, 9026 Győr, Hungary; szabo.attila@sze.hu
[4] Department of General Surgery, School of Public Health, University of Warmia and Mazury in Olsztyn, 10-957 Olsztyn, Poland; jadwiga.snarska@uwm.edu.pl
* Correspondence: podstawskirobert@gmail.com

Abstract: Background: Some neonates are assessed for the risk of atypical psychomotor development at birth and are referred for reflex locomotion therapy using the Vojta method. **Aim**: The aim of this study was to analyze the relationships between spontaneous motor activity (SMA), ideal movement patterns (IMPs), central coordination disorders (CCDs), vital signs at birth, involuntary reflexes, and postural asymmetry in infants. **Methods**: This study involved 90 female and 107 male subjects in the age interval of 1–16 months (4.15 ± 2.18). Their psychomotor development was assessed using the Vojta method. Age-appropriate involuntary reflexes were evaluated, and both parameters were correlated with perinatal risk factors. **Results**: Males scored significantly higher than females (difference of −0.7, $p = 0.022$) in the SMA test. In both genders, SMA ($p < 0.001$ in both genders) and IMP scores improved significantly with age. In male infants, higher CCD scores were associated with significantly lower SMA and IMP scores ($p = 0.017$ and $p < 0.001$, respectively). Significantly higher CCD scores were noted in female subjects with the Moro reflex and postural asymmetry ($p = 0.003$ and $p = 0.002$, respectively). In males, the Moro reflex was significantly correlated with the Vojta reaction ($p = 0.012$) and the Collis vertical suspension reflex ($p < 0.001$). **Conclusions**: Vital signs at birth, including birth weight, Apgar score, and type of delivery, can predict motor development disorders but do not clearly differentiate infants that require neurodevelopmental therapy.

Keywords: physical therapy diagnosis; motor disorders; coordination of the central nervous system; postural reflexes; spontaneous motor activity

1. Introduction

In physical therapy practice, an accurate diagnosis is essential for initiating effective treatment in all age groups. Any deviations or delays in the psychomotor development of infants and young children should be immediately addressed to initiate early therapeutic interventions and prevent psychomotor disorders in later life [1]. However, children younger than 12 months are challenging to diagnose because their central nervous system is not yet fully developed [2,3]. In some cases, delayed myelination of nerve fibers can disrupt neural and muscular coordination, and these symptoms can be misdiagnosed [4]. For this reason, infants with prenatal or perinatal risk factors should receive specialized care immediately after birth and should be subjected to a full range of diagnostic tests.

Children **2025**, *12*, 976 https://doi.org/10.3390/children12080976

Early psychomotor development and disorders of the central nervous system (CNS) are diagnosed with the use of advanced imaging methods, including magnetic resonance imaging (MRI), transfontanellar ultrasound (TFUS), and electroencephalography (EEG) [5,6]. These imaging techniques enable early detection of developmental defects and neonatal encephalopathy, facilitating quick initiation of therapeutic interventions [7]. In neonates, physical therapists also assess primitive reflexes, gross motor skills, positional preferences, and spontaneous movements and posture [8,9]. The most popular diagnostic methods include Vojta therapy [10,11], the Bobath concept (neurodevelopmental treatment, NDT-Bobath) [12–14], Prechtl's method [15,16], and the Munich Functional Developmental Diagnostics (MFDR) scale [17,18].

Vojta therapy is a widely used diagnostic tool in clinical practice that relies on developmental kinesiology and reflex locomotion principles. The Vojta method can be used to diagnose and treat neurophysiological disorders from birth to the achievement of bipedal locomotion [19,20]. This approach examines spontaneous movement patterns, automatic involuntary motor reactions, and seven postural reactions in young children. The development of the CNS influences these reactions and movement patterns. In Vojta therapy, special attention is given to spontaneous motor activity (SMA), postural reactions, the level of maturity of the central nervous system, and, above all, ideal movement patterns (IMPs) [21,22]. In this approach, other reflexes involved in postural control and SMA are also evaluated based on observations of the child's primitive reflexes and automatic reactions, including head control, the uprighting and anti-gravity mechanisms of different body segments, and the ability to prop up on the hands or elbows for support in a prone or sitting position. These milestones follow a predictable sequence in successive neurodevelopmental stages, with contextual variations in the external output that guide the diagnosis [23]. The diagnosis provides information about non-retained disorders of the nervous system that can be effectively resolved through physical therapy involving neurophysiological methods [24].

Atypical psychomotor development of infants exposed to various risk factors during the prenatal period, delivery, and the perinatal period has been explored in numerous studies. Research has shown that perinatal risk factors can lead to neurological disorders and can be captured by the deviations in the output observed in a neurophysiological test conducted using the Vojta method [22,23]. However, the relationships between central coordination disorders (CCDs) in infants diagnosed with the Vojta method and perinatal risk factors such as gestation length, type of delivery, birth weight, Apgar score, and primitive reflexes have never been found in the literature. These links should be identified to facilitate the early detection of psychomotor anomalies in infants and to assist neonatologists and pediatricians in implementing therapeutic approaches that can significantly contribute to the healthy development of children.

Therefore, this study aimed to identify the relationships between the psychomotor skills of infants assessed with the Vojta method based on their SMA, IMP, and CCD scores and perinatal risk factors, involuntary reflexes, and postural asymmetry.

2. Materials and Methods

2.1. Participants

This study involved 197 infants at risk of atypical psychomotor development who were patients of the Rehabilitation Clinic of the Center for Rehabilitation and Education in Szczytno and were referred for Vojta physiotherapy by a physician (a rehabilitation consultant) to confirm or rule out developmental disorders. The study group consisted of 107 male subjects aged 4.15 ± 2.18 months and 90 females aged 3.84 ± 2.12 months (1–16 months). The inclusion criteria were complications during pregnancy and delivery, preterm birth, a low Apgar score in the first minutes after birth, a low birth weight, postural asymmetry (at 7 weeks of age), atypical muscle tone, delayed psychomotor development, and non-age-appropriate involuntary reflexes. During the study, all children were healthy and did not present with any symptoms of infection. Children with genetic disorders were excluded from the study.

2.2. Ethical Statement

This study was conducted in accordance with the guidelines and policies of the Health Science Council and the Declaration of Helsinki. The study received approval from the Ethics Committee of the Medical University of Poznań (179/2012). Each child's parent was provided with detailed information about the study's purpose, potential risks, procedures, and relevant matters. All parents gave voluntary informed consent to participate in the study and agreed to the publication of anonymous data.

2.3. Procedures, Data Collection, and Equipment

The psychomotor development of the studied infants, including potential disorders, was assessed. Before the tests, information regarding the progression of pregnancy, maternal diseases, gestation length, type of delivery (spontaneous or with surgical intervention), the child's birth weight, Apgar score, and adaptation to life in the first days after birth was collected from the parents.

Spontaneous motor activity was evaluated in both supine and prone positions, based on the number of presented skills. Ideal movement patterns were evaluated in the supine position during rolling, sitting, toddling, standing up, and walking. Special attention was placed on postural asymmetry. Any deviations in the alignment of different body parts relative to the midline axis were evaluated in supine and prone positions. Postural asymmetry was diagnosed based on the tilt of the head towards the shoulder girdle (always the same shoulder), obliquity of the shoulder and pelvic girdles, and clear preference for holding the head rotated or the body always towards one side only. The same criteria were applied to diagnose postural asymmetry in sitting and standing positions. In the next stage, primitive reflexes were assessed considering the child's age and CNS development. The test involved evaluating spinal and tonic reflexes, as well as assessing the ability to support the head and control head movements, maintain an upright position and balance, and prop up on the hands or elbows for support in both prone and sitting positions. The child's reactions to and specific behaviors in each test were registered.

Assessment Involving the Vojta Method

The rate of motor development was assessed using the seven postural reactions proposed by Vojta for neuromotor screening [25]. In healthy children, these reactions correspond to typical stages of ontogenic development of postural and locomotive skills during the first year of life [11]. These skills evolve with age and follow a predictable sequence in successive stages of psychomotor development [25]. Atypical reactions that deviate from the pattern described by Vojta are referred to as CCDs. The severity of CCDs is evaluated on a four-point scale based on the number of atypical postural reactions:

1. Very mild—1–3 atypical postural reactions;
2. Mild—4–5 atypical postural reactions;
3. Moderate—6–7 atypical postural reactions;
4. Severe—7 atypical postural reactions [26,27].

The infants' involuntary and automatic reactions to changes in body position were evaluated during the test, and all children received a CCD score based on the above rating scale. Support and extension postures, changes in muscle tone, alignment of the spine and enarthroses, and stages of postural and movement output were assessed in the postural reaction test.

The assessments were conducted by a certified Vojta therapist in the presence of the parents. Each test was conducted under identical, optimal conditions at constant temperature and in a quiet room. Most of the examined infants participated in neurodevelopmental therapy after the study. The children were evaluated for the achievement of age-specific developmental milestones (the age of pre-term infants was adjusted accordingly) and for the presence of typical or atypical postural reactions. The motor skills and CCD scores of male and female participants were compared separately. The presence of significant relationships between vital signs at birth, SMA, IMPs, the severity of CCDs, involuntary reflexes, and postural asymmetry was determined.

2.4. Statistical Analysis

The significance of the differences between means was determined by Student's t-test for independent variables. The relationships between quantitative traits were analyzed by calculating Pearson correlation coefficients (r). The chi-square test was used to analyze the relationships between nominal (category) features. The gamma (γ) coefficient numerically equivalent to Pearson's r was also calculated. The results were processed statistically in Statistica PL v. 13.0 at a significance level of $p < 0.05$.

3. Results

The examined infants were born between 24 and 42 weeks of pregnancy. On average, male subjects were born at 37.5 ± 3.5 weeks, and females were born at 38.4 ± 2.7 weeks. Birth weights were similar in both genders, with an average of 3118.5 ± 859.2 g in males and 3078.4 ± 783.2 g in females. Neonates were evaluated on the 10-point Apgar test in the first minute after birth. The average score was 8.9 ± 2.0 in males and 9.3 ± 1.4 in females. The study population is characterized in Table 1.

Table 1. Characteristics of the studied male and female infants.

Variable	Male n = 107				Female n = 90				t	p
	Mean	SD	Min	Max	Mean	SD	Min	Max		
Gestation length [weeks]	37.5	3.5	24	42	38.4	2.7	26	42	−1.92	0.055
Birth weight [g]	3118.5	859.2	666	4900	3078.4	783.2	660	4450	0.34	0.734
Apgar score * [points]	8.9	2.0	1	10	9.3	1.43	2	10	−1.70	0.091
Age [months]	4.2	2.2	1	16	3.8	2.1	1	11	0.99	0.324

Notes: *—in the first minute after birth.

Male subjects received significantly higher scores than females (difference of −0.7, p = 0.022) only in the assessment of SMA. No significant differences in CCD or IMP scores were observed between the genders (p = 0.151 and p = 0.321, respectively) (Table 2).

In both genders, SMA ($p < 0.001$ in both genders) and IMP ($p < 0.001$ in both genders) scores improved significantly with age. In female subjects, a higher birth weight and higher Apgar scores were associated with significantly higher SMA and IMP scores ($p < 0.05$) (Table 3). In both genders, gestation length was not significantly correlated with SMA or IMP scores.

Table 2. Scores received by male and female infants in CCD, SMA, and IMP tests.

Variable	Male n = 107			Female n = 90			t	p	D-Cohen's
	Mean	SD	Min–Max	Mean	SD	Min–Max			
CCDs	4.61	2.17	0–7	5.06	2.18	0–7	−1.44	0.151	0.202
SMA	3.42	2.02	0–11	2.74	2.07	0–9	2.31	**0.022**	**0.332**
IMPs	1.68	2.01	0–8	1.39	2.05	0–8	0.99	0.321	0.143

Notes: CCDs—central coordination disorders, SMA—spontaneous motor activity, IMPs—ideal movement patterns, bold font—statistically significant difference.

Table 3. Relationships between SMA and IMP scores and vital signs at birth in male and female infants.

Variable		Male (n = 107)		Female (n = 89)	
		r	p	r	p
SMA	Gestation length [weeks]	−0.06	ns	0.12	ns
	Birth weight [g]	−0.04	ns	**0.24**	**0.023**
	Apgar score [points]	−0.12	ns	**0.22**	**0.048**
	Age [months]	**0.71**	**<0.001**	**0.76**	**<0.001**
IMP	Gestation length [weeks]	0.07	ns	0.14	ns
	Birth weight [g]	0.06	ns	**0.27**	**0.011**
	Apgar score [points]	−0.02	ns	**0.24**	**0.025**
	Age [months]	**0.64**	**<0.001**	**0.75**	**<0.001**

Notes: ns—not significant, bold font—statistically significant correlation.

In the study population, CCD scores were not significantly correlated with vital signs at birth or the infant's age on the day of the assessment (Table 4).

Table 4. Relationships between CCD scores and vital signs at birth in male and female infants.

Variable		Male (n = 107)		Female (n = 89)	
		r	p	r	p
CCD	Gestation length [weeks]	0.09	ns	−0.05	ns
	Birth weight [g]	0.04	ns	−0.11	ns
	Apgar score [points]	0.01	ns	−0.14	ns
	Age [months]	−0.09	ns	0.17	ns

Notes: ns—not significant.

The relationships between CCD, SMA, and IMP scores are presented in Table 5. Significant correlations were found only in male subjects. In males, a significant inverse correlation was noted between the CCD score and the SMA and IMP scores ($p = 0.017$ and $p < 0.001$, respectively).

Potential relationships between the number of atypical postural reactions (CCD score) and the type of delivery (spontaneous or with surgical intervention), involuntary motor reflexes, and postural asymmetry were determined in a detailed analysis (Table 6). Female infants with the Moro reflex and postural asymmetry received significantly higher CCD scores ($p = 0.003$ and $p = 0.002$, respectively). The number of atypical postural reactions (CCD score) was also significantly higher in males with the palmar grasp reflex and postural asymmetry ($p = 0.049$ and $p < 0.001$, respectively). In the group of male and female infants born by cesarean section, CCD scores were significantly higher in females ($p = 0.018$).

Table 5. Relationships between the CCD score and SMA and IMP scores in male and female infants.

Variable		Male (n = 107)		Female (n = 89)	
		r	p	r	p
CCD	SMA	**−0.23**	**0.017**	−0.05	ns
	IMP	**−0.36**	**<0.001**	−0.11	ns

Notes: ns—not significant, bold font—statistically significant difference.

Table 6. Relationships between CCD scores, involuntary motor reflexes, postural asymmetry, and type of delivery in male and female infants.

Variable		Male				Female				Differences	
		n	Mean	SD	Min–Max	n	Mean	SD	Min–Max	t	p
Gender		107	4.61	2.17		90	5.06	2.18		1.44	ns
Type of delivery	Spontaneous	20	4.90	1.71	2–7	16	5.07	2.32	0–7	0.24	ns
	C-section	36	4.14	2.37	0–7	26	5.54	2.04	0–7	**2.43**	**0.018**
	t (p)			ns				ns			
Palmar grasp reflex	Absent	41	4.17	2.17	0–7	30	4.33	2.23	0–7	0.31	ns
	Present	52	4.81	2.11	0–7	46	5.34	2.16	0–7	1.25	ns
	t (p)			ns			**1.99 (0.049)**				
Moro reflex	Absent	44	4.30	2.18	0–7	28	5.14	2.12	0–7	1.62	ns
	Present	19	6.00	1.45	3–7	18	5.17	2.41	0–7	1.29	ns
	t (p)		**3.11 (0.003)**					ns			
Postural asymmetry	Absent	16	3.13	2.22	0–7	13	3.15	2.48	0–7	0.03	ns
	Present	88	4.87	2.06	0–7	73	5.45	1.95	0–7	1.78	ns
	t (p)		**3.12 (0.002)**				**3.75 (<0.001)**				

Notes: ns—not significant, bold font—statistically significant difference.

The results of the analysis examining the relationships between the Moro reflex and seven postural reactions (CCD score) are presented in Table 7. In males, the presence of the Moro reflex was significantly correlated only with the Vojta reaction ($p = 0.012$) and the Collis vertical suspension response ($p < 0.001$). In male infants, the relationship between the Moro reflex and the Landau reaction was on the borderline of statistical significance ($p = 0.053$). In female subjects, postural reactions (CCD score) were not significantly correlated with the Moro reflex ($p > 0.05$). Only the correlation between the Moro reflex and the pull-to-sit (traction) reflex was on the borderline of statistical significance ($p = 0.056$) (Table 7).

Table 7. Relationships between the Moro reflex and seven postural reactions in the CCD test.

Variable/Category		Male		Female	
		Present (n = 19)	Absent (n = 44)	Present (n = 18)	Absent (n = 28)
Pull-to-sit test		$\chi^2 = 1.28, \gamma = 0.42, p = 0.258$		$\chi^2 = 3.65, \gamma = 0.58, p = 0.056$ *	
0	*fo*	2	10	7	4
	fo–fe	−1.62	1.62	2.70	−2.70
1	*Fo*	17	34	11	24
	fo–fe	1.62	−1.62	−2.70	2.70

Table 7. *Cont.*

Variable/Category		Male		Female	
		Present (n = 19)	Absent (n = 44)	Present (n = 18)	Absent (n = 28)
Landau reaction		$\chi^2 = 3.74, \gamma = 0.63, p = 0.053$ *		$\chi^2 = 0.01, \gamma = 0.04, p = 0.917$	
0	*fo*	2	15	3	5
	fo–fe	−3.13	3.13	−0.13	0.13
1	*fo*	17	29	15	23
	fo–fe	3.13	−3.13	0.13	−0.13
Auxiliary suspension test		$\chi^2 = 0.75, \gamma = 0.27, p = 0.385$		$\chi^2 = 1.96, \gamma = 0.47, p = 0.161$	
0	*fo*	4	14	3	10
	fo–fe	−1.43	1.43	−2.09	2.09
1	Fo	15	30	15	18
	fo–fe	1.43	−1.43	2.09	−2.09
Vojta reaction		$\mathbf{\chi^2 = 6.37, \gamma = 0.73, p = 0.012}$		$\chi^2 = 0.01, \gamma = 0.02, p = 0.953$	
0	*fo*	2	19	5	8
	fo–fe	−4.33	4.33	−0.09	0.09
1	*fo*	17	25	13	20
	fo–fe	4.33	−4.33	0.09	−0.09
Collis horizontal suspension test		$\chi^2 = 2.81, \gamma = 0.44, p = 0.094$		$\chi^2 = 0.12, \gamma = 0.11, p = 0.732$	
0	Fo	6	24	6	8
	fo–fe	−3.05	3.05	0.52	−0.52
1	*fo*	13	20	12	20
	fo–fe	3.05	−3.05	−0.52	0.52
Peiper-Isbert suspension test		$\chi^2 = 3.18, \gamma = 0.60, p = 0.074$		$\chi^2 = 0.23, \gamma = 0.17, p = 0.632$	
0	*fo*	2	14	4	8
	fo–fe	−2.83	2.83	−0.70	0.70
1	*fo*	17	30	14	20
	fo–fe	2.83	−2.83	0.70	−0.70
Collis vertical suspension test		$\mathbf{\chi^2 = 12.43, \gamma = 0.90, p < 0.001}$		$\chi^2 = 0.10, \gamma = 0.10, p = 0.754$	
0	*fo*	1	23	5	9
	fo–fe	−6.24	6.24	−0.48	0.48
1	*fo*	18	21	13	19
	fo–fe	6.24	−6.24	0.48	−0.48

Notes: * Borderline significant; *fo*—frequency observed; *fe*—frequency expected, ns—not significant, bold font—statistically significant relationship.

The results of the analysis examining the relationship between the palmar grasp reflex and postural reactions in the CCD test are presented in Table 8. In females, the palmar grasp reflex was significantly correlated only with the pull-to-sit reflex and the Landau reaction ($p = 0.006$ and $p = 0.035$, respectively). In both genders, the palmar grasp reflex was not significantly correlated with the results of the remaining motor tests (Table 8).

Table 8. Relationships between the palmar grasp reflex and seven postural reactions in the CCD test.

Variable/Category		Male		Female	
		Present (n = 52)	Absent (n = 41)	Present (n = 46)	Absent (n = 30)
Pull-to-sit test		$\chi^2 = 2.63, \gamma = 0.38, p = 0.105$		$\mathbf{\chi^2 = 7.57, \gamma = 0.61, p = 0.006}$	
0	*fo*	9	13	8	14
	fo–fe	−3.30	3.30	−5.32	5.32
1	*fo*	43	28	38	16
	fo–fe	3.30	−3.30	5.32	−5.32

Table 8. *Cont.*

Variable/Category		Male		Female	
		Present (n = 52)	Absent (n = 41)	Present (n = 46)	Absent (n = 30)
Landau reaction		$\chi^2 = 2.71, \gamma = 0.37, p = 0.010$		$\boldsymbol{\chi^2 = 4.42, \gamma = 0.56, p = 0.035}$	
0	*fo*	11	15	5	9
	fo–fe	−3.54	3.54	−3.47	3.47
1	*fo*	41	26	41	21
	fo–fe	3.54	−3.54	3.47	−3.47
Auxiliary suspension test		$\chi^2 = 0.93, \gamma = 0.22, p = 0.335$		$\chi^2 = 1.09, \gamma = 0.28, p = 0.296$	
0	*fo*	13	14	9	9
	fo–fe	−2.10	2.10	−1.89	1.89
1	*fo*	39	27	37	21
	fo–fe	2.10	−2.10	1.89	−1.89
Vojta reaction		$\chi^2 = 2.37, \gamma = 0.32, p = 0.124$		$\chi^2 = 2.69, \gamma = 0.38, p = 0.101$	
0	*fo*	16	19	13	14
	fo–fe	−3.57	3.57	−3.34	3.34
1	*fo*	36	22	33	16
	fo–fe	3.57	−3.57	3.34	−3.34
Collis horizontal suspension test		$\chi^2 = 0.05, \gamma = 0.05, p = 0.829$		$\chi^2 = 0.13, \gamma = 0.09, p = 0.715$	
0	*fo*	28	23	15	11
	fo–fe	−0.52	0.52	−0.74	0.74
1	*fo*	24	18	31	19
	fo–fe	0.52	−0.52	0.74	−0.74
Peiper-Isbert suspension test		$\chi^2 = 1.14, \gamma = 0.24, p = 0.286$		$\chi^2 = 0.96, \gamma = 0.24, p = 0.326$	
0	*fo*	18	10	12	11
	fo–fe	2.34	−2.34	−1.92	1.92
1	*fo*	34	31	34	19
	fo–fe	−2.34	2.34	1.92	−1.92
Collis vertical suspension test		$\chi^2 = 2.73, \gamma = 0.34, p = 0.099$		$\chi^2 = 0.74, \gamma = 0.21, p = 0.390$	
0	*fo*	19	22	14	12
	fo–fe	−3.92	3.92	−1.74	1.74
1	*fo*	33	19	32	18
	fo–fe	3.92	−3.92	1.74	−1.74

Notes: *fo*—frequency observed, *fe*—frequency expected, ns—not significant, bold font—statistically significant relationship.

4. Discussion

In the first year of life, SMA serves as a window into the development and functional state of the CNS. Neurodevelopmental disorders should be diagnosed with the use of standardized tools based on the results of thorough observations to identify potential correlations between a child's spontaneous behavior and motor reflexes.

In the present study, an attempt was also made to analyze the relationships between vital signs at birth, the infants' motor skills, IMPs, and CCDs. In physical therapy practice, the identified correlations could facilitate diagnosis and shorten the time from diagnosis to treatment. This study revealed significant correlations only for some vital signs at birth; in no case were they observed simultaneously in both genders. These findings suggest that the identified relationships may indicate a risk of neurodevelopmental disorders; however, they cannot serve as definitive predictors of such atypical conditions.

The analyzed relationships indicate that vital signs at birth, including birth weight and Apgar score, as well as the infant's age during the examination, can be associated with developmental anomalies in females but do not play a key role because they proceed differently in both genders. In turn, SMA and IMPs are related to CCDs in male infants. The analyses that we conducted indicated that, in males, there was an interdependence between the CCD assessments and SMA, as well as between CCDs and IMPs, which appeared to be influenced by delayed neurological maturation. In female subjects, no such interdependence was observed. In females, CCDs did not significantly affect the development of spontaneous motor activity or movement patterns. Despite the presence of these disorders, the studied infants continued to acquire subsequent motor skills, although they did not always display the ideal movement patterns. Male and female subjects differed in baseline characteristics; therefore, it might be more informative to compare the deficits or gains in psychomotor skills relative to the infant's gestational age rather than the raw data. This approach could provide a clearer picture of the differences in neurological maturation between the genders.

This observation suggests that newborns who have not achieved motor development milestones or whose motor skills deviate from the physiological standard should be diagnosed for CNS disorders and referred for neurodevelopmental therapy as soon as possible.

In the current study, the risk of CCD was not correlated with gestation length, birth weight, or Apgar score. The above could be attributed to the fact that these associations were explored across the entire study population without division into subgroups characterized by short (up to 37 weeks) and typical gestation lengths (40 weeks), low birth weight (up to 2500 g) and macrosomia (birth weight higher than 4000 g), or low Apgar scores ($\leq$4 points). Therefore, further and more detailed research is needed to explore potential differences between these subgroups.

In many review and cohort studies conducted in Denmark, Italy, and Canada, perinatal parameters (such as birth weight, gestational age, and complications) had no significant impact on the development of CCDs/DCD [28–30]. A similar phenomenon was described in systematic reviews [31]; only in cases of extremely low birth weight, some factors (such as the male gender) had predictive value, but, overall, negative findings were reported in the literature [32]. Parameters such as birth weight and Apgar score assess perinatal conditions, which do not necessarily reflect the neurological status of the newborn. In contrast, the Vojta assessment is an independent diagnostic tool evaluating the state and maturity of the central nervous system. Furthermore, when assessing the neurophysiological development of preterm infants, the child's chronological age is corrected for the number of weeks missing to reach full-term pregnancy. As a result, corrected age itself may not always serve as a predictive factor for the development of preterm infants.

Lipińska et al. [33] examined potential correlations between the progression of pregnancy and hyperactivity in children and adolescents aged 7–17 years. They found that the risk of neurodevelopmental disorders was higher in children who received an Apgar score of 0–4 points at 1 min and 5 min after birth. In turn, Kubisa [34] evaluated the psychomotor development of preterm infants and reported no significant correlations ($p > 0.05$) between the Apgar score at 1, 3, 5, and 10 min after birth and the psychomotor development of infants in the first year of life. The present study revealed a significant correlation between the Apgar score ($p < 0.05$) and the psychomotor abilities (SMA and IMPs) of females, but not males. These observations suggest that the Apgar score is not always a reliable predictor of typical or atypical psychomotor development; therefore, the decision to refer infants for motor skills therapy should not be based solely on this parameter.

In a cohort study examining infants aged up to 5 months, Kwong et al. [35] attempted to identify diagnostic tools for evaluating SMA and capturing the activity repertoire of newborns who were later diagnosed with cerebral palsy. The cited authors conducted a thorough analysis of the literature to identify studies investigating the SMA of infants using Prechtl's General Movements Assessment. They concluded that the SMA and motor skills of infants are strong predictors of neurodevelopmental disorders and cerebral palsy. The cited authors also attempted to demonstrate that motor skills and IMPs are associated with CNS disorders in newborns. They found that male infants' scores in the SMA and IMP tests deteriorated substantially with an increase in the number of atypical postural reactions in the CCD test. Espel et al. [36] conducted a cohort study of 232 mothers and their term newborns (50.4% males) who were assessed at three time points in the first postnatal year. An analysis of the relationship between gestation length and the child's cognitive and motor development revealed that a longer pregnancy, even in children that were born at full term, promotes mental and motor development and that preterm infants show persisting impairments in cognitive function, school achievement, and brain development. In turn, Zachwieja [37] investigated the psychomotor development of 283 preterm children and found that the risk of pediatric cerebral palsy increases with shorter gestational length. The cited studies indicate that the length of pregnancy affects the development and potential anomalies of the CNS in newborns. This observation was not corroborated by the present study, which found no significant correlations between neurodevelopmental disorders and gestational length in male or female infants.

In this study, an attempt was also made to analyze the relationships between the Moro reflex, the palmar grasp reflex, and seven postural reactions. Age-appropriate involuntary reactions were evaluated in each of the seven tested postures. The assessment revealed a significant correlation between both involuntary reactions and the postural reaction. In females, the grasp reflex was significantly correlated with an atypical pull-to-sit reflex and an atypical Landau reaction. Prolonged retention of the grasp reflex is typically related to unusually high muscle tone in the upper limbs, which may explain the postural reactions observed in the study. In male infants, the Moro reflex was correlated with the Vojta reaction and the Collis vertical suspension response. In addition, females and males diagnosed with postural asymmetry were also characterized by higher CCD scores. The above suggests that postural asymmetry is significantly correlated with CCD and could be a predictor of atypical psychomotor development in later life.

Surowińska et al. [38] examined 107 newborns at 3 months of age, with follow-up checks at 9 and 16 months, and they found that qualitative assessments were better predictors of developmental milestones than any of the reflexes, excluding walking, which is strongly predicted by the Babkin reflex. Chinello et al. [39] observed that the persistence of primitive reflexes, including the sucking reflex and palmar and plantar grasp reflexes, can be promising early indicators of autism spectrum disorders in children. The clinical significance of palmar and plantar grasp reflexes was also demonstrated by Futagi et al. [40]. The cited researchers concluded that these reflexes are sensitive and clinically significant predictors of atypical neural development, particularly in children with spastic cerebral palsy.

Neurodevelopmental assessments of neonates should be conducted as early as possible, especially in children at risk of developmental anomalies. The risk factors that predispose infants to neurodevelopmental disorders include obstructed labor, maternal hygiene and lifestyle, maternal medical history, and maternal physical activity [41,42], which were not considered in the current study. These assessments can be conducted using numerous diagnostic tools that were discussed in the study. These tools should be carefully selected based on the examiner's skills and experience, as well as the child's age, to ensure that neonates' psychomotor development is evaluated objectively and that the results of the assessment can be reliably used to choose the optimal treatment.

The clinical observations and scientific analyses presented in this publication clearly indicate that the persistence of infantile reflexes may serve as a predictive factor for atypical motor development. Confirmation of this diagnosis can be supported by assessment using the Vojta method, which is an effective tool for diagnosing and treating infants; however, its effectiveness depends on the timing of the intervention and the specificity of the underlying problems. In pediatric practice, it has been consistently observed that early identification and therapy with the Vojta method provide measurable developmental and psychosocial benefits with a long-term impact.

5. Strengths and Limitations

The strength of this study lies in the comprehensive analysis of the correlations between numerous variables, including separate assessments of perinatal factors in each gender. The principal limitation, however, is that the study population was not stratified into age subgroups defined by specific risk factors, such as preterm birth, low birth weight, or low Apgar scores. Additional age-based stratification would have substantially broadened the scope of the analysis, thus increasing the length of the manuscript. Furthermore, age-based stratification could lead to insufficient numbers of subjects within certain age categories, potentially necessitating the exclusion of newborns from specific groups, thereby reducing the overall sample size.

6. Conclusions

Vital signs at birth, including birth weight, Apgar score, and type of delivery, can be useful predictors of motor development disorders but do not clearly discriminate infants who require neurodevelopmental therapy. The grasp reflex, the Moro reflex, and postural asymmetry are significantly correlated with CCDs and could be indicative of potential irregularities in the psychomotor development of infants. Special attention should be paid to the prolonged retention of motor reflexes to diagnose neonates at risk of atypical psychomotor development and to initiate appropriate treatment as early as possible.

Author Contributions: Conceptualization: R.P. and K.B.-J.; Data curation: K.B.-J.; Formal analysis: K.B.; Funding acquisition: R.P. and J.S.; Investigation: K.B.-J., R.P., and J.S.; Methodology: K.B. and R.P.; Validation: K.B.; Project administration: R.P.; Software: K.B.; Supervision: R.P.; Writing—original draft: R.P., K.B., K.B.-J., A.S., and J.S.; Writing—review and editing: R.P., K.B., and A.S.; Visualization: R.P.; Resources: R.P. All authors have read and agreed to the published version of the manuscript.

Funding: This research received no external funding.

Institutional Review Board Statement: This study was performed in compliance with the guidelines and policies of the Health Science Council and the Declaration of Helsinki. This study was conducted upon the prior consent of the Ethics Committee of the Medical University of Poznań, Poland (179/2012), approval date: 2 February 2012.

Informed Consent Statement: This study involved volunteer children whose parents provided written informed consent.

Data Availability Statement: The access to Excel data generated during this study has been restricted by the Ethics Committee of the UWM in Olsztyn to protect the participants' privacy. Researchers who meet the criteria for access to confidential data can submit a data request by email to podstawskirobert@gmail.com.

Acknowledgments: The authors would like to express their gratitude to the parents whose children participated in the study.

Conflicts of Interest: The authors declare no conflicts of interest.

Abbreviations

The following abbreviations are used in this manuscript:

SMA	spontaneous motor activity
IMPs	ideal movement patterns
CCDs	central coordination disorders
MRI	magnetic resonance imaging

References

1. Brown, K.A.; Parikh, S.; Patel, D.R. Understanding basic concepts of developmental diagnosis in children. *Transl. Pediatr.* **2020**, *9* (Suppl. 1), S9–S22. [CrossRef] [PubMed]
2. Izett, E.; Rooney, R.; Prescott, S.L.; De Palma, M.; McDevitt, M. Prevention of Mental Health Difficulties for Children Aged 0-3 Years: A Review. *Front. Psychol.* **2021**, *29*, 500361. [CrossRef] [PubMed]
3. Joseph, H.M.; Lorenzo, N.E.; Fisher, N.; Novick, D.R.; Gibson, C.; Rothenberger, S.D.; Foust, J.E.; Chronis-Tuscano, A. Research Review: A systematic review and meta-analysis of infant and toddler temperament as predictors of childhood attention-deficit/hyperactivity disorder. *J. Child. Psychol. Psychiatry* **2023**, *64*, 715–735. [CrossRef]
4. Grotheer, M.; Rosenke, M.; Wu, H.; Kular, H.; Querdasi, F.R.; Natu, V.S.; Yeatman, J.D.; Grill-Spector, K. White matter myelination during early infancy is linked to spatial gradients and myelin content at birth. *Nat. Commun.* **2022**, *13*, 997. [CrossRef]
5. De Vries, L.S.; Verboon-Maciolek, M.A.; Cowan, F.M.; Groenendaal, F. The role of cranial ultrasound and magnetic resonance imaging in the diagnosis of infections of the central nervous system. *Early Hum. Dev.* **2006**, *82*, 819–825. [CrossRef]
6. Shen, W.; Pan, J.H.; Chen, W.D. Comparison of transcranial ultrasound and cranial MRI in evaluations of brain injuries from neonatal asphyxia. *Int. J. Clin. Exp. Med.* **2015**, *8*, 18319–18326.
7. Bokiniec, R.; Bekesińska-Figatowska, B.; Rudzińska, I.; Borszewska-Kornacka, M.K. Sonographic and MRI findings in neonates following selective cerebral hypothermia. *Ginekol. Pol.* **2014**, *85*, 933–938. [CrossRef]
8. Malak, R.; Torzyńska, P.; Żółkiewska, J.; Matecka, M.; Samborski, W. Assessment of motor development in children with postural asymmetry and the application of neurodevelopmental-based improvement methods. *Rheumatol. Forum* **2024**, *10*, 194–206. [CrossRef]
9. Pecuch, A.; Gieysztor, E.; Wolańska, E.; Telenga, M.; Paprocka-Borowicz, M. Primitive Reflex Activity in Relation to Motor Skills in Healthy Preschool Children. *Brain Sci.* **2021**, *11*, 967. [CrossRef]
10. De-La-Barrera-Aranda, E.; Gonzalez-Gerez, J.J.; Saavedra-Hernandez, M.; Fernandez-Bueno, L.; Rodriguez-Blanco, C.; Bernal-Utrera, C. Vojta Therapy in Neuromotor Development of Pediatrics Patients with Periventricular Leukomalacia: Case Series. *Medicina* **2021**, *57*, 1149. [CrossRef] [PubMed]
11. Strojek, K.; Wójtowicz, D.; Kowalska, J. Assessment of the Emotional State of Parents of Children Starting the Vojta Therapy in the Context of the Physical Activity-A Pilot Study. *Int. J. Env. Res. Public Health* **2022**, *19*, 10691. [CrossRef]
12. Bobath, K.; Bobath, B. The Neuro-Developmental Treatment of Cerebral Palsy. *Phys. Ther.* **1967**, *47*, 1039–1043. [CrossRef]
13. Te Velde, A.; Morgan, C.; Finch-Edmondson, M.; McNamara, L.; McNamara, M.; Paton, M.C.B.; Stanton, E.; Webb, A.; Badawi, N.; Novak, I. Neurodevelopmental Therapy for Cerebral Palsy: A Meta-analysis. *Pediatrics* **2022**, *149*, e2021055061. [CrossRef] [PubMed]
14. Ungureanu, A.; Rusu, L.; Rusu, M.R.; Marin, M.I. Balance Rehabilitation Approach by Bobath and Vojta Methods in Cerebral Palsy: A Pilot Study. *Children* **2022**, *9*, 1481. [CrossRef] [PubMed]
15. Apaydın, U.; Erol, E.; Gücüyener, K.; Yıldız, A.; Elbasan, B.; Yıldız, R.; Acar, S.-S.; Gücüyener, K.; Elbasan, B. The use of neuroimaging, Prechtl's general movement assessment and the Hammersmith infant neurological examination in determining the prognosis in 2-year-old infants with hypoxic ischemic encephalopathy who were treated with hypothermia. *Early Hum. Dev.* **2021**, *163*, 105487. [CrossRef] [PubMed]
16. Darsaklis, V.; Snider, L.M.; Majnemer, A.; Mazer, B. Predictive validity of Prechtl's Method on the Qualitative Assessment of General Movements: A systematic review of the evidence. *Dev. Med. Child Neurol.* **2011**, *53*, 896–906. [CrossRef]
17. Pazera, G.; Młodawska, M.; Kukulska, K.; Młodawski, J. The Assessment of Psychomotor Development in Full-Term Children at 12 Months of Age with Munich Functional Development Diagnostics Depending on the Feeding Method: A Cross-Sectional Study. *Pediatr. Rep.* **2023**, *15*, 381–389. [CrossRef]
18. Pazera, G.; Młodawska, M.; Młodawski, J.; Klimowska, K. Principal Component Analysis of Munich Functional Developmental Diagnosis. *Pediatr. Rep.* **2021**, *13*, 227–233. [CrossRef]
19. Sánchez-González, J.L.; Sanz-Esteban, I.; Menéndez-Pardiñas, M.; Navarro-López, V.; Sanz-Mengíbar, J.M. Critical review of the evidence for Vojta Therapy: A systematic review and meta-analysis. *Front. Neurol.* **2024**, *15*, 1391448. [CrossRef]

20. Costi, G.C.; Radice, C.; Raggi, A.; Kron, A.M.; Angrisano, A.; Busato, E.; Montrasio, G.; Perfetti, C.; Pissacroia, C. Vojta's seven postural reactions in the detection of neuromotor disorders in infants. Experience with 2382 subjects. *Pediatr. Med. Chir.* **1983**, *5*, 59–65. [PubMed]
21. Vojta, V. *Die Entdeckung der Idealen Motorik*; Pflaum Verlag: München, Germany, 2009.
22. Menéndez-Pardiñas, M.; Alonso-Bidegaín, M.; Santonja-Medina, F.; Sánchez-González, J.L.; Sanz-Mengibar, J.M. Effects of Vojta Therapy on the Motor Function of Children with Neuromotor Disorders: Study Protocol for a Randomized Controlled Trial. *J. Clin. Med.* **2023**, *12*, 7373. [CrossRef]
23. Polczyk, A.E. Early Use of Vojta Therapy in Children with Postural Asymmetry, at Risk of Hip Dysplasia. *Pediatr. Ther.* **2018**, *8*, 339. [CrossRef]
24. Jung, M.W.; Landenberger, M.; Jung, T.; Lindenthal, T.; Philippi, H. Vojta therapy and neurodevelopmental treatmentin children with infantile postural asymmetry: A randomised controlled trial. *Phys. Ther.* **2017**, *29*, 301–306. [CrossRef]
25. Vojta, V. Frühbehandlung der CP-Risikokonder Analyse der Endresultate. *Mschr. Kinderhelik.* **1973**, *121*, 271–273.
26. Vojta, V. Lokomotorische Prognose der CP-Kinder bei Behandlung mit Refleks-Lokomoti-onssystemen. In Proceedings of theVortag, Jahreskongres der Zentralverbandes der Krankengymnastik, Mainz, Germany, 5 May 1985.
27. Vojta, V. The postural activity and reactivity and its stages of ontogenical maturation. In *Neurological Lesions in Infancy*; Bottos, M., Ed.; Liviana: Padova, Italy, 1989; pp. 45–52.
28. van Hoorn, J.F.; Schoemaker, M.M.; Stuive, I.; Dijkstra, P.U.; Rodrigues Trigo Pereira, F.; van der Sluis, C.K.; Hadders-Algra, M. Risk factors in early life for developmental coordination disorder: A scoping review. *Dev. Med. Child Neurol.* **2021**, *63*, 511–519. [CrossRef] [PubMed]
29. Faebo Larsen, R.; Hvas Mortensen, L.; Martinussen, T.; Nybo Andersen, A.M. Determinants of developmental coordination disorder in 7-year-old children: A study of children in the Danish National Birth Cohort. *Dev. Med. Child Neurol.* **2013**, *55*, 1016–1022. [CrossRef]
30. Caravale, B.; Herich, L.; Zoia, S.; Capone, L.; Voller, F.; Carrozzi, M.; Chiandotto, V.; Balottin, U.; Lacchei, M.; Croci, I.; et al. Risk of Developmental Coordination Disorder in Italian very preterm children at school age compared to general population controls. *Eur. J. Paediatr. Neurol.* **2019**, *23*, 296–303. [CrossRef]
31. Tuñón-Domínguez, I.; Cuesta-Gómez, A.; Molina-Rueda, F.; Juárez-Vela, R.; Ruiz de Viñaspre-Hernández, R.; Santolalla-Arnedo, I.; Sánchez-González, J.L.; Carratalá-Tejada, M. The influence between gestational age and postural control, a systematic review. *Front. Pediatr.* **2022**, *10*, 883218. [CrossRef]
32. Hua, J.; Gu, G.; Jiang, P.; Zhang, L.; Zhu, L.; Meng, W. The prenatal, perinatal and neonatal risk factors for children's developmental coordination disorder: A population study in mainland China. *Res. Dev. Disabil.* **2014**, *35*, 619–625. [CrossRef]
33. Lipińska, E.; Słopień, A.; Pytlińska, N.; Słopień, R.; Wolańczy, T.; Bryńska, A. The role of factors associated with the course of pregnancy and childbirth in attention deficit hyperactivity disorder (ADHD). *Psychiatr. Pol.* **2021**, *55*, 659–673. [CrossRef]
34. Kubisa, A. Ocena Rozwoju Psychoruchowego u Dzieci po Zastosowaniu Selektywnego Chłodzenia Mózgu. Ph.D. Thesis, Wroclaw Medical University of the Piasts of Silesia, Wroclaw, Poland, 2021. [CrossRef]
35. Kwong, A.K.L.; Fitzgerald, T.L.; Doyle, L.W.; Cheong, J.L.Y.; Spittle, A.J. Predictive validity of spontaneous early infant movement for later cerebral palsy: A systematic review. *Dev. Med. Child Neurol.* **2018**, *60*, 480–489. [CrossRef]
36. Espel, E.V.; Glynn, L.M.; Sandman, C.A.; Davis, E.P. Longer gestation among children born full term influences cognitive and motor development. *PLoS ONE* **2014**, *9*, e113758. [CrossRef] [PubMed]
37. Zachwieja, J. Psychomotor Development of Children Born Prematurely. Ph.D. Thesis, Medical university of Silesia in Katowice, Katowice, Poland, 2021.
38. Surowińska, J.; Sobieska, M.; Gajewska, E. Qualitative assessment in the third month of life allows for a better prognosis of the achievement of motor milestones versus assessment of pathological reflexes- prospective studies on Polish children. *Front. Public Health* **2023**, *11*, 1253137. [CrossRef] [PubMed]
39. Chinello, A.; Di Gangi, V.; Valenza, E. Persistent primary reflexes affect motor acts: Potential implications for autism spectrum disorder. *Res. Dev. Disabil.* **2018**, *83*, 287–295. [CrossRef] [PubMed]
40. Futagi, Y.; Toribe, Y.; Suzuki, Y. The grasp reflex and moro reflex in infants: Hierarchy of primitive reflex responses. *Int. J. Pediatr.* **2012**, *2012*, 191562. [CrossRef]
41. Luoto, R.; Mottola, M.F.; Hilakivi-Clarke, L. Pregnancy and lifestyle: Short- and long-term effects on mother's and her children's health. *J. Pregnancy* **2013**, *2013*, 537526. [CrossRef]
42. Bagherzadeh, R.; Gharibi, T.; Safavi, B.; Mohammadi, S.Z.; Karami, F.; Keshavarz, S. Pregnancy; an opportunity to return to a healthy lifestyle: A qualitative study. *BMC Pregnancy Childbirth* **2021**, *21*, 751. [CrossRef]

MDPI AG
Grosspeteranlage 5
4052 Basel
Switzerland
Tel.: +41 61 683 77 34

Children Editorial Office
E-mail: children@mdpi.com
www.mdpi.com/journal/children

www.ingramcontent.com/pod-product-compliance
Lightning Source LLC
Chambersburg PA
CBHW061608210926
51850CB00009B/2254
9783725878475